Video Atlas of Neuromusculoskeletal Ultrasound

Reza Salman Roghani • Jose Juan Diaz
Editors

Video Atlas of Neuromusculoskeletal Ultrasound

Springer

Editors
Reza Salman Roghani
Department of Physical Medicine and Rehabilitation
Larkin Community Hospital, Nova Southeastern University
Miami, FL, USA

Jose Juan Diaz
Department of Physical Medicine and Rehabilitation
Larkin Community Hospital, Nova Southeastern University
Miami, FL, USA

Integrative Spine and Sport
Fort Lauderdale, FL, USA

ISBN 978-3-031-81036-7 ISBN 978-3-031-81037-4 (eBook)
https://doi.org/10.1007/978-3-031-81037-4

This Springer imprint is published by the registered company Springer Nature Switzerland AG
The registered company address is: Gewerbestrasse 11, 6330 Cham, Switzerland

To my parents, Shamsolmoluk and Abbas, whose constant support and encouragement have guided every stage of my journey. To my beloved wife, Padideh, for her boundless love, patience, and understanding throughout this endeavor. To my cherished daughter, Helia, whose happiness and inquisitiveness inspire me daily. And to Professor Diaz, my mentor and program director, whose unwavering trust and insightful guidance have empowered me to pursue my passion in the USA. This book is as much a reflection of you as it is of me.

—Reza Salman Roghani

We cannot separate the path of this book and the Larkin Community Hospital's Physical Medicine and Rehabilitation Residency. They are intricately woven together. To Rob Gotlin, DO, who mentored the Larkin Community Hospital's Physical Medicine and Rehabilitation Residency into existence and whom we mourn for his untimely death. To the AOCPMR board members, who supported the Larkin Community Hospital's Physical Medicine and Rehabilitation Residency program while we were under construction. To Jack Michel, MD, the heart and soul of Larkin Community Hospital and who supports all our endeavors. To all the hard-working attendings and residents who worked on this project and are Larkin PMR. To my mother Aurea and sister Maria: my backbone until I could build my own. To my wife Lissandra and children Eli, Mateo, Beba, Gabi, and Rafael, who replenish the love I give to the world every day. To my brother, Reza, who suddenly appeared in my life.

—Jose Juan Diaz

Preface

The expanding role of ultrasound in evaluating and treating neuromusculoskeletal (NMSK) conditions has fundamentally transformed how healthcare professionals approach patient care. As a real-time, non-invasive imaging modality, ultrasound enables clinicians to diagnose, treat, and monitor a wide range of musculoskeletal and nerve disorders with unmatched precision and efficiency. This capability allows for more dynamic and immediate insights into patient conditions, enabling more accurate and timely interventions. From acute injuries to chronic pain syndromes, ultrasound has become an indispensable tool in enhancing both diagnostic and therapeutic outcomes. In response to the increasing demand for ultrasound expertise, this book was conceived as a comprehensive visual guide to the evolving field of NMSK ultrasound.

The *Video Atlas of Neuromusculoskeletal Ultrasound* represents our ongoing dedication to residents, fellows, and students—past and present—who have sought to deepen their understanding of musculoskeletal ultrasound. It is through their enthusiasm, questions, and pursuit of knowledge that we have been motivated to create this detailed resource. Designed as both a learning tool and clinical reference, this book offers detailed guidance for mastering ultrasound techniques, making it valuable for those new to the field as well as experienced clinicians looking to refine their skills. Each chapter provides in-depth coverage of specific anatomical regions and pathologies, with a focus on real-world scenarios commonly encountered in clinical practice. Through this approach, we aim to make the material immediately applicable to daily clinical workflows.

In this edition, the core principles of NMSK scanning have been meticulously covered. Each image is paired with specific details on patient positioning, probe placement, and schematic anatomy illustrations derived from MRI or CT cross-sections to aid in understanding sono-anatomy. This combination of visual aids and written guidance ensures that readers not only understand the theory behind the scans but also feel confident in applying these techniques in practice. Additionally, each technique is accompanied by a video with step-by-step image analysis, providing deeper insight into the procedures. We have also explained ultrasound-guided injections in detail, including images and videos that outline each step, such as needle insertion, preferred planes, and optimal target points. This integrative approach allows readers to visualize anatomical structures more clearly, correlate ultrasound images with other imaging modalities, and ultimately improve diagnostic accuracy and procedural confidence.

Our goal in developing this atlas was to bridge the gap between theoretical knowledge and hands-on application. The inclusion of dynamic imaging and video content sets this work apart, allowing readers to observe real-time procedures that are essential for mastering NMSK ultrasound. Whether you are just beginning your journey into ultrasound or seeking to refine and perfect your skills, we hope this atlas will enhance your practice and contribute to better patient outcomes.

It is our sincere hope that this book will serve as a valuable resource for years to come, helping clinicians achieve more accurate diagnoses and deliver more effective treatments in the rapidly advancing field of neuromusculoskeletal ultrasound.

Miami, FL, USA Reza Salman Roghani

Fort Lauderdale, FL, USA Jose Juan Diaz

Acknowledgments

The completion of the *Video Atlas of Neuromusculoskeletal Ultrasound* has been a collaborative effort, and we are deeply grateful to all those who contributed to its realization.

First and foremost, we would like to thank our residents, fellows, and students—past and present—whose curiosity and dedication to learning inspired this work. Their questions, enthusiasm, and pursuit of excellence have driven us to expand our knowledge and understanding, shaping the content and direction of this book.

We are immensely grateful to our co-authors and collaborators, whose expertise and insights have enriched this atlas. Their contributions were vital in ensuring the accuracy and comprehensiveness of the material presented.

Special thanks go to our colleagues and mentors who have supported us throughout our careers. Their guidance has been invaluable, both in our professional development and in the creation of this book.

A special acknowledgment goes to Dr. Jack Michelle, founder and president of Larkin Health System, for his leadership and continued support. His commitment to advancing healthcare has been instrumental in fostering the environment that allowed this project to come to life.

We also wish to extend our sincere thanks to the Springer publisher staff, especially Lee Klein, for his professional guidance, encouragement, and invaluable support throughout the publication process. His expertise has been key in bringing this book to fruition.

Additionally, we would like to thank Nicole Schneider for her exceptional work in video creation and Niloofar Nejad Darab for her artistic contributions to the drawings featured in this book.

Finally, we extend our gratitude to the patients who have entrusted us with their care. Their stories and experiences have been the foundation of our work, providing us with the insights necessary to continually improve and evolve in the field of neuromusculoskeletal ultrasound.

AI-assisted tools were used to improve clarity, uniformity, and academic readability, ensuring consistency throughout the text.

Thank you to everyone who has been a part of this journey.

Contents

Contributors

Mina Abadir, MD Ross University School of Medicine, Miramar, FL, USA

Padideh Baran, RDMS Imaging Department, University of Miami, Miami, FL, USA

Seungwoo Chai, MD Surgery Department, Robert Packer Hospital, Guthrie Clinic, Sayre, PA, USA

Jose Juan Diaz, DO Department of Physical Medicine and Rehabilitation, Larkin Community Hospital, Nova Southeastern University, Miami, FL, USA
Integrative Spine and Sports, Fort Lauderdale, FL, USA

Ghazaleh Ebrahimi Department of Physical Medicine and Rehabilitation, Larkin Community Hospital, Nova Southeastern University, Miami, FL, USA

Yashar Eshraghi, MD Division of Pain Medicine, Department of Anesthesiology and Critical Care Medicine, Ochsner Health System, University of Queensland Ochsner Medical School, New Orleans, LA, USA

Sina Davari Farid, MD Division of Pain Medicine, Department of Anesthesiology and Critical Care Medicine, George Washington University, Washington, DC, USA

Amirhossein Foroughianyazdi Department of Science, Toronto Metropolitan University, Toronto, ON, Canada

Jorge E. Garcia-Negron, MD Department of Physical Medicine and Rehabilitation/Pain Medicine, West Palm Beach VA Healthcare System, U.S. Department of Veterans Affairs, West Palm Beach, FL, USA

Ceci Guerrero, DO Department of Physical Medicine and Rehabilitation, Larkin Community Hospital, Nova Southeastern University, Miami, FL, USA

Shravan Gupta Coastal Interventional Pain & Spine Center, Seminole, FL, USA

Tariq Islam, MD Ross University School of Medicine, Miramar, FL, USA

Naffiseh Jafarian, MD Department of Physical Medicine and Rehabilitation, Shohada Hospital, Shahid Beheshti University of Medical Science, Tajrish, Tehran, Iran

Lynn Kohan, MD Pain management division, Department of Anesthesia, University of Virginia School of Medicine, Charlottesville, VA, USA

Megan McGuire, MD Pohlman Pain Associates, Coral Springs, FL, USA

Natasha Mehta, DO Division of Pain Medicine, Department of Anesthesia, Larkin Community Hospital, Nova Southeastern University, South Miami, FL, USA

John Melendez-Benabe, MD Pain Medicine Division, Department of Physical Medicine and Rehabilitation, West Palm Beach VA Healthcare System, US Department of Veterans Affairs, West Palm Beach, FL, USA

Andrew M. Mendelson, DO Pain Management Division, Department of Anesthesia, University of Virginia School of Medicine, Charlottesville, VA, USA

Richard Morgan, DO Department of Physical Medicine and Rehabilitation, Miami Neuroscience Institute, Baptist Health, Miami, FL, USA

Joseph Mouhanna, MD Division of Pain Medicine, Department of Anesthesiology, Larkin Community Hospital, Nova Southeastern University, South Miami, FL, USA

Mihir Nakrani, DO Department of Physical Medicine and Rehabilitation, Larkin Community Hospital, Nova Southeastern University, Miami, FL, USA

Mohammad R. Nezamabadi, MD Neshat Pain Clinic, Fardis, Karaj, Iran

Brian Palacios, DO Department of Physical Medicine and Rehabilitation, Larkin Community Hospital, Nova Southeastern University, Miami, FL, USA

Geet Paul, MD Division of Pain Medicine, Department of Anesthesiology and Critical Care Medicine, George Washington University, Washington, DC, USA

Reza Salman Roghani, MD, PhD Department of Physical Medicine and Rehabilitation, Larkin Community Hospital, Nova Southeastern University, Miami, FL, USA

Nicole Schneider, DO Dr. Kiran C. Patel College of Osteopathic Medicine, Nova Southeastern University, Fort Lauderdale, FL, USA

Jasmine Sidhu, MD Department of Physical Medicine and Rehabilitation, Larkin Community Hospital, Nova Southeastern University, Miami, FL, USA

Hein Linn Thant, MD Department of Physical Medicine and Rehabilitation, Larkin Community Hospital, Nova Southeastern University, Miami, FL, USA

Ronald Tolchin, DO Department of Physical Medicine and Rehabilitation, Miami Neuroscience Institute, Baptist Health, Miami, FL, USA

Somayeh Younesian, MD Department of Physical Medicine and Rehabilitation, Broward Health North Hospital, Pompano Beach, FL, USA

Basics and Knobology

1

Jose Juan Diaz, Reza Salman Roghani,
Padideh Baran, and Mohammad R. Nezamabadi

1.1 Ultrasound Modes

Common ultrasound modes in NMSK are B, M, and Doppler (color and power modes) [1].

B-mode, also known as "brightness mode," displays structural information in a 2D image using grayscale levels (i.e., brightness) and is the most widely utilized mode in neuromusculoskeletal ultrasound [1] (Fig. 1.1).

The brightness of an image, known as echogenicity, is determined by the reflection of sound waves. It is influenced by the characteristics of the sound beam and the density of the tissue.

Hyperechoic: When echoes return with a high amplitude, they appear brighter than the surrounding tissue.

J. J. Diaz
Department of Physical Medicine and Rehabilitation, Larkin Community Hospital, Nova Southeastern University, Miami, FL, USA

Integrative Spine and Sports, Fort Lauderdale, FL, USA

R. S. Roghani (✉)
Department of Physical Medicine and Rehabilitation, Larkin Community Hospital, Nova Southeastern University, Miami, FL, USA

P. Baran
Imaging Department, University of Miami, Miami, FL, USA
e-mail: Pxb646@miami.edu

M. R. Nezamabadi
Neshat Pain Clinic, Fardis, Karaj, Iran

Hypoechoic: When there are very few echoes, the structure appears darker than the surrounding tissue.

Anechoic: When a structure does not reflect sound waves, the corresponding area appears dark or black on the ultrasound image.

M-mode, also known as motion mode, is a type of ultrasonography that records returning echoes in a single line of the B-mode image displayed over time. Real-time M-mode is frequently used in ultrasound to locate moving body parts like the heart and its compartments, such as in echocardiography (Fig. 1.2) [1].

Color Doppler: Color-flow ultrasound is a mode that applies to the machine to convert sound waves to coded colors, which are then superimposed on a matching B-mode picture to color-code blood flow and tissue mobility (Fig. 1.3) [2].

Power Doppler: This mode detects movement in different flow levels without investigating the flow direction or speed. It provides additional information for chronic inflammation conditions like lateral epicondylitis and rheumatoid diseases (Fig. 1.4) [2].

R. S. Roghani, J. J. Diaz (eds.), *Video Atlas of Neuromusculoskeletal Ultrasound*,
https://doi.org/10.1007/978-3-031-81037-4_1

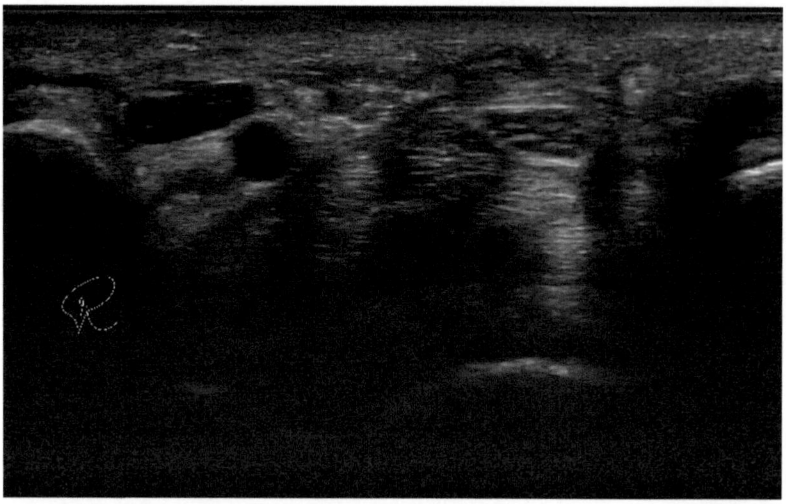

Fig. 1.1 B-mode: An ultrasound image in B-mode showing a cross-sectional view of the carpal tunnel. The image displays varying shades of gray, indicating different tissue densities. A small, dark circular area is visible, representing a fluid-filled space; ulnar artery. The background texture is grainy, typical of ultrasound imaging. (© Reza Roghani 2024. All Rights Reserved)

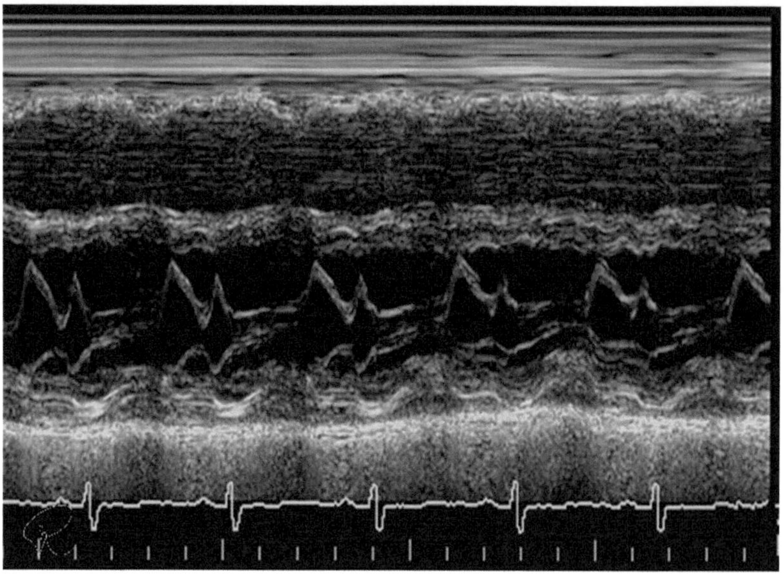

Fig. 1.2 M-mode: An ultrasound M-mode image of the heart, displaying rhythmic wave patterns representing cardiac motion. Below the ultrasound, a green electrocardiogram (ECG) line shows corresponding heartbeats with regular intervals. The image illustrates the synchronization between heart motion and electrical activity. (© Reza Roghani 2024. All Rights Reserved)

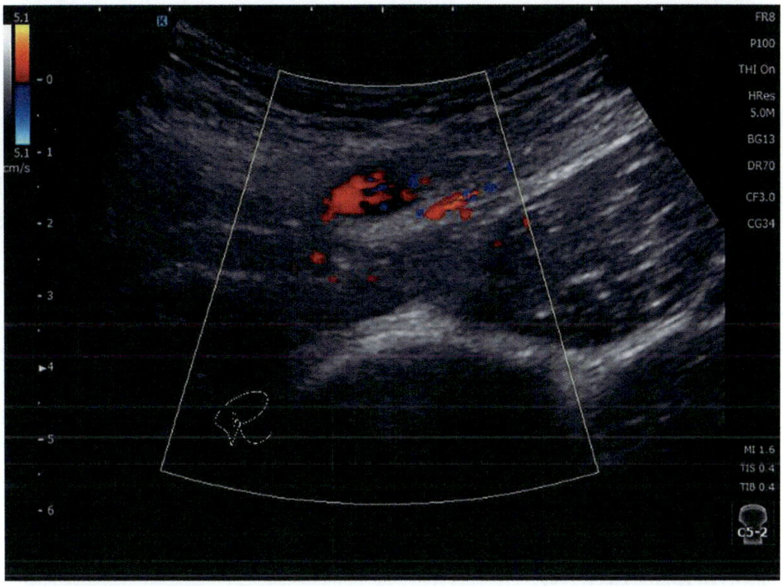

Fig. 1.3 An ultrasound image showing a cross-sectional view of internal body structures. The image includes color Doppler signals, with red and blue areas indicating blood flow direction and velocity. A color scale on the left representing the flow velocity. (© Reza Roghani 2024. All Rights Reserved)

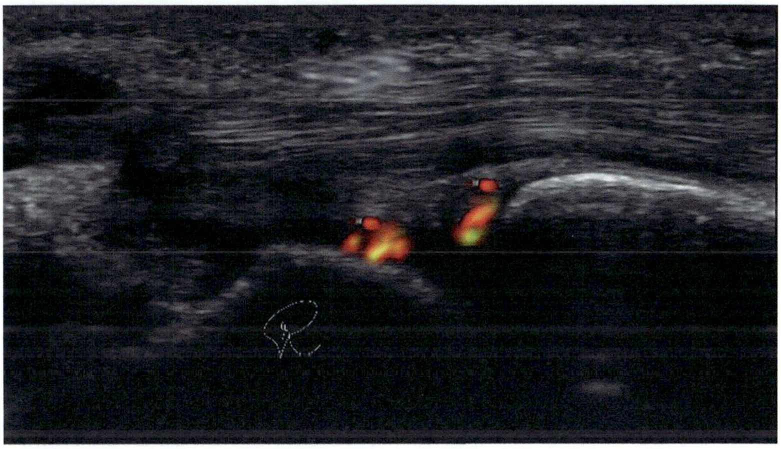

Fig. 1.4 Power Doppler: Hyperemia in a CMC joint affected by inflammation in rheumatoid arthritis is detected using power Doppler. This technique identifies increased blood flow but does not measure flow direction or speed. (© Reza Roghani 2024. All Rights Reserved)

1.2 Ultrasound Probes

Linear, curved, and hockey stick probes are commonly used transducers in the NMSK field [3] (Fig. 1.5).

Linear probes: These transducers produce flat, straight, high-frequency (7–15 MHz) square waves and are widely used for musculoskeletal and vascular sonography, superficial soft tissue structure assessment, and procedure guidance.

Curved probes: These low-frequency (1–5 MHZ) probes produce sector-shaped images with curved footprints, mainly used for deep tissue and spine sonography.

Hokey stick probes: These are high-frequency (7–15 MHz) ultrasound linear probes with a smaller footprint, used for smaller parts like toes and fingers.

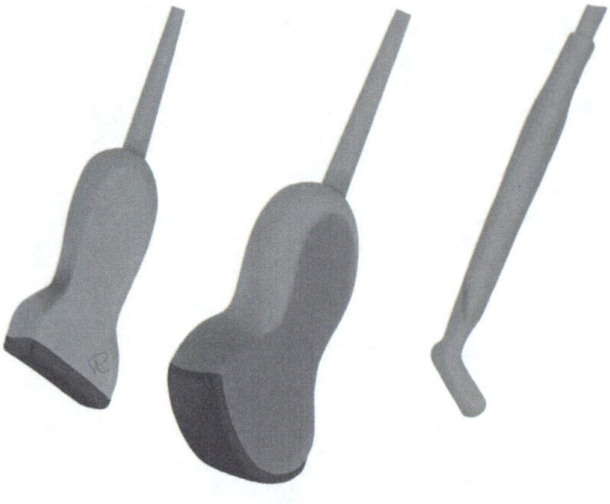

Fig. 1.5 Ultrasound probes: Three different types of ultrasound probes are shown: a linear probe with a flat surface, a curved probe with a rounded surface, and an hokey stick probe with a smaller footprint. Each probe has a handle and a cable extending from it. (© Reza Roghani 2024. All Rights Reserved)

1.3 Anatomical Plane

There are three different ways to slice or divide the body: sagittal, transverse (also called horizontal), and coronal (also called frontal). The sagittal plane divides the body into left and right halves, the transverse plane divides it into upper and lower halves, and the coronal plane divides it into front and back halves. These three principal planes run perpendicular to each other [3] (Fig. 1.6).

Sagittal Plane: When patients lie flat on their back, an imaginary line runs vertically along the body's midline, separating the left and right sides. This line is perpendicular to the ground.

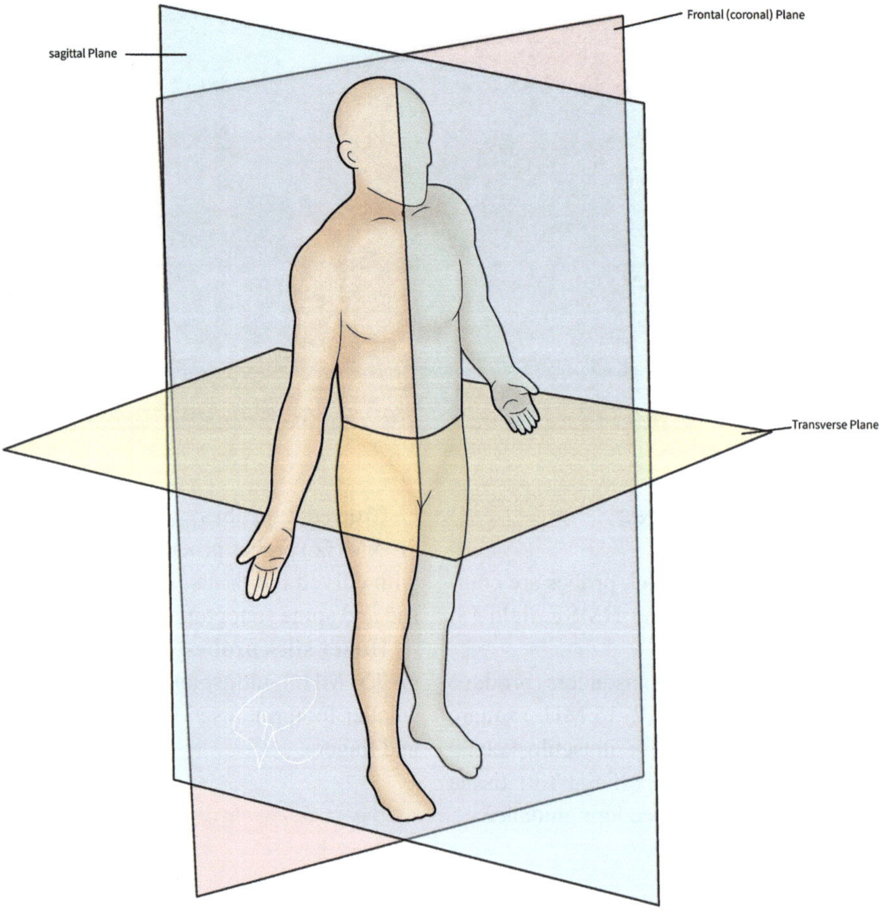

Fig. 1.6 Anatomical planes: Illustration of a human figure intersected by three anatomical planes: sagittal, frontal (coronal), and transverse. The sagittal plane divides the body into left and right sections, the frontal plane divides it into front and back sections, and the transverse plane divides it into upper and lower sections. Each plane is labeled accordingly. (© Reza Roghani 2024. All Rights Reserved)

Transverse Plane: (axial plane or cross-sectional)—Runs perpendicular to the ground in the supine patient and separates the head from the feet or superior from inferior.

Coronal plane: (frontal plane)—When a patient is lying down, a horizontal line runs along the body's midline divides the front (anterior) from the back (posterior).

The oblique plane is a type of anatomical plane that divides the body at an angle, neither parallel to the sagittal, coronal, nor transverse planes. It combines elements of two or more of these planes, cutting through the body diagonally. The oblique plane can be useful in imaging and surgical contexts where the body needs to be viewed from non-standard angles, allowing for more complex or detailed visualization of structures.

1.4 Probe Manipulation

Slide: This refers to the process of scanning tissue along a single line, parallel to the probe's long axis. The ultrasound probe is moved along the body, maintaining alignment with its lengthwise orientation, enabling longitudinal imaging of the tissue. This technique provides a continuous scan, capturing the full length of structures such as muscles, tendons, ligaments, or nerves (Fig. 1.7).

Sweep: Movement of the probe along its short axis to adjust the ultrasound image field and optimize visualization (Fig. 1.8).

Compression: The movement of the probe is achieved by pressing it while maintaining contact and keeping it perpendicular to the target area.

Rotation: Rotate the probe clockwise or counterclockwise, ensuring the center remains fixed on

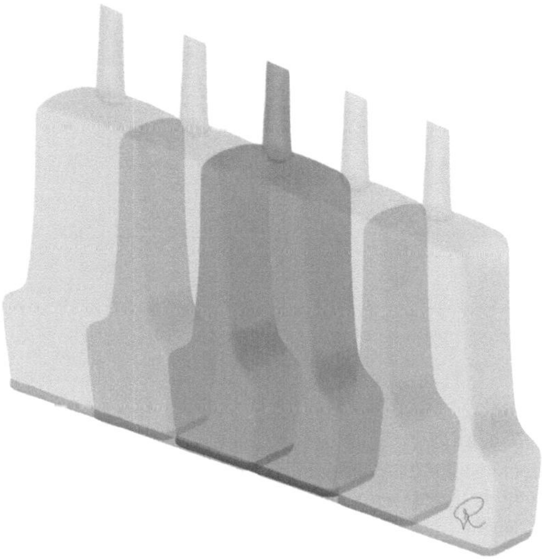

Fig. 1.7 Probe slide: A sequence of five overlapping, semi-transparent probes arranged in a line, illustrating probe sliding. (© Reza Roghani 2024. All Rights Reserved)

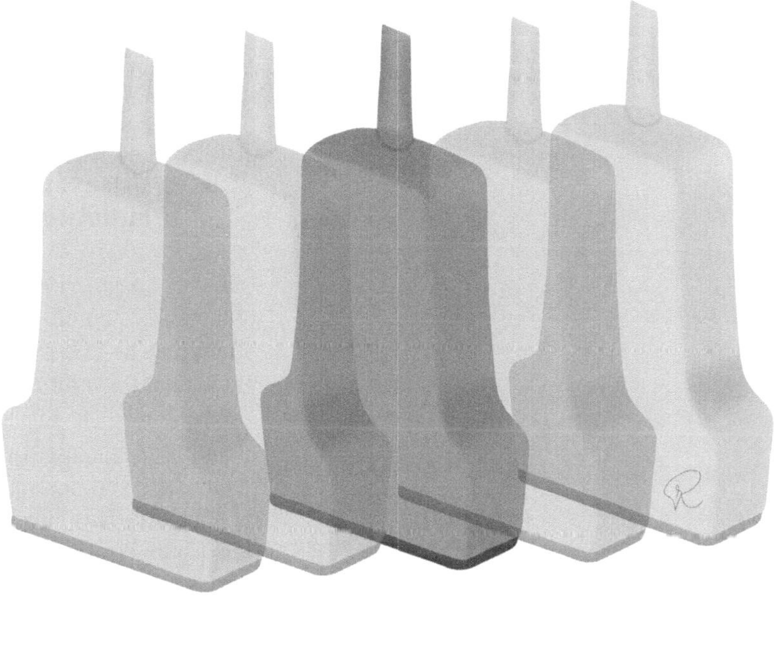

Fig. 1.8 Probe sweep: A series of five probe images, each aligned along the same short axis, illustrating the probe sweep movement. (© Reza Roghani 2024. All Rights Reserved)

the center of the image, while the probe's footprint stays in contact with the body's surface (Fig. 1.9).

Rocking: refers to a technique where the ultrasound probe is gently tilted or rocked back and forth around its central axis. This movement can be used to adjust the angle of insonation or to better visualize structures, particularly in areas with irregular contours or difficult angles. Rocking the probe can help optimize image quality, ensure better coverage of the area being scanned, and capture a more accurate representation of the tissue or structure (Fig. 1.10).

Fanning: Adjust the probe's angle along its short axis without changing its point of contact with the body's surface (Fig. 1.11).

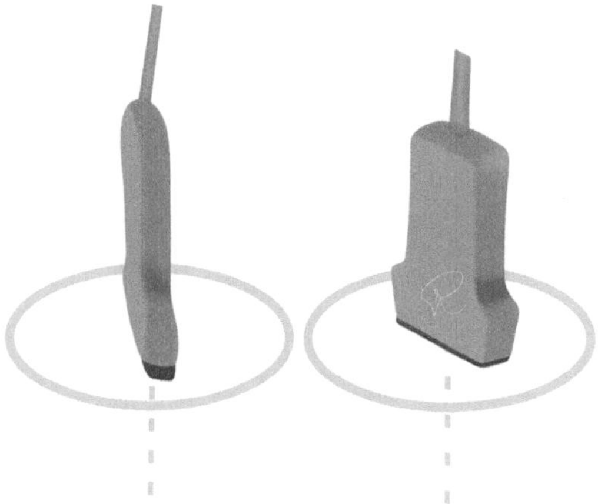

Fig. 1.9 Probe rotation: A series of two probe images demonstrate the counterclockwise rotation of the probe, with the center remaining fixed in the same spot.

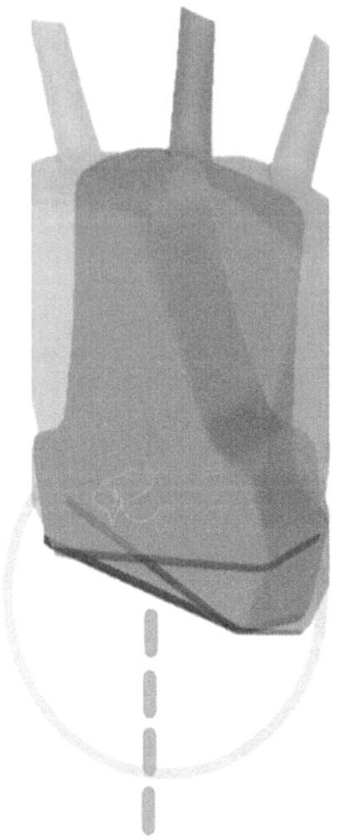

Fig. 1.10 Probe rocking: A sequence of three probe images demonstrates the heel–toe maneuver, with the probe maintaining contact with the body to illustrate probe rocking.

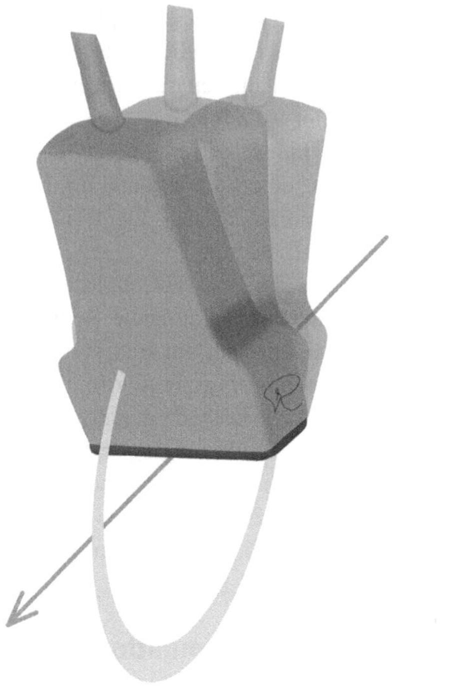

Fig. 1.11 Probe fanning: A series of three images showing the probe tilting around its long axis while maintaining its point of contact, effectively illustrating the process of probe fanning.

1.5 Ultrasound Machine Functions

This section provides an overview of the essential functions of an ultrasound machine. These functions may be accessed through physical or digital keys, and the information provided is kept broad to ensure its relevance to most devices. Familiarizing oneself with these functions is crucial when working with ultrasound machines [4].

On/Off: This function lets the user turn the device on or off. Many devices also have a sleep mode.

Select/Change Probes: Choose the patient, probe, and exam type.

Scroll: A scrolling feature, such as a trackball, allows you to move the cursor around an image or menu. The scroll ball will enable you to cycle through the final few seconds of imagery after an image has been frozen.

Freeze: This key stops the ultrasound from working and fixes the currently visible image.

Save: Saves a picture or video clip to your hard disk.

Gain: It modifies the total power of returning echoes, affecting image brightness.

Time Gain Compensation (TGC): Adjusts the intensity of echoes returning at different depths to create an evenly illuminated ultrasound image.

Mode Change: When you push the M-mode button on the machine, it will switch to M-mode. Similarly, pressing the Doppler button will change the mode to color Doppler, and so on. Typically, when different modes are selected (such as B-mode along with Doppler or M-mode), most computers are set up to display a "dual" screen.

Depth: To adjust the depth of the ultrasonic beam, you can increase or decrease it as needed.

Focus: Altering or adding focal zones improves image quality at specific depths.

1.6 Artifacts

Ultrasound images captured by machines can display things that do not exist, known as artifacts. These artifacts may either aid or hinder the interpreter's visual understanding of the image. Below are some examples of common artifacts that are frequently observed [5].

Shadowing: Sound-absorbing structures can either reflect entirely or partially absorb sound, resulting in a weaker signal returning from a strong reflector or absorptive structure (Fig. 1.12).

Edge Shadowing: When using ultrasound imaging, the margins of circular structures, such as cystic formations or large vessels, often appear unclear due to a thin acoustic shadow. This occurs because sound waves are tangentially reflected by the curved surface or cystic wall, allowing only a few echoes to return to the transducer (Fig. 1.13).

Posterior enhancement: A phenomenon in ultrasound imaging where structures located behind a fluid-filled area, such as a cyst or blood vessel, appear brighter (hyperechoic) due to reduced attenuation of the ultrasound waves. Since fluid allows sound waves to pass through with minimal resistance, more energy reaches the deeper tissues, leading to increased echogenicity in the posterior region. This artifact is commonly observed in simple cysts and other

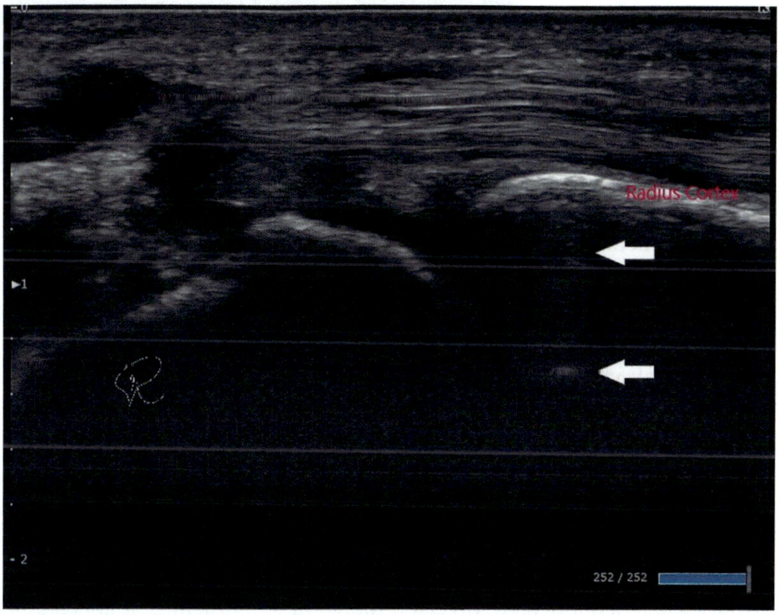

Fig. 1.12 Shadowing: An ultrasound image showing the cross-section of a forearm. The text "Radius Cortex" is labeled in pink, indicating the location of the radius bone. Two white arrows point the reflections beneath the bone cortex, where sound waves cannot penetrate, demonstrating the shadowing artifact. (© Reza Roghani 2024. All Rights Reserved)

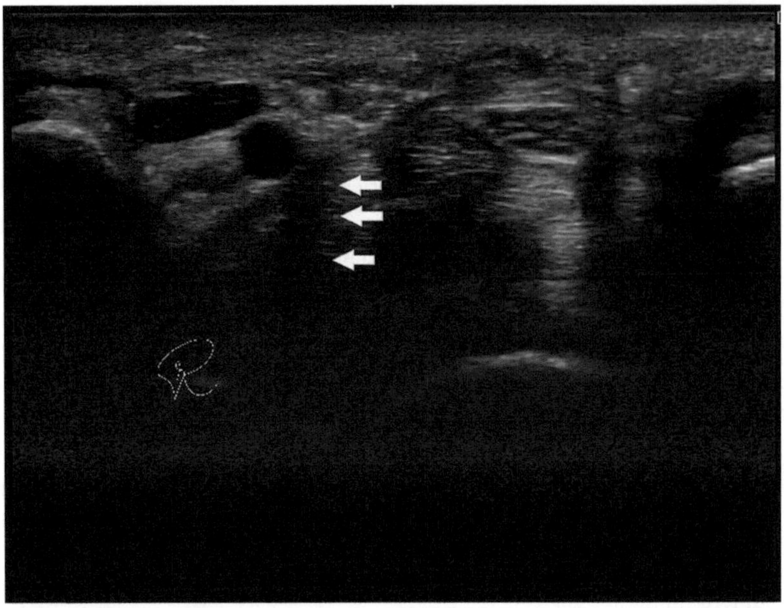

Fig. 1.13 Edge shadowing: An ultrasound image displaying a cross-sectional view of the carpal tunnel tissue, with three white arrows highlighting a thin acoustic shadow beneath the edge of the ulnar artery. This illustrates the edge shadowing artifact. (© Reza Roghani 2024. All Rights Reserved)

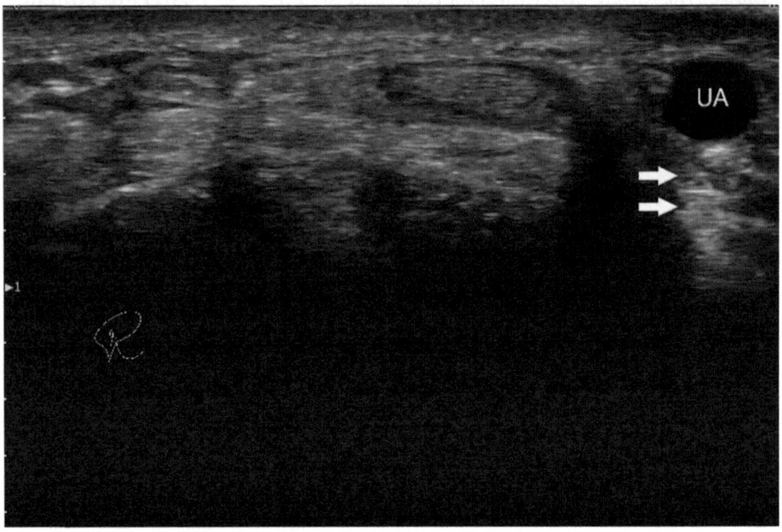

Fig. 1.14 Posterior enhancement: An ultrasound image showing a cross-sectional view of the distal forearm with a dark circular area labeled "UA" on the right side, indicating the ulnar artery. Two white arrows point to hyperechoic lines below the ulnar artery. (© Reza Roghani 2024. All Rights Reserved)

anechoic structures, aiding in their identification and differentiation from solid masses (Fig. 1.14).

Reverberation: When sound waves hit highly reflective layers before returning to the transducer, they bounce back and forth between the two layers, causing echoes and reverberations. An example is the reverberation that occurs when a needle is inserted into tissue for injection (Fig. 1.15).

Comet tail: It is like an echo in the front and back of a powerful reflector, such as a bullet.

Mirroring effect: A common ultrasound artifact where a duplicated, reversed image of a structure appears on the opposite side of a strong reflector, such as the bone cortex. This occurs when sound waves bounce off a highly reflective surface before returning to the transducer, creating the illusion of an additional structure beyond the actual anatomical boundary (Fig. 1.16).

Anisotropy: A common artifact in musculoskeletal ultrasound where the echogenicity of a structure, such as a tendon or ligament, changes depending on the angle of the ultrasound beam. When the transducer is perpendicular to the structure, it appears bright (hyperechoic), but as the angle deviates, the structure becomes darker

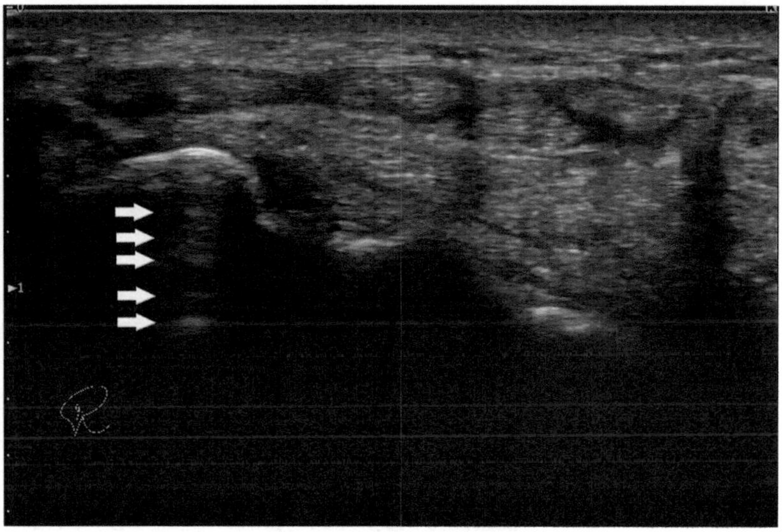

Fig. 1.15 Reverberation: An ultrasound image showing a cross-sectional view of the wrist with five white arrows pointing to a ladder-like structure that appears brighter on ultrasound, with darker areas in between located below the bone's cortex. (© Reza Roghani 2024. All Rights Reserved)

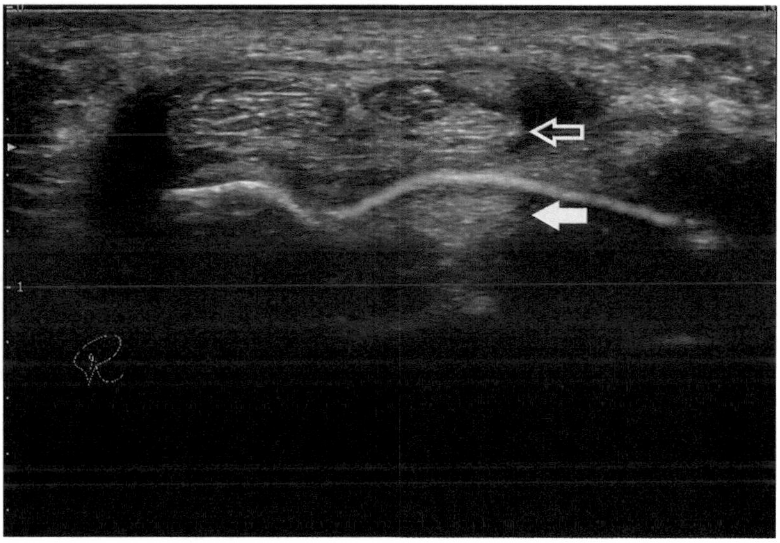

Fig. 1.16 Mirroring effect: An ultrasound image showing a cross-sectional view of the wrist, with two white arrows—one hollow indicating the flexor digitorum profundus tendon and one solid pointing to its mirror image beneath the cortex of the radius bone. (© Reza Roghani 2024. All Rights Reserved)

(hypoechoic), potentially mimicking pathology. This artifact is particularly notable in tendons, ligaments, and nerves, requiring careful probe positioning to ensure accurate interpretation.

1.7 Echogenicity

Echogenicity is a term used to describe how well a tissue reflects or transmits ultrasound waves to other tissues. Based on its echogenicity, a structure can be classified as hyperechoic (appearing white on the screen due to more reflection), hypoechoic (appearing gray on the screen due to more transmission), or anechoic (appearing black on the screen) [6]. Different musculoskeletal structures exhibit varying echogenicities on ultrasound due to their composition and ability to reflect sound waves.

Bone: Appears as a bright (hyperechoic) cortical line with complete shadowing beneath due to high acoustic impedance (Fig. 1.17).

It is worth noting that ultrasonography can only assess the outer surfaces of bones in minor

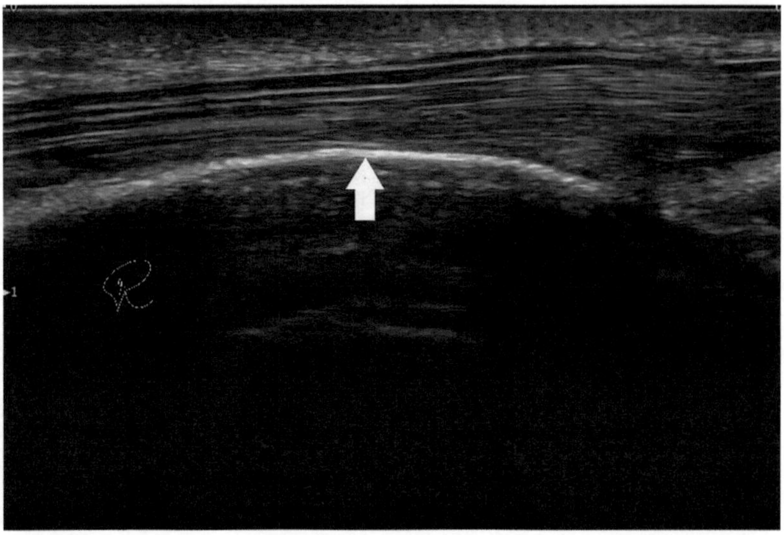

Fig. 1.17 Bone echogenicity: An ultrasound image displaying a longitudinal view of the distal radius in the forearm. A white arrow highlights the bone cortex, which appears as a bright, hyperechoic line with posterior acoustic shadowing. (© Reza Roghani 2024. All Rights Reserved)

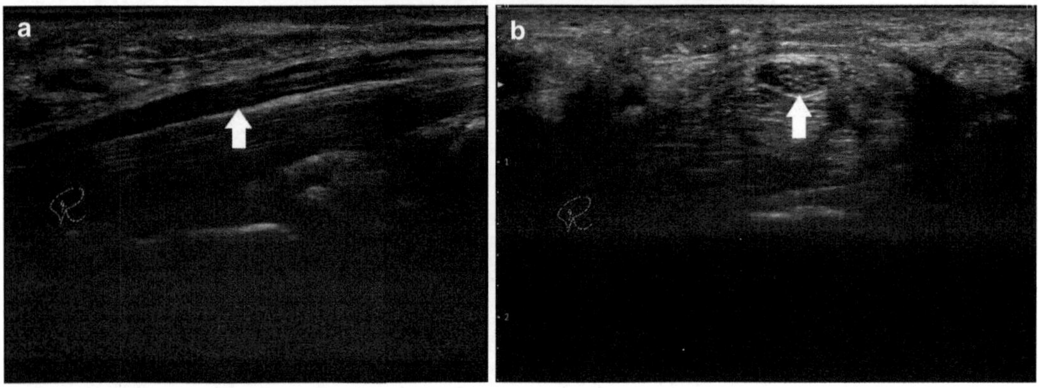

Fig. 1.18 Nerve echogenicity: Two ultrasound images, labeled (**a**) and (**b**), display the long-axis and short-axis views of the carpal tunnel, with solid white arrows highlighting the median nerve. (© Reza Roghani 2024. All Rights Reserved)

fractures that exhibit a clear break in the hyperechoic line. Nevertheless, recent research has demonstrated that ultrasonography is reliable for detecting joint bone erosions. In some cases, ultrasonography has even been found to identify more erosions than radiography.

Nerves: When scanned axially, nerves can appear as linear patches arranged in parallel patterns on ultrasound imaging. These patches are known as neuronal fascicles, which are distinguishable from the surrounding tissue due to their hypoechoic nature. They appear darker in comparison to the surrounding tissue. They are separated by hyperechoic (brighter) bands corresponding to connective tissue layers. When viewed in cross-section, nerves have a honeycomb appearance consisting of spherical hypoechoic regions surrounded by a hyperechoic background (Fig. 1.18).

Tendons: In ultrasound imaging, tendons exhibit a characteristic fibrillar pattern. On the longitudinal plane, they appear as parallel hyperechoic lines (collagen fibers) within an intermediate echogenic background (proteoglycan matrix). On the transverse plane, tendons are bright, stippled spots within a hyperechoic, circular to, ovoid structure. Due to their anisotropic nature, tendon echogenicity varies with the angle of the ultrasound beam. Optimal visualization requires the beam to be perpendicular to the tendon fibers, unlike nerves, which maintain their echogenicity more consistently across different angles (Fig. 1.19).

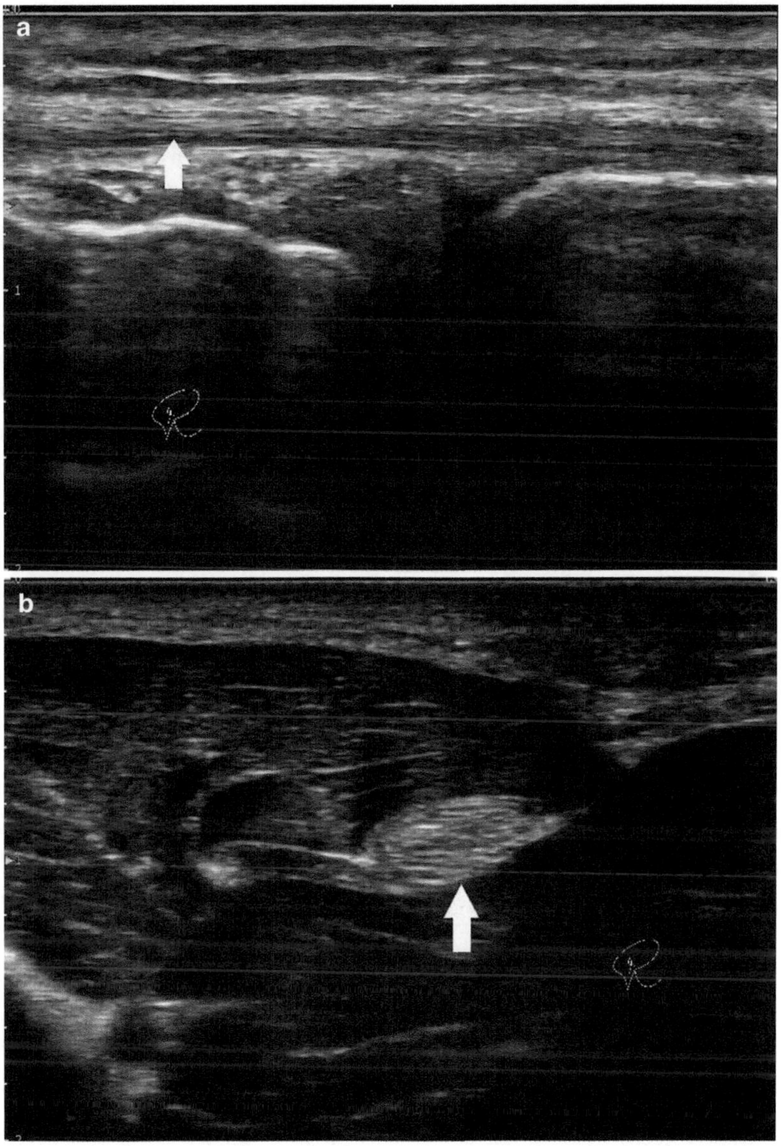

Fig. 1.19 Tendon echogenicity: Two ultrasound images, labeled (**a**) and (**b**), display the thenar eminence of the hand. In image (**a**), an arrow highlights the flexor pollicis longus tendon in the long axis, while in image (**b**), the same tendon is shown in the short axis. (© Reza Roghani 2024. All Rights Reserved)

Muscle fibers: When viewed longitudinally, the muscles appear less reflective on ultrasound (hypoechoic) and show linear echogenic bands of the perimysium. On transverse images, these bands appear as echogenic dots that resemble a starry night (Fig. 1.20). Due to the variable orientation of muscle fibers, they are susceptible to anisotropy errors, much like tendons.

Vessels and liquid cysts: In ultrasound imaging, vessels typically appear as anechoic (dark) structures with well-defined borders, with arteries showing pulsatile flow and veins demonstrating compressibility under pressure. Doppler ultrasound is often used to visualize blood flow, revealing color patterns that differentiate arterial and venous flow (Fig. 1.21). Liquid cysts, such as synovial or ganglion cysts, are also anechoic and typically appear round or oval with smooth borders, often exhibiting posterior acoustic enhancement due to the low attenuation of sound waves passing through the fluid. These cysts are usually devoid of internal echoes unless complicated by hemorrhage or infection.

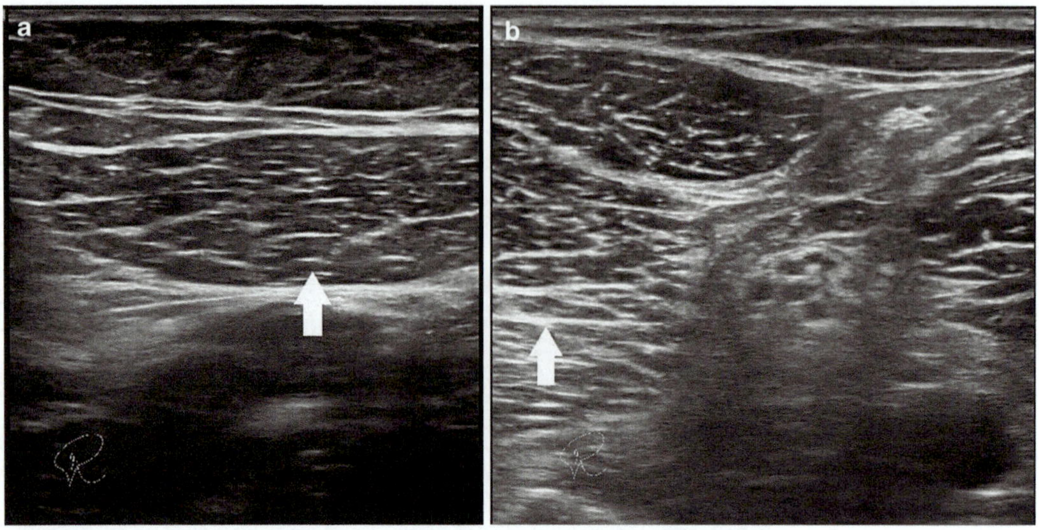

Fig. 1.20 Muscle echogenicity: Two ultrasound images, labeled (**a**) and (**b**), show different views of muscle tissue. In image (**a**), arrows highlight hypoechoic muscle fibers in the long axis, while in image (**b**), the perimysium surrounding the muscle fibers appears prominently in a "starry night" pattern in the short axis. (© Reza Roghani 2024. All Rights Reserved)

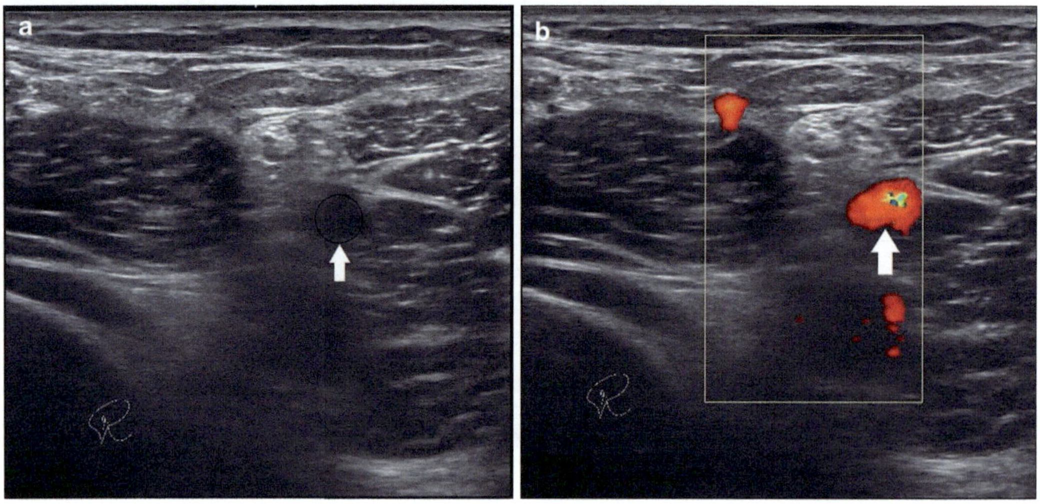

Fig. 1.21 Vessels echogenicity: Two ultrasound images, labeled (**a**) and (**b**), show the popliteal region. Image (**a**) is a B-mode image displaying a circled area with a white arrow pointing to the popliteal artery. Image (**b**) uses color Doppler imaging to highlight blood flow in red and yellow within the same circled region, again marked by a white arrow. (© Reza Roghani 2024. All Rights Reserved)

References

1. Edelman SK. Understanding ultrasound physics. 4th ed. E.S.P. Ultrasound; 2012.
2. Grogan SP, Mount CA. Ultrasound physics and instrumentation. In: StatPearls. StatPearls Publishing; 2024.
3. Jacobson JA. Fundamentals of musculoskeletal ultrasound. 3rd ed. Elsevier; 2017.
4. Rumack CM, Levine D, editors. Diagnostic ultrasound. 6th ed. 2-volume set. Elsevier; 2024.
5. Baston CM, Moore C, Krebs EA, Dean AJ, Panebianco N. Physics and knobology. In: Pocket guide to POCUS: point-of-care tips for point-of-care ultrasound. McGraw-Hill Education; 2018.
6. Hendee WR, Ritenour ER. Diagnostic ultrasound imaging: Inside out. 2nd ed. Elsevier; 2012.

Shoulder

2

Lynn Kohan, Reza Salman Roghani, Jose Juan Diaz, Richard Morgan, Ronald Tolchin, Mina Abadir, and Tariq Islam

2.1 Introduction

This chapter, Shoulder, provides a comprehensive overview of ultrasound imaging techniques for evaluating the complex structures of the shoulder. The shoulder complex consists of three primary joints—the sternoclavicular, acromioclavicular, and glenohumeral joints—each contributing to its extensive range of motion. The stability of the glenohumeral joint is maintained by bony congruency, ligamentous support, and the joint capsule's vacuum-like pressure. Additionally, dynamic stabilization is provided by the rotator cuff muscles, including the subscapularis, supraspinatus, infraspinatus, and teres minor (SSIT) [1, 2]. Through high-resolution ultrasound imaging, this chapter explores the echogenic characteristics of these structures and their clinical significance in diagnosing common pathologies such as rotator cuff tears, tendinopathy, bursitis, impingement syndromes, adhesive capsulitis, and glenohumeral instability. Key ultrasound techniques, probe positioning, patient positioning, and common artifacts encountered in shoulder imaging are discussed to enhance diagnostic accuracy. A structured shoulder scan protocol is presented to ensure a systematic sonographic evaluation. The anterior scan focuses on the biceps tendon and subscapularis muscle. The superior scan includes the acromioclavicular joint, supraspinatus, and suprascapular nerve, while the posterior scan evaluates the glenohumeral (GH) joint. Proper patient positioning and probe placement techniques are detailed for each scanning approach to optimize image acquisition. Additionally, the chapter provides comparative raw and highlighted ultrasound images to help practitioners distinguish different

Supplementary Information The online version contains supplementary material available at https://doi.org/10.1007/978-3-031-81037-4_2.

L. Kohan
Pain management division, Department of Anesthesia, University of Virginia School of Medicine, Charlottesville, VA, USA
e-mail: lrk9g@uvahealth.org

R. S. Roghani (✉)
Department of Physical Medicine and Rehabilitation, Larkin Community Hospital, Nova Southeastern University, Miami, FL, USA

J. J. Diaz
Department of Physical Medicine and Rehabilitation, Larkin Community Hospital, Nova Southeastern University, Miami, FL, USA

Integrative Spine and Sports, Fort Lauderdale, FL, USA

R. Morgan · R. Tolchin
Department of Physical Medicine and Rehabilitation, Miami Neuroscience Institute, Baptist Health, Miami, FL, USA
e-mail: ronaldbt@baptisthealth.net

M. Abadir · T. Islam
Ross University School of Medicine, Miramar, FL, USA
e-mail: MinaAbadir@mail.rossmed.edu; tariqislam@mail.rossmed.edu

R. S. Roghani, J. J. Diaz (eds.), *Video Atlas of Neuromusculoskeletal Ultrasound*,
https://doi.org/10.1007/978-3-031-81037-4_2

structures in an image. Furthermore, this chapter delves into common ultrasound-guided interventions, offering a step-by-step guide to performing precise and effective procedures for shoulder disorders. Each intervention is described in detail, including indications, patient positioning, probe selection, needle guidance techniques, and post-procedural considerations. To enhance understanding, this chapter is supplemented with 46 high-resolution images, probe placements, and procedural techniques. Additionally, 7 instructional videos provide dynamic demonstrations of scanning techniques, patient positioning, real-time ultrasound-guided interventions, and needle visualization methods, equipping practitioners with practical, hands-on knowledge. By integrating anatomical insights with practical sonographic applications, this chapter aims to improve diagnostic accuracy and procedural success in both evaluation and intervention for shoulder pathologies.

2.1.1 Shoulder Scan Protocol

Anterior

- **Sagittal Plane**:
  - Evaluate the **long head of the biceps tendon** in its long axis.
  - Assess the **subscapularis tendon** in its short axis.
- **Transverse Plane**:
  - Visualize the **biceps tendon** in its short axis and the **bicipital sheath** for potential injection.
  - Evaluate the **subscapularis tendon** in its long axis and tendon sheath for potential injection guidance.

Superior

- **Coronal Plane**:
  - Assess the **acromioclavicular (AC) joint** for structural integrity and guide AC joint injections.
  - Identify the **suprascapular nerve** for targeted nerve block.
- **Coronal Oblique Plane**:
  - Evaluate the **supraspinatus tendon** and the **subacromial-subdeltoid (SASD) bursa** and guide therapeutic injections.
- **Sagittal Oblique Plane**:
  - Visualize the **rotator cuff interval**, including assessment of the biceps pulley and adjacent structures.

Posterior

- **Transverse Oblique Plane**:
  - Access the **glenohumeral (GH) joint** for diagnostic evaluation and guided injection.

2.2 Anterior Shoulder

2.2.1 Biceps Tendon

2.2.1.1 Anatomy

The biceps brachii muscle has two components: the long head and the short head. The long head originates from the supraglenoid tubercle and passes through the biceps groove, while the short head originates from the coracoid process of the scapula. These two heads converge to form a single muscle and a tendon, which inserts in the radial tuberosity—innervated by the musculocutaneous nerve from the lateral cord of the brachial plexus (C5–7) [2, 3]. The primary action of the biceps brachii is supination and flexion of the forearm. In the cross-sectional view, the anatomy of the biceps region reveals the long head of the biceps tendon (LHBT) situated within the bicipital groove of the proximal humerus, bordered medially by the lesser tuberosity and laterally by the greater tuberosity. The tendon is encased by the synovial sheath, which facilitates smooth gliding movement. Anteriorly, the deltoid muscle overlays the region, appearing as a homogenous soft tissue structure, while the subcutaneous fat layer separates it from the skin. The biceps pulley complex, composed of the superior glenohumeral ligament and coracohumeral ligament, stabilizes the tendon within the groove. Deep to the tendon, the humeral head is visible with its cortical surface appearing as a bright, hyperechoic line on ultrasound. Adjacent structures include the pectoralis major tendon inserting onto the humerus, and laterally, the supraspinatus tendon transitioning toward its insertion at the greater tuberosity. Posteriorly, the infraspinatus and teres minor muscles contribute to shoulder stability. This cross-sectional perspective is essential for evaluating tendon

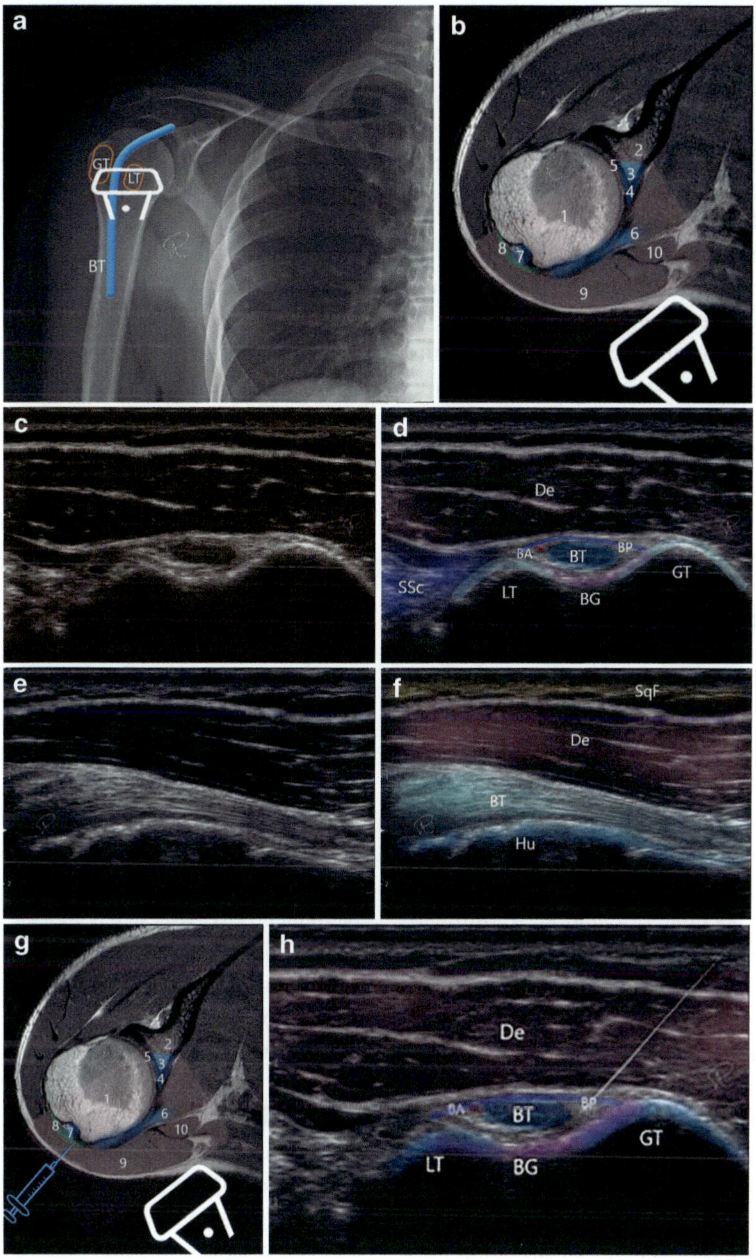

Fig. 2.1 Biceps tendon long head scan and injection technique. The image consists of multiple panels illustrating the biceps tendon scan and injection technique. Panel (**a**) is an X-ray demonstrating patient and probe positioning, highlighting the humerus, biceps tendon, and shoulder joint, with labeled anatomical structures: BT (biceps tendon), LT (lesser tuberosity), and GT (greater tuberosity). Panel (**b**) presents a MRI scan cross-section of the shoulder, with highlighted structures and numbered annotations corresponding to features visible in an ultrasound image: (1) humerus head, (2) glenoid, (3) labrum, (4) glenohumeral joint capsule, (5) humerus head cartilage, (6) subscapularis, (7) biceps tendon, (8) biceps tendon pulley, (9) deltoid, and (10) short head of the biceps. Panels (**c**) and (**d**) feature ultrasound images of the biceps tendon in the short axis, displayed in raw format and with highlighted annotations of key anatomical landmarks: De (deltoid), BT (biceps tendon), BP (biceps pulley), BA (biceps arteriole), LT (lesser tuberosity), GT (greater tuberosity), BG (biceps groove), and SSC (subscapularis). Panels (**e**) and (**f**) further illustrate long-axis views of the biceps tendon, presented in both raw and enhanced formats with labeled structures: De (deltoid), BT (biceps tendon), SqF (subcutaneous fat), and Hu (humerus). Panels (**g**) and (**h**) replicate the content of (**b**) and (**d**), with the addition of needle insertion, trajectory, and the target point for ultrasound-guided biceps tendon injection in the short-axis. ()

integrity, detecting inflammation, effusion, or pathology such as tendinopathy, tears, or subluxation (Fig. 2.1b).

2.2.1.2 Scan (Video 2.1)

Patient position: The patient is positioned seated upright with the ipsilateral elbow flexed at 90°, the arm supinated, and the dorsum of the hand resting on the ipsilateral thigh. This positioning allows for optimal exposure of the bicipital groove and the long head of the biceps tendon, minimizing muscle tension and ensuring a clear ultrasound window for accurate imaging (Fig. 2.1a).

Probe position: Position the probe in the transverse plane proximal to the axillary fold (Fig. 2.1a) until the biceps tendon is visualized within the bicipital groove. Make fanning motions with the probe until it becomes perpendicular to the tendon to minimize anisotropy and optimize visualization of the tendon fibers, ensuring clear imaging and accurate assessment of the tendon's integrity.

Scanning: The transducer should be perpendicular to the biceps tendon, displaying a short-axis view of the tendon at the groove (Fig. 2.1c). In this orientation, the greater and lesser tuberosities can be clearly visualized adjacent to the bicipital groove, providing critical anatomical landmarks for accurate orientation. Additionally, the biceps pulley, deltoid muscle, and biceps arteriole can also be visualized, offering a more comprehensive view of the shoulder anatomy. Begin the scanning process proximally, about the axillary fold, and progressively move distally along the short axis of the biceps tendon. With dynamic, continuous fanning of the probe, make sure the tendon's fibers remain sharply defined throughout the scan, allowing for the detection of any variations in echogenicity or structural integrity. This technique helps assess the entire length of the tendon while minimizing anisotropy. This approach is key in evaluating the tendon's morphology and is particularly effective for identifying pathologies such as tears, tendinopathy, or inflammation. Pay close attention to any irregularities in the tendon's appearance, as well as any changes in the biceps pulley, deltoid muscle, or biceps arteriole. Additionally, observe for any fluid around the tendon, which may indicate bursitis, tenosynovitis, or other inflammatory conditions, warranting further clinical investigation (Fig. 2.1c, d). To obtain a long-axis view of the biceps tendon, center the tendon in the image and rotate the transducer 90° from the short-axis orientation. This adjustment allows for the visualization of the tendon's longitudinal fibers, providing a detailed view of its structure across its full width. Ensure that the probe is aligned parallel to the tendon and perpendicular to the target for optimal clarity and consistent imaging. Slide the probe from medial to lateral to capture the full width of the tendon fibers. This technique is essential for evaluating the tendon, helping to identify any abnormalities such as tears, tendinopathy, or inflammation. Maintain consistent pressure and adjust the transducer angle as needed to minimize anisotropy, ensuring the tendon is clearly visualized and any potential issues are accurately detected (Fig. 2.1e, f).

Dynamic assessment for biceps tendon subluxation or dislocation involves positioning the probe in a short-axis view over the bicipital groove, ensuring a clear visualization of the biceps tendon in its normal alignment. Then, instruct the patient to perform controlled internal and external shoulder rotation while continuously monitoring the tendon's position. Observe for any displacement from the bicipital groove, which may indicate subluxation or dislocation. This dynamic technique is essential for evaluating tendon stability and detecting conditions such as biceps tendon instability or injury, which can contribute to shoulder dysfunction.

2.2.1.3 Injection

This injection is indicated for refractory pain secondary to biceps tendinopathy or partial tear. Following the standard scan, adjust the optimal short-axis view in the mid-screen. Insert the needle in-plane relative to the transducer from the lateral (Fig. 2.1g) with the needle tip placed deep on the biceps sheath but not into the tendon (Fig. 2.1h). Color flow (CF) Doppler is recommended to identify the bicipital arteriol. A 1.5-in. 25-gauge needle is appropriate to deliver 1 cc of local anesthetic and 1 cc of steroid or platelet rich plasma.

*Alternatively, in a long-axis view, the needle can be introduced in-plane relative to the transducer, approaching the tendon from distal to proximal and targeting the tendon sheath. This technique is particularly effective for isolated bicipital tendinitis, whereas the lateral approach is preferred when there is concomitant joint involvement, as the joint can be accessible in this view with one insertion.

2.2.2 Subscapularis Tendon

2.2.2.1 Anatomy

In a cross-sectional anatomical view, the subscapularis muscle is located on the anterior surface of the scapula, occupying the subscapular fossa. It is a thick, triangular muscle that extends laterally to insert onto the lesser tuberosity of the humerus, with its fibers running obliquely before converging into a strong tendon near insertion. Anteriorly, the pectoralis major and pectoralis minor muscles lie superficial to the subscapularis, forming part of the anterior shoulder structure. The short head of the biceps brachii originates from the coracoid process and runs medial to the long head of the biceps, positioned anterior to the subscapularis. The coracobrachialis muscle also originates from the coracoid process and runs adjacent to the short head of the biceps. The subscapularis bursa, situated between the tendon and the anterior glenohumeral joint capsule, facilitates smooth movement. Laterally, the subscapularis contributes to the rotator cuff, functioning alongside the supraspinatus, infraspinatus, and teres minor muscles to stabilize the shoulder joint (Fig. 2.2b). It is innervated by the subscapular nerve from the posterior cord of the brachial plexus (C5–6) [2]. The subscapularis's primary action is the humerus's internal rotation.

2.2.2.2 Scan (Video 2.2)

Patient position: The patient is seated upright with the ipsilateral arm supinated, the shoulder externally rotated, and the elbow flexed at 90°. This positioning allows optimal access for imaging or examination of the subscapularis muscle and its associated structures. The external rotation of the shoulder and supination of the forearm help bring the subscapularis tendon into view, particularly for ultrasound assessment or dynamic evaluation of the muscle's function. Keeping the elbow flexed at 90° ensures a stable position, minimizing movement artifacts while maintaining the natural anatomical alignment of the glenohumeral joint (Fig. 2.2a).

Probe position: Probe position: Place the transducer in a transverse plane slightly superior to the axillary fold, ensuring proper contact with the skin. Identify the biceps tendon within the bicipital groove and the subscapularis tendon as it inserts onto the lesser tuberosity. Ensure the probe is perpendicular to the biceps tendon to optimize imaging clarity and minimize anisotropy. Then, slide the probe medially to visualize the subscapularis myotendinous junction, ensuring a comprehensive assessment of its structure and integrity. Adjust the angle and pressure as needed to maintain a clear and stable view of the structures (Fig. 2.2a).

Scanning: When positioning the transducer transversely over the anterior shoulder, it's crucial to identify the biceps tendon within the bicipital groove as a landmark. From this point, slide the probe medially to visualize the lesser tuberosity, where the subscapularis tendon inserts. To obtain an optimal long-axis view of the subscapularis tendon (Fig. 2.2b), ensure that the probe is aligned parallel to the tendon fibers. This alignment is key to reducing anisotropy and improving image clarity. Since the subscapularis tendon is highly anisotropic due to its oblique orientation, instruct the patient to externally rotate the arm while maintaining a stable probe position (Fig. 2.2c, d). This maneuver stretches the tendon, enhances fiber definition, and minimizes dropout artifacts caused by anisotropy. Additionally, the external rotation allows for better visualization of most of the tendon, a portion of the subscapularis muscle, and the myotendinous junction, providing a more comprehensive assessment of the structure. In this position, assess the integrity of the tendon by sliding the probe along tendon length, identifying any pathological changes such as tendinosis, partial tears, or calcifications. Proper probe angulation is crucial to differentiate normal tendon architecture from pathological findings. To ensure complete evaluation, sweep the probe from proximal to distal and vice versa, scanning the entire tendon width. This movement helps detect focal abnor-

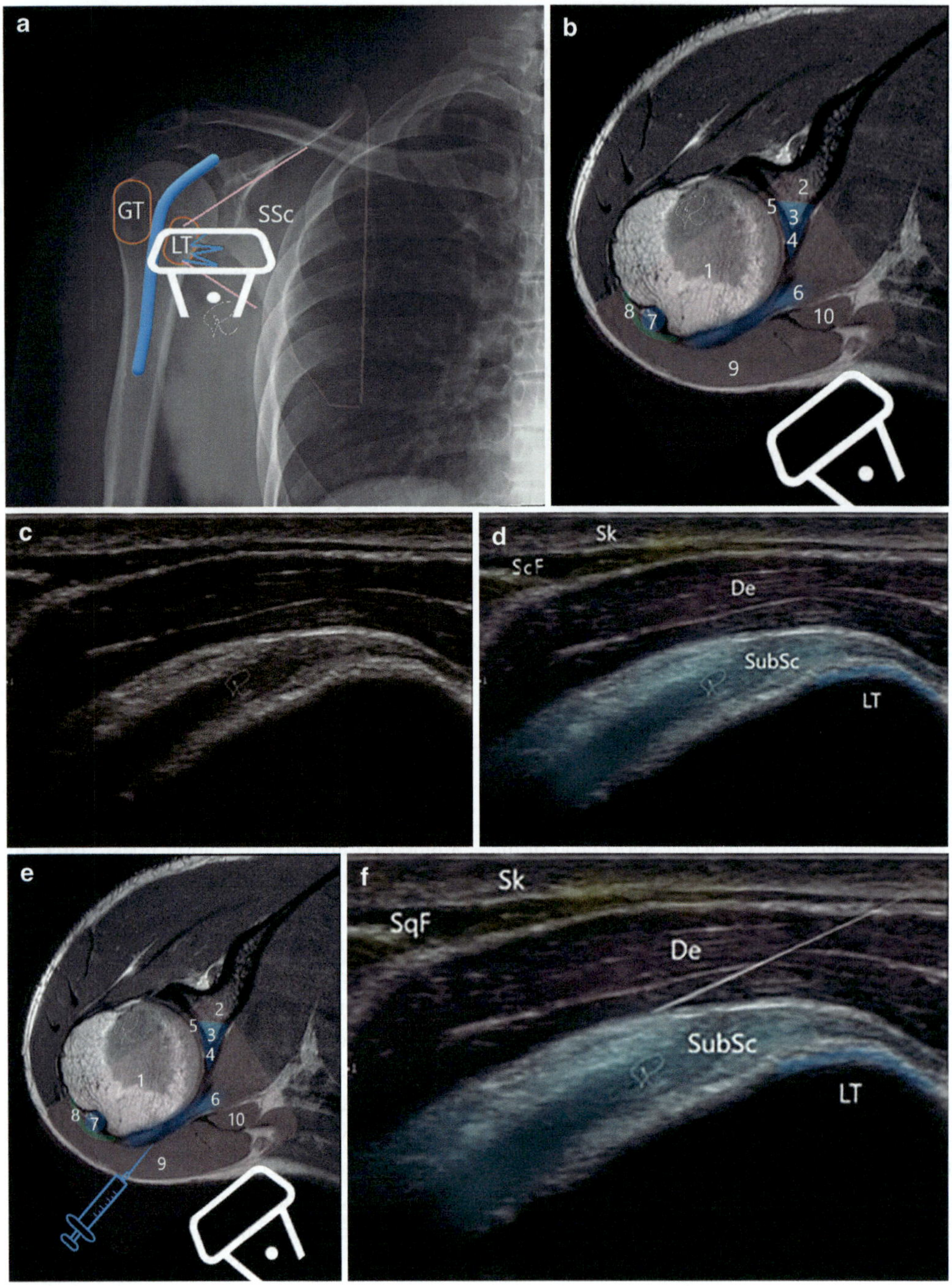

Fig. 2.2 Subscapularis tendon scan and injection: The image consists of six panels showing medical imaging of a shoulder joint. Panel (**a**) is an X-ray highlighting the patient and probe positions, with anatomical landmarks such as the greater tuberosity (GT), lesser tuberosity (LT), and subscapularis (SSc). Panel (**b**) is an MRI scan showing the subscapularis tendon cross-section, with labels for various structures: (1) humerus head, (2) glenoid, (3) labrum, (4) glenohumeral joint capsule, (5) humerus head cartilage, (6) infraspinatus, (7) biceps tendon, (8) biceps tendon pulley, (9) deltoid, and (10) the short head of the biceps. Panel (**c**) shows an ultrasound image of the subscapularis tendon and muscle, displaying the tendon's structure and surrounding tissues. Panel (**d**) is the same ultrasound image as (**c**), but with color-enhanced imaging that identifies the skin (Sk), deltoid (De), subcutaneous fat (ScF), lesser tuberosity (LT), and subscapularis (SubSc). Panel (**e**) is the same as (**b**), but with needle insertion and injection approach added, showing the positioning of the needle relative to the subscapularis tendon. Panel (**f**) is the same as (**d**), with the addition of the needle trajectory and target point, illustrating the intended path for the injection.

malities that might be missed in a static view, such as partial-thickness tears or calcifications. But don't stop there. Dynamic assessment with shoulder internal and external rotation can further help evaluate tendon function, gliding motion, and potential impingement. It's the final touch that ensures a comprehensive evaluation. After obtaining a long-axis view of the subscapularis tendon, rotate the transducer 90° to achieve a short-axis view. This perspective provides a cross-sectional image of the subscapularis, allowing for a detailed assessment of its fibrillar structure and overall integrity. The short-axis view is especially useful for evaluating tendon thickness, detecting focal pathologies such as tears, tendinosis, or calcifications, and assessing the relationship between the tendon and surrounding structures. In this orientation, it is important to position the probe perpendicular to the tendon to reduce anisotropy and achieve a uniform echotexture. The biceps tendon can serve as an additional landmark, as its medial border is closely related to the lateral portion of the subscapularis. Applying gentle pressure with the transducer can also help differentiate the tendon from adjacent structures. Performing a dynamic assessment in this plane, with internal and external rotation of the arm, can further aid in evaluating the entire length of the tendon. This approach helps observe tendon mobility and identify any impingement or abnormal displacement of surrounding tissues.

To assess for sub-coracoid impingement of the Subscapularis Tendon, follow these steps. First, place the transducer in a transverse plane over the biceps tendon and scan medially until you locate the coracoid. Next, identify the subscapularis tendon just inferior and lateral to the coracoid in the long-axis view. Then, move the arm into internal and external rotation to check for impingement or bursal fluid. The tendon should move smoothly beneath the coracoid process. If there is pooling of bursal fluid next to the coracoid, it is another sign of impingement [4, 5].

2.2.2.3 Injection

Refractory pain resulting from subscapularis tendinopathy or partial tears is the primary indication for this injection. Start with a standard ultrasound scan to obtain an optimal long-axis view of the subscapularis tendon, ensuring that the tendon is centered on the screen. Insert the needle in-plane from the lateral aspect, advancing it medially toward the tendon sheath (Fig. 2.2e). Carefully track the needle tip in real time until it successfully pierces the sheath (Fig. 2.2f). For the injection, use a 25-gauge needle to administer 1–2 cc of local anesthetic and 1 cc of corticosteroid. Alternatively, platelet-rich plasma (PRP) can be considered as a regenerative treatment option [6].

Safety considerations: If significant resistance is encountered during needle advancement, reposition the needle, as it may be embedded within the subscapularis tendon rather than within the sheath [7].

2.3 Superior Shoulder

2.3.1 Acromioclavicular (AC) Joint

2.3.1.1 Anatomy

The acromioclavicular (AC) joint is a synovial joint formed by connecting the clavicle's lateral end and the scapula's acromion process. The acromioclavicular ligament, the coracoclavicular ligament, and other supporting structures stabilize it. The AC joint is encased in a fibrous capsule lined with a synovial membrane, allowing smooth movement. On cross-sectional imaging, the joint appears as a space between the acromion and the clavicle. The acromion is triangular and located laterally on the scapula, while the clavicle runs horizontally across the top of the chest (Fig. 2.3a) [8]. The muscles surrounding the AC joint include the deltoid, supraspinatus, and trapezius. The deltoid muscle lies antrolaterally and covers the shoulder joint, including part of the AC joint. It is responsible for arm abduction and is seen as a thick, triangular muscle on cross-sectional imaging. The supraspinatus muscle lies inferiorly to the AC joint, originating from the supraspinous fossa of the scapula and inserted into the greater tuberosity of the humerus. It is part of the rotator cuff group of muscles and plays a key role in shoulder abduction and stabilization. Pathologies such as arthritis, ligament tears, or joint dislocations can lead to joint dysfunction, which is visible on imaging.

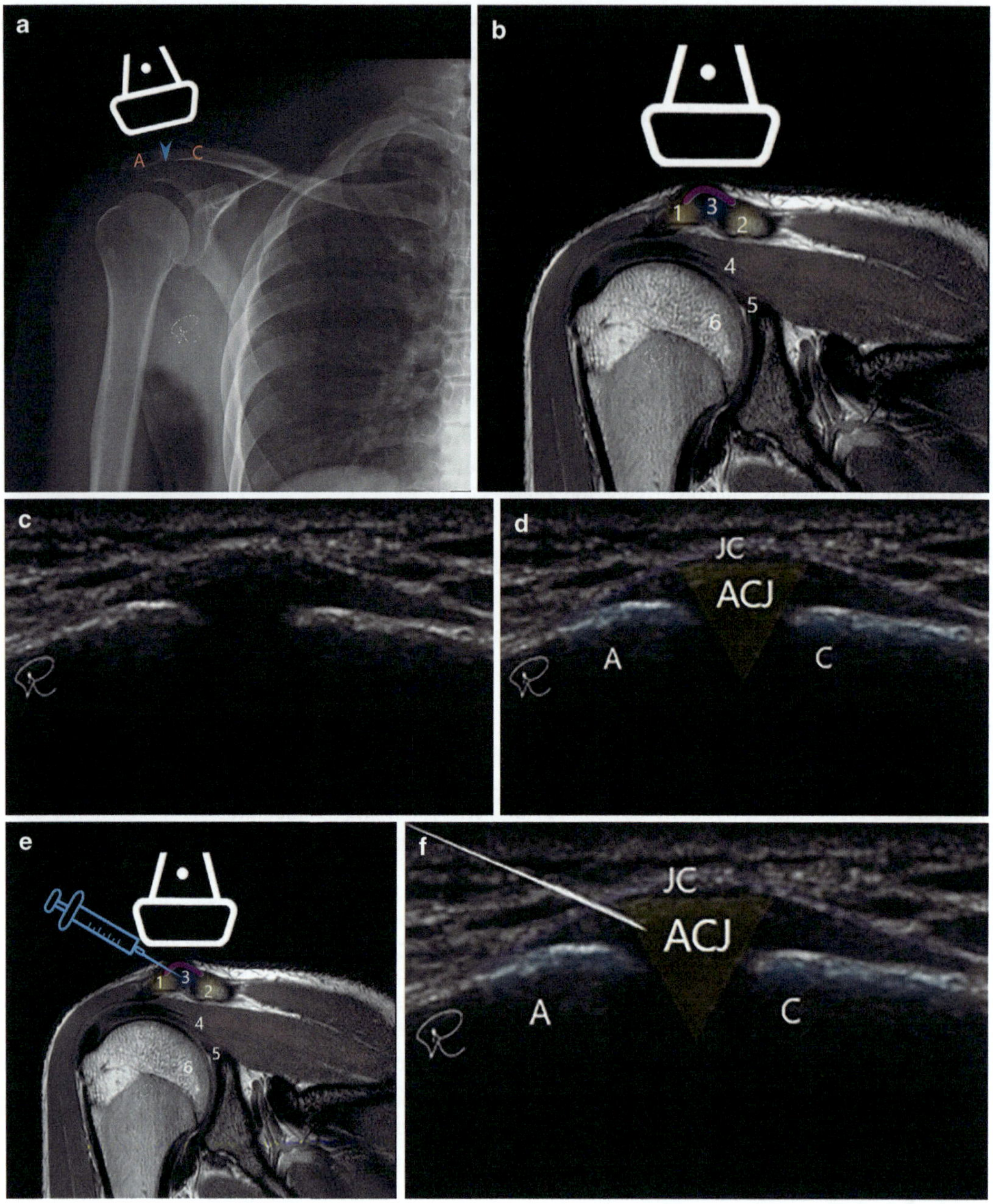

Fig. 2.3 Acromioclavicular joint scan and injection: The image consists of six panels that demonstrate various imaging techniques for assessing the acromioclavicular (AC) joint. Panel (**a**) features an X-ray of the shoulder, showing the patient and probe position with labeled points for the acromion (A) and clavicle (C). Panel (**b**) presents an MRI scan highlighting the AC joint anatomy, with numbered regions identifying different anatomical structures: (1) acromion, (2) clavicle, (3) AC joint, (4) supraspinatus tendon, (5) glenohumeral joint (GH joint), and (6) head of the humerus. Panel (**c**) displays an ultrasound image of the AC joint, offering a detailed view of the joint's structures. Panel (**d**) is the same ultrasound image as (**c**) but with additional labels highlighting the joint capsule (JC), acromioclavicular joint (ACJ), acromion (A), and clavicle (C). Panel (**e**) is similar to panel (**b**) but includes a syringe icon to demonstrate the needle insertion point for intervention. Panel (**f**) is an extension of panel (**d**), showing the needle trajectory and target point for injection.

2.3.1.2 Scan (Video 2.3)

Patient Position: For an acromioclavicular (AC) joint ultrasound, position the patient in a comfortable seated position with their back supported, ensuring the shoulder is relaxed and the arm resting naturally by the side to minimize muscle tension. The examiner should stand behind or beside the patient, depending on scanning hand preference (Fig. 2.3b).

Probe Position: Palpate the clavicle to identify anatomical landmarks, then place the transducer in a transverse plane along the superior border of the clavicle, and slide it laterally over the acromion for optimal visualization. To assess joint space and alignment, keep the patient's arm in a neutral position, while dynamic assessment can be performed by asking the patient to horizontally adduct the arm across the chest to evaluate joint movement, detect subtle separations, and assess for joint stiffness. The probe should be aligned with the clavicle and acromion to obtain a clear long-axis view of the joint space, capsule, and ligaments (Fig. 2.3a).

Scanning: Scan laterally along the clavicle toward the acromion until the "V-shaped" AC joint becomes visible (Fig. 2.3c). Within the scan, identify two hyperechoic structures: the acromion cortex on one side and the clavicle cortex on the other side. The middle V shape is the AC joint, while on top is a hyperechoic dome-shaped structure comprising the joint capsule, the subcutaneous fat, and skin layers (Fig. 2.3d). Scanning in both transverse and longitudinal planes ensures a comprehensive evaluation of the joint, detecting any degenerative changes, joint effusion, or ligament injuries.

2.3.1.3 Injection

AC joint injection is indicated for persistent superior shoulder pain secondary to AC joint arthritis that does not respond to conservative treatments, including physical therapy, NSAIDs, and activity modification. The procedure begins with an ultrasound scan to visualize the AC joint and confirm the presence of synovial hypertrophy, joint effusion, or osteophytes. Using an in-plane approach, the needle is inserted from lateral to medial under direct ultrasound guidance to ensure precise placement within the joint capsule (Fig. 2.3e, f). The injection technique involves a 25–30-gauge needle to deliver 0.5 mL of local anesthetic and 0.5 mL of injectable corticosteroid into the joint. Utilize Color Flow (CF) Doppler to monitor and confirm the distribution of the injected fluid in real-time, ensuring accurate delivery within the joint space. If standard corticosteroid injections fail, alternative treatments such as platelet-rich plasma (PRP) or viscosupplementation may be considered to promote joint healing and long-term symptom relief.

2.3.2 Supraspinatus

2.3.2.1 Anatomy

The supraspinatus is a small but crucial muscle of the rotator cuff located in the supraspinous fossa of the scapula. It originates from the medial two-thirds of this fossa and extends laterally, passing beneath the acromion before inserting into the superior facet of the greater tuberosity of the humerus. The supraspinatus is primarily responsible for initiating arm abduction and plays a key role in stabilizing the glenohumeral joint. On coronal cross-sectional imaging, the supraspinatus muscle appears as a well-defined structure superior to the scapular spine, extending laterally from the scapula toward the greater tuberosity (Fig. 2.4a, b). The muscle belly is located in the supraspinous fossa, while its tendon courses beneath the acromion within the subacromial space. Surrounding structures include the acromion and the subacromial-subdeltoid bursa superiorly and the glenohumeral joint capsule inferomedially. The close relationship between the supraspinatus tendon and the acromion makes it susceptible to impingement and degeneration, which are common causes of shoulder pain and dysfunction. It is innervated by the suprascapular nerve of the superior trunk of the brachial plexus (C5–6). The primary action of the supraspinatus is abduction of the humerus, predominantly between 0° and 15° [9].

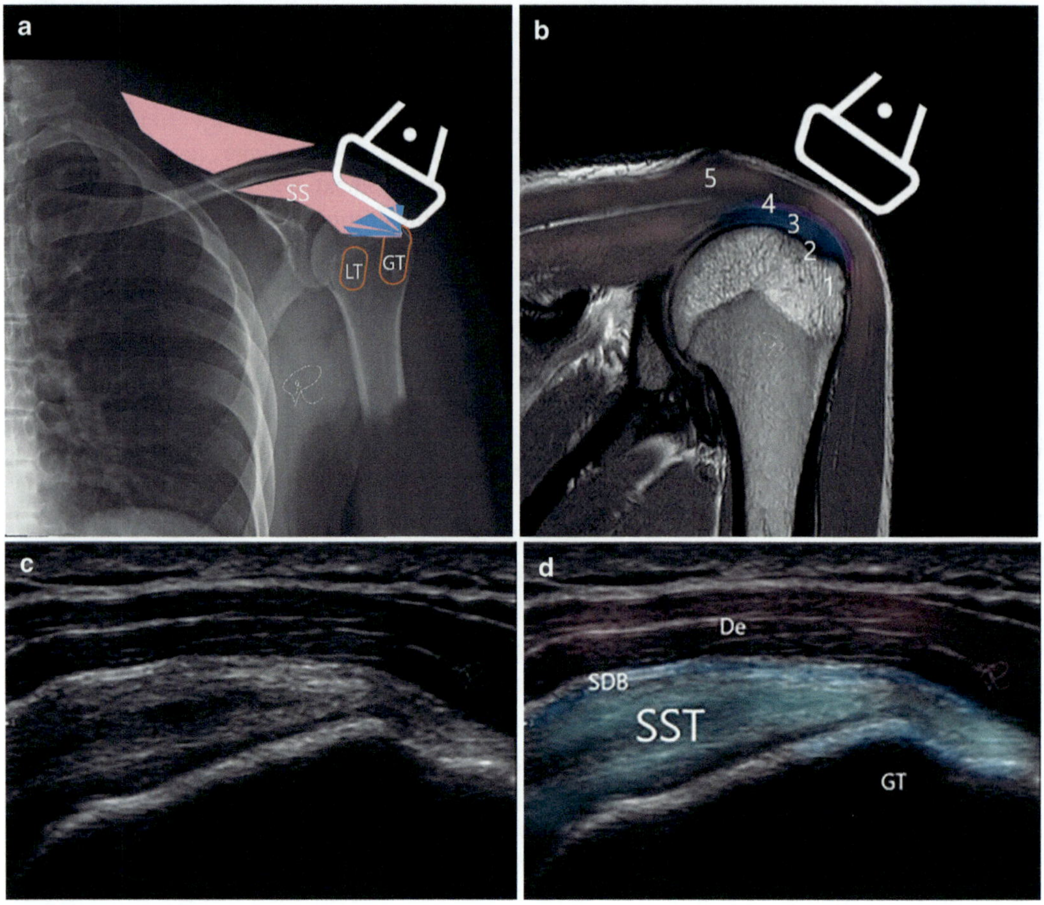

Fig. 2.4 Supraspinatus tendon scan: Composite image displaying shoulder anatomy and ultrasound visualization using multiple imaging modalities. (**a**) X-ray image of the shoulder with highlighted regions in pink and blue, illustrating the location of the supraspinatus muscle and tendon. The supraspinatus originates from the supraspinous fossa of the scapula, passes laterally beneath the acromion, and inserts onto the greater tuberosity of the humerus. The image demonstrates patient and probe positioning with labeled anatomical landmarks: SS (supraspinatus), GT (greater tuberosity), and LT (lesser tuberosity). (**b**) A coronal MRI slice of the shoulder with numbered regions 1–5, highlighting key anatomical structures. (1) The greater tuberosity (GT), situated on the lateral aspect of the proximal humerus, acts as the insertion point for the supraspinatus tendon. (2) The glenohumeral (GH) joint capsule. (3) The supraspinatus tendon (SST). (4) The subdeltoid bursa (SDB). (5) The deltoid muscle (De). (**c**) A raw ultrasound image of the supraspinatus tendon presents a hyperechoic fibrillar pattern that spans from the muscle belly to its insertion on the greater tuberosity. This image effectively highlights the tendon's position in relation to the greater tuberosity, which tapers to resemble the shape of a bird's beak. It serves as a valuable reference for assessing the structural integrity of the tendon, identifying potential tears, and evaluating bursitis. (**d**) The same (**c**) ultrasound image highlighted with different colors, labeling SST (supraspinatus tendon), SDB (subdeltoid bursa), De (deltoid), and GT (greater tuberosity), providing enhanced visualization of these anatomical structures and their spatial relationships. (© Reza Roghani 2024. All Rights Reserved)

2.3.2.2 Scan (Video 2.4)

Patient Position: For an optimal supraspinatus ultrasound scan, position the patient in a seated position with their arm placed in slight internal rotation and extension, commonly referred to as the modified Crass or "hand behind the back" position. This posture moves the supraspinatus tendon out from under the acromion, allowing better visualization and reducing anisotropy (Fig. 2.4a).

Probe Position: Place the transducer in a longitudinal plane along the supraspinatus muscle, aligning it parallel to the humeral head. The probe should be positioned anterior to the acromion and angled slightly posteriorly (toward patient neck) to follow the course of the tendon as it inserts onto the greater tuberosity. To obtain a short-axis view, rotate the probe 90° perpendicular to the tendon. Adjusting the probe angle and applying gentle pressure can further enhance image quality and minimize acoustic shadowing from the overlying acromion.

Scanning: After proper positioning scan slightly inferolateral until the supraspinatus tendon insertion onto the greater tuberosity is viewed in the long axis (Fig. 2.4b). The footprint of the supraspinatus tendon will exhibit a "bird's beak" appearance on the long axis (Fig. 2.4c, d). This allows for an optimal long-axis view, where the tendon appears as a fibrillar structure running toward its insertion. To assess the entire tendon width sweep the probe anterior to posterior, from the biceps tendon to the supraspinatus-infraspinatus junction. To scan the tendon completely, capturing the full extent of the tendon and any potential abnormalities, rotate the transducer 90° to obtain a short-axis view of the supraspinatus tendon. Then, slide the probe from medial to lateral to ensure full tendon coverage. Scan in all four directions—superior-inferior and medial-lateral—to thoroughly assess the tendon fibers and ensure complete visualization of the tendon. This approach guarantees a comprehensive scan of the supraspinatus tendon. Always ensure that your probe is perpendicular to the tendon by continuously fanning the probe. This technique helps to minimize anisotropy, improving image clarity and allowing for more accurate visualization of the tendon's structure and any abnormalities. Proper probe alignment is crucial for obtaining high-quality, reliable images during the ultrasound scan.

To assess subacromial impingement of the supraspinatus tendon, begin by palpating the acromion. Then, position the transducer in the coronal plane and align the medial portion of the transducer over the acromion. You should be able to see the hyperechoic fibers of the supraspinatus tendon, which are visible lateral to the acromion and medial to the tendon insertion site on the greater tuberosity. Next, move the arm into the abduction and check for bursal fluid and impingement of the tendon-bursa complex. Key indicators include increased bursal fluid accumulation between the supraspinatus tendon and acromion, which can become more pronounced with shoulder movement, especially in abduction. Compression of the tendon between the acromion and humeral head may be visualized, often leading to tendon flattening or deformation. Osteophytes on the acromion or AC joint may become more prominent during motion, irritating the tendon and bursa. Additionally, the proximal migration of the humeral head or narrowing of the subacromial space during shoulder elevation can suggest impingement. Tendon tears or fissures may also become more apparent as the arm moves, providing real-time evidence of tendon dysfunction [5].

2.3.3 Subacromial-Subdeltoid (SASD) Bursa

2.3.3.1 Anatomy

The subacromial-subdeltoid (SASD) bursa is an anatomical structure characterized as a synovial fluid-filled cavity. It is strategically located beneath the acromion process, functioning as a cushion between the rotator cuff tendons, the overlying coracoacromial ligament, and the deltoid muscle. This bursa plays a crucial role in reducing friction between these anatomical components during shoulder movements (Fig. 2.4b). Under normal conditions, the bursa has a thin, compressible appearance, with a regular thickness of less than 2 mm, making it challenging to visualize on ultrasound in the absence of pathology [2, 9]. In instances of inflammation, impingement, or overuse injuries, the bursa may become distended with fluid, which can be readily identified through ultrasound imaging. This often appears as a hypoechoic or anechoic area located between the deltoid muscle and the supraspinatus tendon. Pathological thickening or excessive fluid accumulation within the subacromial/subdeltoid (SASD) bursa is frequently linked to conditions such as subacromial bursitis, rotator cuff

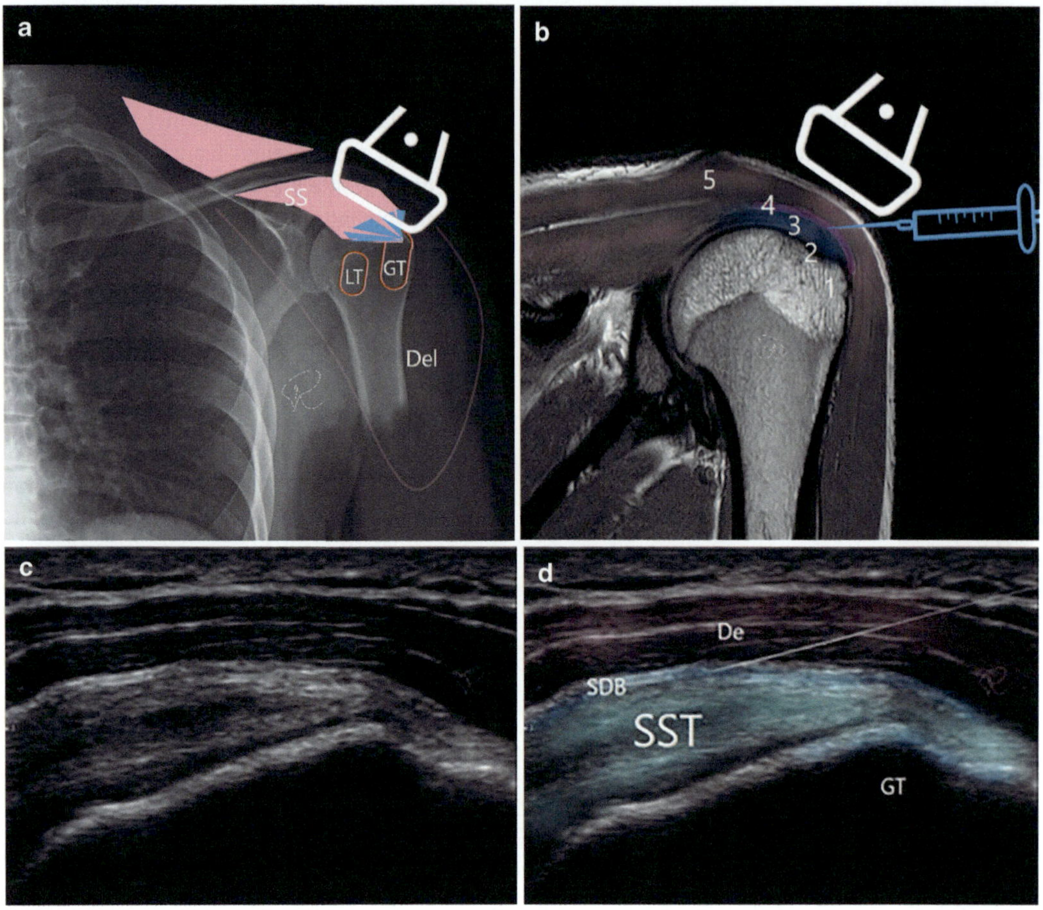

Fig. 2.5 Subacromial-subdeltoid (SASD) bursa scan and injection technique: Composite image showing shoulder anatomy, ultrasound, and SASD injection technique. Panel (**a**) X-ray of the shoulder demonstrates patient and probe positioning with labeled structures, including SS (supraspinatus), LT (lesser tuberosity), GT (greater tuberosity), and Del (deltoid). Panel (**b**) A coronal MRI slice of the shoulder with numbered regions 1– 5, highlighting key anatomical structures. (1) The greater tuberosity (GT), situated on the lateral aspect of the proximal humerus, acts as the insertion point for the (2) glenohumeral (GH) joint capsule, (3) supraspinatus tendon (SST), (4) subdeltoid bursa (SDB), (5) deltoid muscle (De), and probe position and needle insertion point for SASD bursa injection. Panel (**c**) A raw ultrasound image of the supraspinatus tendon presents a hyperechoic fibrillar pattern that spans from the muscle belly to its insertion on the greater tuberosity. Panel (**d**) presents the same ultrasound image as in (**c**) but with color highlights to enhance visualization. It labels key anatomical structures, including the supraspinatus tendon (SST), subdeltoid bursa (SDB), deltoid muscle (De), and greater tuberosity (GT). Additionally, it illustrates the needle trajectory and target point for SASD bursa injection, providing a clearer understanding of the procedural approach and spatial relationships between these structures. (© Reza Roghani 2024. All Rights Reserved)

tendinopathy, or impingement syndrome. Therefore, assessing the bursa plays a vital role in shoulder ultrasound evaluations.

2.3.3.2 Scan

Patient Position: To perform an ultrasound examination of the subacromial-subdeltoid (SASD) bursa, begin by positioning the patient in a relaxed seated posture, with the shoulder gently abducted and the hand resting in the back pocket (Modified Crass position) (Fig. 2.5a).

Probe Position: Place the transducer in a coronal-oblique plane at the anterosuperior aspect of the shoulder, just below the acromion, directing it toward the neck. For optimal visualization, utilize the fanning technique to ensure that the probe is perpendicular to the target area, specifically the supraspinatus tendon (Fig. 2.5a).

Scanning: On the ultrasound screen, the SASD bursa will typically appear as a thin, hypoechoic, or anechoic space located between the supraspinatus tendon (SST) and the deltoid muscle. The footprint of the supraspinatus tendon will exhibit a "bird's beak" appearance on the long axis. The subdeltoid bursa separates this tendon from the overlying deltoid muscle, and in case of inflammation, it enlarges with fluid (Fig. 2.4c, d). If any abnormalities are suspected, such as fluid accumulation, measure the width of the bursa and evaluate for any signs of tendon damage or inflammation in the surrounding tissues. Color Doppler imaging may also be helpful in assessing increased vascularity, which could indicate inflammation. Finally, dynamic scanning with shoulder movement (such as abduction) can help identify any changes in the bursa's size or fluid accumulation during motion, which can assist in diagnosing impingement or rotator cuff pathology.

2.3.3.3 Injection

The subacromial-subdeltoid (SASD) bursa injection is indicated for refractory pain after a trial of conservative treatment for bursitis or impingement. Begin the procedure using the scanning protocol mentioned above. Align the optimum view in the mid-screen. Insert the needle in plane from lateral to medial and into the distended bursa (Fig. 2.5d). Use color flow to visualize the fluid spread linearly within the bursa space. The injection technique involves a 25-gauge needle to deliver 1 mL of local anesthetic and 1 mL of injectable corticosteroid into the bursa. Platelet-rich plasma is an alternative treatment option [6].

Safety consideration(s): Reposition the needle if significant resistance is encountered, as the needle tip may be embedded within the supraspinatus tendon [7].

2.3.4 Rotator Cuff Interval

2.3.4.1 Anatomy

The rotator cuff consists of a crucial group of four muscles and their associated tendons, which play a vital role in stabilizing the shoulder joint and enabling movement. These muscles—subscapularis, supraspinatus, infraspinatus, and teres minor—originate from the scapula and insert into the greater or lesser tuberosity of the humerus. Their coordinated action allows for a wide range of shoulder movements, including abduction, internal rotation, and external rotation, while also ensuring dynamic stabilization of the glenohumeral joint. A significant anatomical feature within the rotator cuff is the rotator cuff interval (RCI), a triangular space situated between the supraspinatus and subscapularis tendons. The RCI is traversed by the long head of the biceps brachii tendon as it extends from the superior glenoid tubercle and passes beneath the transverse humeral ligament. This interval also contains the coracohumeral and superior glenohumeral ligaments, which provide additional stability to the shoulder. A comprehensive understanding of rotator cuff anatomy is essential for ultrasound scanning, diagnosis, and management of conditions like tears, tendinopathy, and impingement syndromes (Fig. 2.6b) [2].

2.3.4.2 Scan (Video 2.5)

Patient position: For the ultrasound evaluation of the rotator cuff interval, the patient should be positioned either seated or supine, with the arm resting in a neutral position, the elbow flexed at 90 degrees, and the forearm adequately supported. This positioning facilitates optimal visualization of the interval structures while avoiding excessive tension on surrounding tissues (Fig. 2.6a).

Probe position: The probe is initially placed in a transverse orientation over the anterior shoulder, just medial to the greater tuberosity, to visualize the long head of the biceps tendon within the bicipital groove.

Scanning: From this position, the probe is gently swept proximally and tilted to make the groove shallow and continue until it disappears,

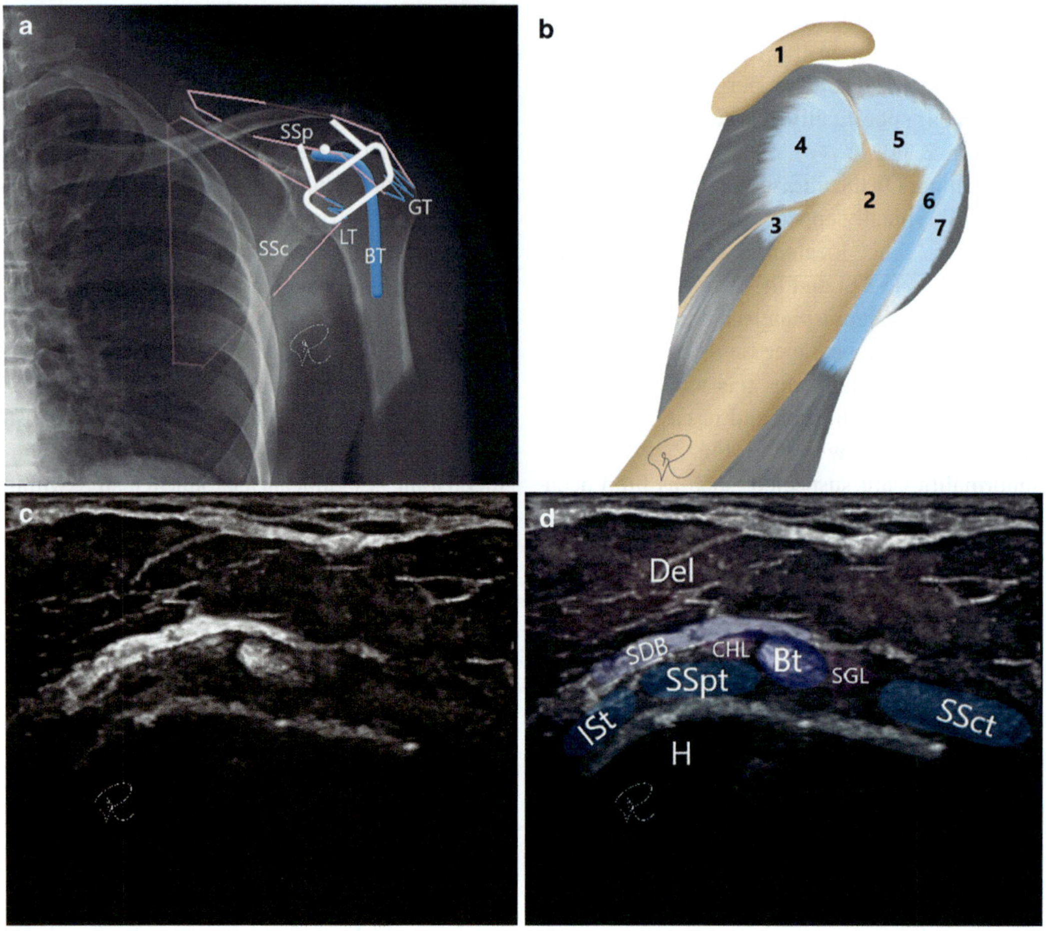

Fig. 2.6 Rotator cuff interval scan: The image consists of four panels illustrating shoulder anatomy. Panel (**a**) shows an X-ray of a shoulder with labeled anatomical landmarks: SSp (supraspinatus), SSc (subscapularis), GT (greater tuberosity), LT (lesser tuberosity), and BT (biceps tendon). Panel (**b**) is a diagram of a shoulder joint with numbered muscle and tendon areas: (1) acromion, (2) humerus (H), (3) teres minor, (4) infraspinatus (ISt), (5) supraspinatus (SSpt), (6) biceps tendon (Bt), and (7) subscapularis (SSct). Panel (**c**) displays an ultrasound image of the rotator cuff, highlighting muscle layers and tendons. Panel (**d**) is another ultrasound image with labeled structures: Del (deltoid), SDB (subdeltoid bursa), CHL (coraco humeral ligament), Bt (biceps tendon), SGL (superior glenoid ligament), ISt (infraspinatus tendon), and SSct (subscapularis tendon), SSpt (supraspinatus tendon) showing detailed rotator cuff ultrasound anatomy. ()

tilted, and then rotate the transducer 20–30° to capture the rotator cuff interval, which is located between the supraspinatus and subscapularis tendons and biceps tendon is sandwiched between the coracohumeral and superior glenoid ligaments. To enhance imaging, the transducer should be dynamically fanned to maintain perpendicular alignment to the biceps tendon, thereby minimizing anisotropy and improving image clarity. By sliding the probe posteriorly, the remaining rotator cuff tendons—including the infraspinatus and teres minor—can be visualized, providing a comprehensive assessment of the shoulder structures (Fig. 2.6c, d). Rotator cuff pathologies commonly detected on ultrasound include tendinosis, partial-thickness or full-thickness tears, calcific tendinopathy, and bursitis. Tendinosis appears as tendon thickening with reduced echogenicity and a heterogeneous texture. Partial-thickness tears are hypoechoic or anechoic defects within the tendon, while full-thickness tears show complete discontinuity with tendon retraction and fluid-filled gaps. Calcific tendinopathy is identified by hyperechoic deposits with or without posterior acoustic shadowing within the tendon. Bursitis, often involving the subacromial-subdeltoid (SASD) bursa, manifests as fluid distension greater than 2 mm, sometimes with increased vascularity on Doppler imaging. Dynamic ultrasound can further assess impingement by observing changes in tendon thickness, bursal distension, or abnormal movement patterns during active shoulder motion.

2.3.5 Suprascapular Nerve

2.3.5.1 Anatomy

The suprascapular nerve arises from the upper trunk of the brachial plexus, originating from the C5 and C6 nerve roots, with occasional contributions from C4. It travels laterally and posteriorly, passing beneath the trapezius muscle toward the suprascapular notch, where it enters the supraspinous fossa by traversing under the transverse scapular ligament. Within the supraspinous fossa, the nerve innervates the supraspinatus muscle before continuing through the spinoglenoid notch into the infraspinous fossa, where it provides motor innervation to the infraspinatus muscle (Fig. 2.7b). Although primarily a motor nerve, it also carries sensory fibers that contribute to the innervation of the glenohumeral and acromioclavicular joints. Due to its anatomical pathway, the suprascapular nerve is vulnerable to compression at the suprascapular or spinoglenoid notch, potentially resulting in suprascapular neuropathy, which is commonly observed in overhead athletes, weightlifters, and individuals engaged in repetitive shoulder movements [9].

2.3.5.2 Scan (Video 2.6)

Patient Position: For a suprascapular nerve ultrasound scan, the patient is typically seated or prone with the shoulder relaxed and slightly flexed (Fig. 2.7a).

Probe Position: The probe is initially placed at the midpoint of the spine of the scapula transversely and then, slowly move the transducer proximally to reach the suprascapular notch, located at the superior border of the scapula, just medial to the acromion process. Placing the ultrasound transducer on the acromion process in the coronal plane and slide it medially is an alternate positioning. This position allows visualization of the suprascapular nerve as it passes beneath the transverse scapular ligament (Fig. 2.7a, b). To further evaluate the nerve, the probe can be moved laterally and posteriorly along the supraspinous fossa to track the nerve's course toward the spinoglenoid notch. To examine its passage through the spinoglenoid notch into the infraspinous fossa, the probe is repositioned more inferiorly and obliquely. Dynamic scanning with gentle shoulder movements can help assess potential entrapment, impingement, or pathology along the nerve's course.

Scanning: Starting with the initially mentioned probe position, gently move the transducer upward along the scapula until the cortical bone comes into view, appearing as a highly reflective, bright line. As you continue your scanning motion, you will encounter a distinctive "U-shaped" depression known as the suprascapular notch. This notch is situated at the superior border of the scapula and is seen as a deep feature within the image (Fig. 2.7a, b). Within this depression, you can identify a smal dark, round structure that represents the pulsatile suprascapular artery. Adjacent to this artery, there is an oval structure with mixed echogenicity that corresponds to the suprascapular nerve, which often presents with a slightly hypoechoic or heterogeneous appearance compared to the surrounding tissues. Above these anatomical features, you will note the suprascapular retinaculum, a ligamentous structure, and just posterior to the retinaculum lie the supraspinatus and trapezius muscles (Fig. 2.7c, d). These muscles are well visualized on ultrasound due to their clearly defined borders and the contrast provided by the surrounding tissues. Identifying the suprascapular nerve structures is essential for evaluating potential impingement, entrapment, or other related issues, especially in shoulder pain or dysfunction cases.

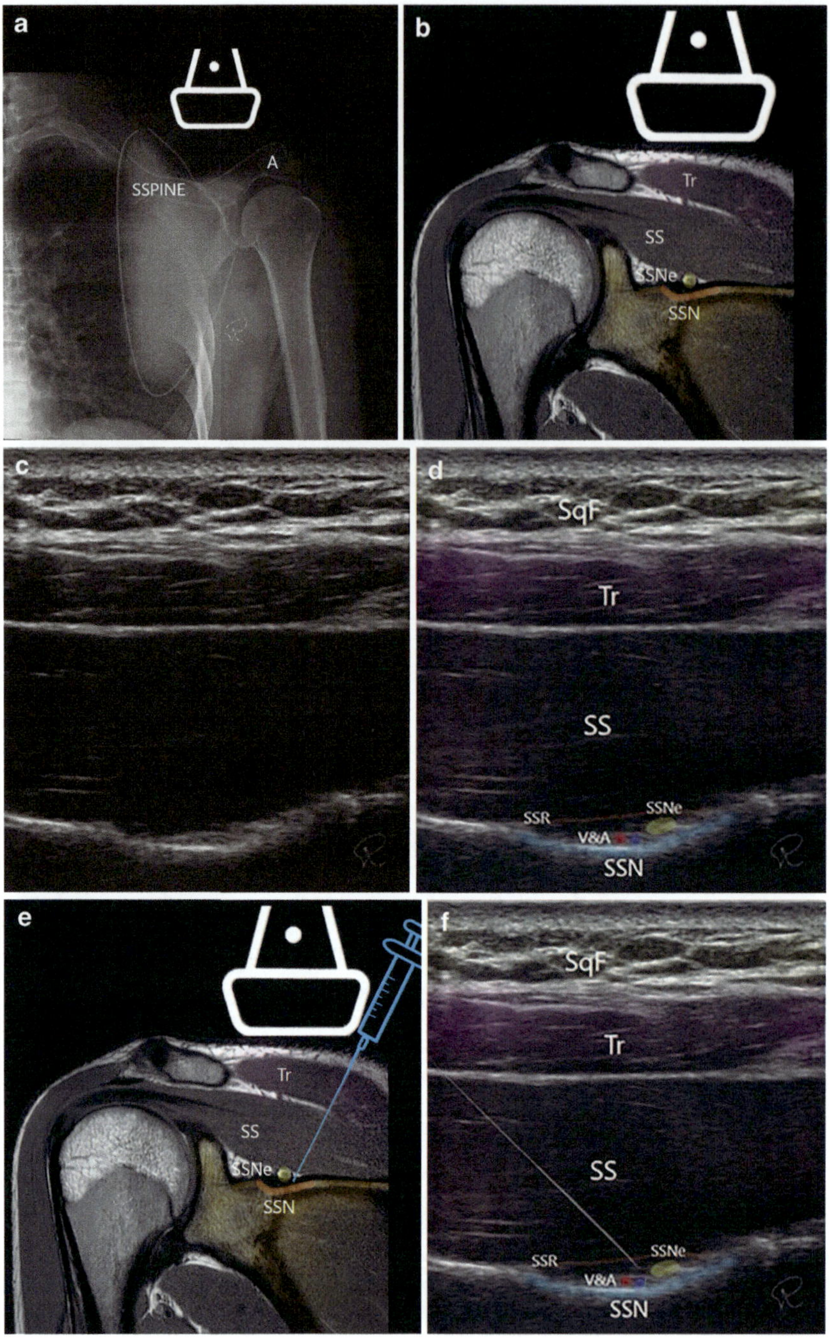

Fig. 2.7 Suprascapular nerve scan and block: A series of six medical images showing different views and techniques for examining suprascapular nerve. Image (**a**): X-ray of a shoulder with labels "SSPINE" and "A" indicating scapular spine and acromion anatomical landmarks for patient and probe position. Image (**b**): A coronal MRI scan slice of a shoulder with labels "Tr, trapezius" "SS, supraspinatus", "SSNe, suprascapular nerve" and "SSN, suprascapular notch" showing detailed anatomy of suprascapular nerve and notch. Image (**c**): Ultrasound image of a suprascapular nerve and notch with no labels. Image (**d**): Is the same (**c**) ultrasound image with highlights and labels SqF, subcutaneous fat; Tr, trapezius; SS, supraspinatus; SSR, suprascapular retinaculum; SSNe, suprascapular nerve; V&A, suprascapular vein and artery; SSN, supra scapular notch. Explaining various ultrasound image anatomical structures. Image (**e**): This image is the same as image (**b**), featuring a syringe illustration that indicates the needle insertion site. Image (**f**): This image is identical to image (**d**) and features an illustration of a needle that indicates both the needle trajectory and the target point.

Injection: It is indicated for post-operative pain control or chronic shoulder pain secondary to rheumatoid arthritis, osteoarthritis, adhesive capsulitis, hemiplegic shoulder pain, or rotator cuff tendinopathies [10, 11]. Following the scanning mentioned above, insert the needle in plane from medial to lateral (Fig. 2.7e). When inserting the needle, aim to pierce the overlying transverse suprascapular ligament near the neurovascular bundle (Fig. 2.7f). Utilize CF Doppler to identify the suprascapular artery. Alternatively, insert the needle out of the plane relative to the transducer, approaching antero-posterior to avoid entering the pleural region, and use CF Doppler to prevent damage to nearby arteries. Through a 25-gauge 2.5-in. needle, deliver 5 ccs of local anesthetic.

Safety consideration: In the alternative method, it is advised not to approach from posterior to anterior as there is a risk of needle advancement, which can result in penetration to the anterior and lung apex [10].

2.4 Posterior Shoulder

2.4.1 Anatomy

2.4.1.1 Glenohumeral Joint

The glenohumeral joint (GHJ) is recognized as the ball-and-socket joint that plays a critical role in connecting the scapula (shoulder blade) to the humerus (upper arm bone). Renowned for being the most mobile joint in the human body, it permits an extensive range of motion across various directions. This joint is anatomically structured by the convex head of the humerus and the concave glenoid cavity of the scapula. Surrounding the glenoid is a fibrocartilaginous ring known as the labrum, which deepens the socket and enhances the stability of the humeral head within it. The stability and mobility of the GHJ are further supported by the rotator cuff muscles, which include the supraspinatus, infraspinatus, teres minor, and subscapularis. These muscles encase the GHJ and their tendons integrate with the joint capsule, playing a crucial role in maintaining the stability of the humeral head as it resides in the shallow glenoid fossa. Additional support is provided by the glenohumeral ligaments—superior, middle, and inferior—contributing to the joint's stability by restricting excessive movements. The joint capsule itself is a robust fibrous tissue structure that encapsulates the entire joint, encasing the glenohumeral space while housing synovial fluid essential for joint lubrication. Moreover, the presence of the subacromial bursa, a sac filled with synovial fluid, is significant as it minimizes friction between the tendon and the adjacent structures. In clinical settings, ultrasound imaging is employed to assess the glenohumeral joint, utilizing specific cross-sectional planes for optimal visualization of essential anatomical components. The longitudinal or sagittal view provides an opportunity to observe the humeral head, labrum, and rotator cuff tendons, facilitating the assessment of their interrelations and identification of potential tears in either the rotator cuff or labrum. Conversely, the transverse or axial view depicts the rounded structure of the humeral head alongside the concave glenoid fossa, allowing for evaluations of the joint itself [12].

2.4.1.2 Glenoid Labrum

The glenoid labrum is a fibrocartilaginous structure that encircles the rim of the glenoid cavity, enhancing the socket's depth and improving the stability of the glenohumeral joint. It serves as an attachment point for the glenohumeral ligaments and the long head of the biceps brachii tendon. Structurally, the labrum consists of dense connective tissue with a triangular cross-section, featuring a firm attachment to the glenoid rim and a looser connection to the joint capsule. The labrum is divided into superior, inferior, anterior, and posterior regions, each contributing to the stabilization of the humeral head during movement. The superior labrum is particularly noteworthy because of its attachment to the biceps tendon, making it vulnerable to SLAP (Superior Labrum Anterior to Posterior) tears. The anterior and posterior portions of the labrum are essential in preventing excessive translation of the humeral head, with the anterior labrum playing a crucial role in stabilizing against anterior dislocations. In the axial (transverse) plane ultrasound imaging, the anterior and posterior labrum can be visualized as a hyperechoic triangular or curved structure adjacent to the glenoid rim. The posterior labrum is best visualized with the probe posi-

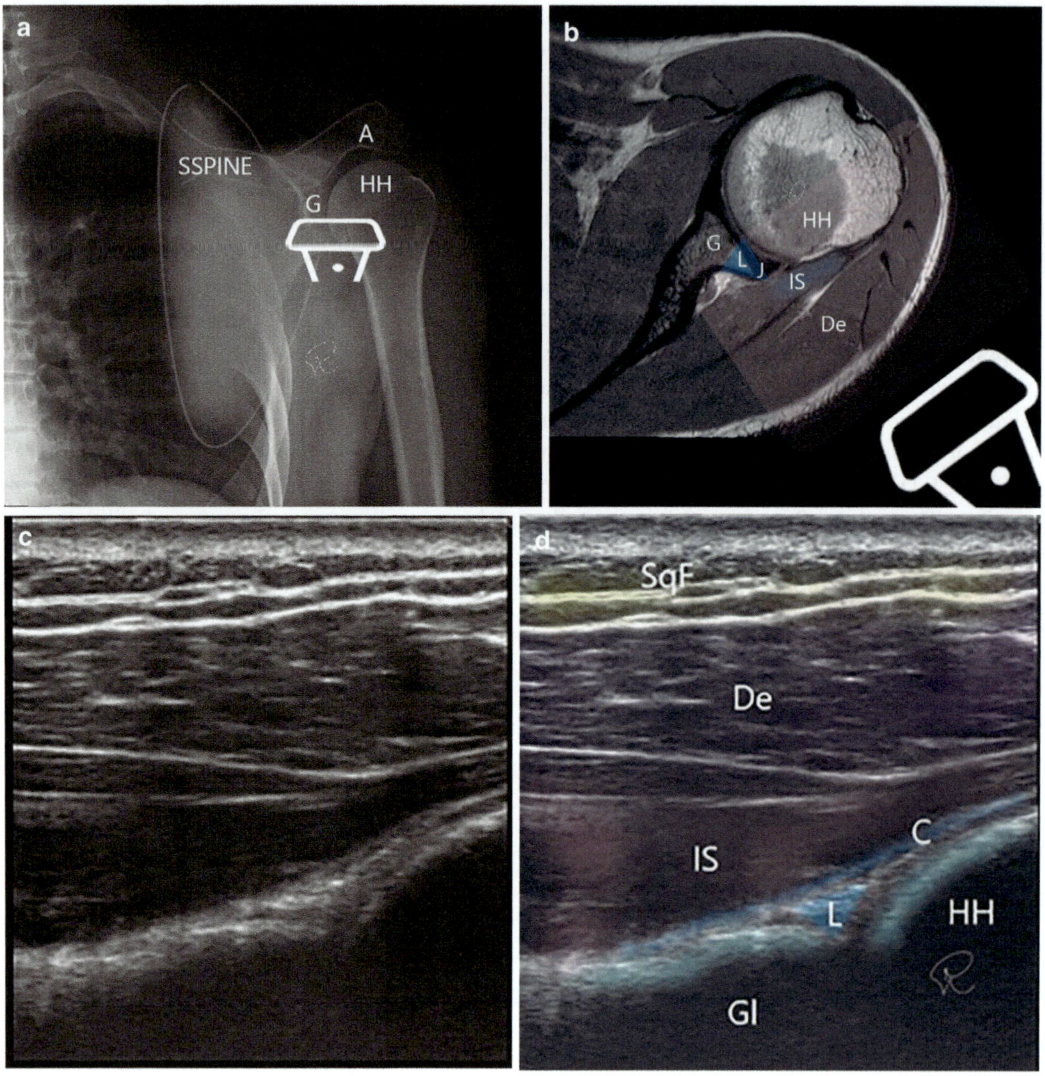

Fig. 2.8 Glenohumeral joint scan. Composite image showing four medical scans of a shoulder. (**a**) Antero-posterior X-ray image of the shoulder demonstrating probe and patient position with labels: SSPINE (scapular spine), A (acromion), G (glenoid), HH (humorous head). (**b**) An axial MRI scan slice resembling cross-sectional anatomy of the glenohumeral joint with labels: G (glenoid), L (labrum), IS (infraspinatus), HH (humorous head), De (deltoid). (**c**) Glenohumeral joint ultrasound image. (**d**) Glenohumeral joint ultrasound image with analysis labels. SqF (subcutaneous fat), De (deltoid), IS (infraspinatus), C (joint capsule), L (labrum), Gl (glenoid), HH (humorous head). (© Reza Roghani 2024. All Rights Reserved)

tioned over the posterior glenohumeral joint, facilitating assessment of tears or detachments. Dynamic ultrasound imaging, including stress maneuvers, may help identify labral instability or impingement, especially in athletes or individuals subjected to repetitive shoulder stress (see Fig. 2.8b) [2].

2.4.1.3 Infraspinatus

The infraspinatus muscle is one of the four rotator cuff muscles, originating from the infraspinous fossa of the scapula and inserting on the middle facet of the greater tuberosity of the humerus. It plays a crucial role in external rotation of the shoulder and contributes to glenohumeral joint stability, particularly in preventing anterior translation of the humeral head. The infraspinatus tendon is a thick, fibrous structure that extends from the muscle belly, passing deep to the deltoid and subcutaneous tissue before inserting onto the greater tuberosity. In cross-sectional ultrasound anatomy, the infraspinatus muscle appears as a hypoechoic, striated structure with a well-defined pennate pattern in the posterior aspect of the shoulder. The infraspinatus tendon is seen as a fibrillar, hyperechoic structure extending toward the greater tuberosity. In the transverse (axial) plane, placing the ultrasound probe over the posterior aspect of the shoulder at the level of the glenohumeral joint reveals the infraspinatus muscle lying posterior to the scapula. As the probe moves laterally, the muscle tapers into its tendon, which inserts onto the middle facet of the greater tuberosity. The posterior labrum and the glenohumeral joint capsule can also be visualized in this plane. In the sagittal (longitudinal) plane, the probe placed along the posterior shoulder aligns with the infraspinatus muscle fibers, providing a clear view of the muscle-tendon transition and its attachment to the greater tuberosity. This view is useful for assessing tendinopathy, partial or full-thickness tears, and fatty infiltration of the muscle [2, 9].

2.4.1.4 Scan (Video 2.7)

Patient Position: For a posterior glenohumeral (GH) joint ultrasound scan, the patient is typically positioned either seated or prone, with their arm held in a neutral or slightly internally rotated position to enhance the visualization of joint structures. The elbow should be flexed at 90 degrees, allowing the forearm to rest on the patient's lap or on an arm support to promote relaxation of the posterior shoulder muscles. In certain cases, positioning the arm across the chest in adduction may facilitate better access to the posterior joint capsule and labrum (Fig. 2.8a).

Probe position: The ultrasound probe is placed in a transverse orientation over the posterior aspect of the shoulder, just inferior and parallel to the scapular spine, then slid laterally towards the acromion. The probe's alignment should be parallel to the glenoid to adequately visualize the posterior aspect of the GH joint.

Scanning: In the transverse (axial) plane, placing the ultrasound probe over the posterior aspect of the shoulder bellow and parallel to the scapular spine, at the level of the glenohumeral joint reveals the infraspinatus muscle lying posterior to the scapula. As the probe slides laterally, the muscle tapers into its tendon, which inserts onto the middle facet of the greater tuberosity. The view at the level of GH joint will display the hyperechoic humeral head and glenoid, the hypoechoic articular cartilage, and the glenoid cavity. As adjustments are made for optimal imaging, the posterior glenoid labrum and posterior joint capsule become clearly identifiable (Fig. 2.8b). Within the image scan, two hyperechoic structures are observed: the round one represents the cortex of the humerus, and the bow-shaped one corresponds to the cortex of the glenoid. A triangular structure is positioned between the glenoid and the humerus head, identified as the labrum. Above the labrum, a hyperechoic line representing the joint capsule is visible. Further above are the infraspinatus and deltoid muscles (Fig. 2.8c, d). For a more comprehensive evaluation of joint dynamics, the probe can be gently swept slightly inferiorly to examine the posterior synovial recess, which may reveal joint effusion, synovial hypertrophy, or indications of posterior glenohumeral instability. A dynamic assessment can be conducted by applying gentle posterior pressure or by instructing the patient to externally and internally rotate the shoulder. This allows for the observation of joint motion and potential pathological findings, such as posterior capsular thickening or labral tears.

2.4.1.5 Injection

Some indications for this injection include adhesive capsulitis, glenohumeral joint arthritis, glenoid labrum tears, and recalcitrant pain after conservative treatment. Following the standard scan above, ensure the joint view is centered on the screen and measure the estimated needle length to the target point (Fig. 2.9c). Insert the

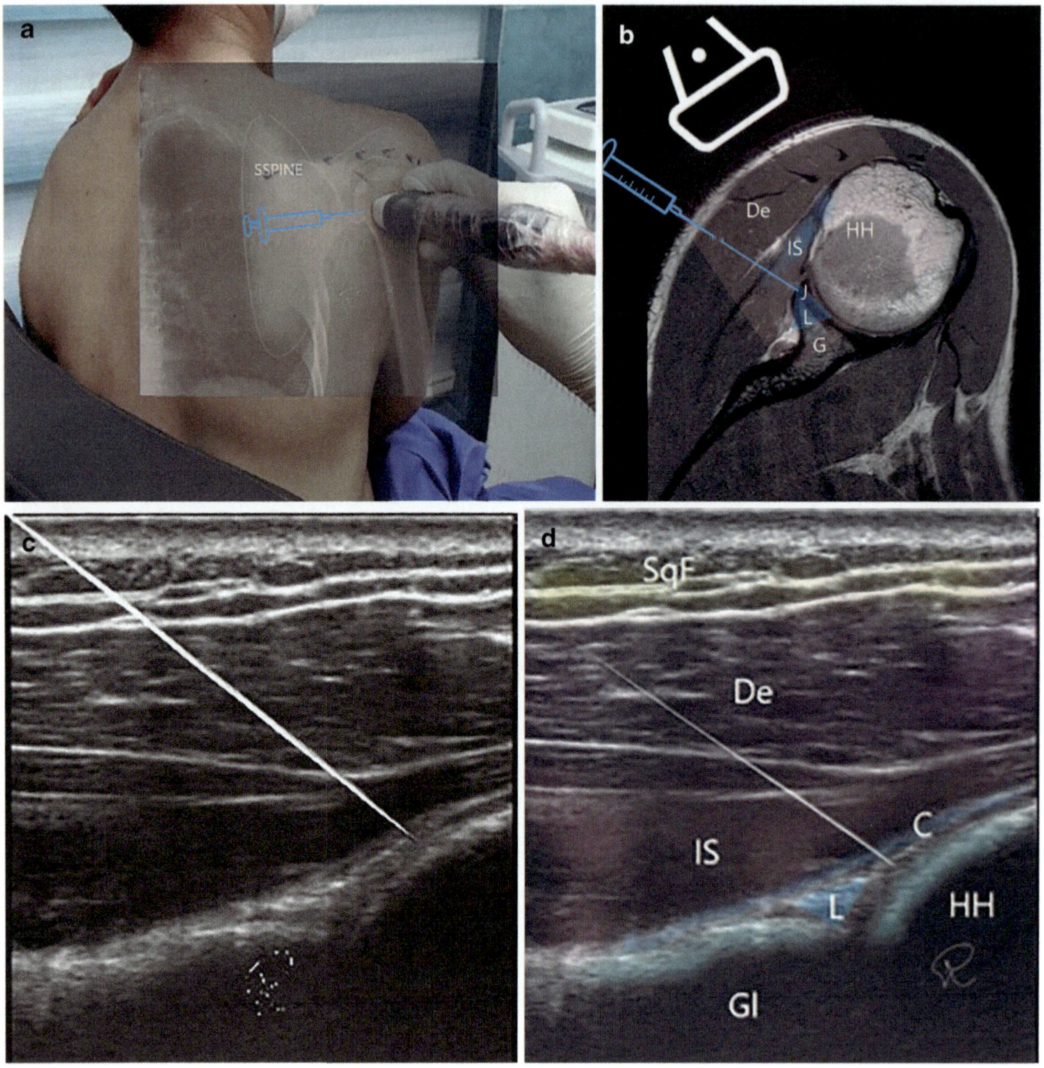

Fig. 2.9 Glenohumeral joint injection. A composite image showing four panels related to shoulder injection techniques. Panel (**a**) depicts a medical professional presenting probe and patient position and performing an injection on a patient's GH joint, with an overlay X-ray showing the shoulder bony structure and a syringe. Panel (**b**) is an MRI scan of a shoulder with labels: De (deltoid), IS (infraspinatus), HH (humeral head), G (glenoid), and L (labrum) demonstrating needle insertion point and trajectory. Panel (**c**) shows an ultrasound image with a needle inserted into tissue showing needle trajectory and target point. Panel (**d**) is another ultrasound image with labeled layers: SqF (subcutaneous fat), De (deltoid), IS (infraspinatus), C (capsule), L (labrum), Gl (glenoid), and HH (humeral head) with needle trajectory and target point. (© Reza Roghani 2024. All Rights Reserved)

needle in plane from medial to lateral until the tip of the needle encroaches on the capsule just superolateral and above the labrum (Fig. 2.9c, d). Use color flow to visualize the linear spread of fluid within the joint space. This injection technique involves a 25-gauge 2.5-in. needle to deliver 1–2 mL of local anesthetic and 1–2 mL of injectable corticosteroid into the joint. Other options include low molecular weight hyaluronic acid and Platelet-rich plasma (PRP) [13, 14].

References

1. Akhtar A, Richards J, Monga P. The biomechanics of the rotator cuff in health and disease—a narrative review. J Clin Orthop Trauma. 2021;18:150–6. https://doi.org/10.1016/j.jcot.2021.04.019.
2. Maruvada S, Madrazo-Ibarra A, Varacallo M. Anatomy, rotator cuff. In: StatPearls. StatPearls Publishing; 2024. http://www.ncbi.nlm.nih.gov/books/NBK441844/.
3. Beitzel K, Mazzocca AD, Arciero RA. Clinical anatomy, biomechanics, physiologic function, history, examination, and radiographic evaluation of the biceps. Oper Tech Sports Med. 2012;20(3):233–7.
4. McKernan MJ, Schickendantz MS, Frangiamore SJ. Diagnosis and management of subcoracoid impingement. J Am Acad Orthop Surg. 2021;29(3):100. https://doi.org/10.5435/JAAOS-D-20-00008.
5. Park J, Chai JW, Kim DH, Cha SW. Dynamic ultrasonography of the shoulder. Ultrasonography. 2018;37(3):190–9. https://doi.org/10.14366/usg.17055.
6. Hamid MSA, Sazlina SG. Platelet-rich plasma for rotator cuff tendinopathy: a systematic review and meta-analysis. PLoS One. 2021;16(5):e0251111. https://doi.org/10.1371/journal.pone.0251111.
7. Lin C-Y, Huang S-C, Tzou S-J, Yin C-H, Chen J-S, Chen Y-S, Chang S-T. A positive correlation between steroid injections and cuff tendon tears: a cohort study using a clinical database. Int J Environ Res Public Health. 2022;19(8):4520. https://doi.org/10.3390/ijerph19084520.
8. Cowan PT, Mudreac A, Varacallo M. Anatomy, back, scapula. In: StatPearls. StatPearls Publishing; 2024. http://www.ncbi.nlm.nih.gov/books/NBK531475/.
9. Vosloo M, Keough N, De Beer MA. The clinical anatomy of the insertion of the rotator cuff tendons. Eur J Orthop Surg Traumatol. 2017;27(3):359–66. https://doi.org/10.1007/s00590-017-1922-z.
10. Schoenherr JW, Flynn DN, Doyal A. Suprascapular nerve block. In: StatPearls. StatPearls Publishing; 2024. http://www.ncbi.nlm.nih.gov/books/NBK580556/.
11. Shanahan EM, Gill TK, Briggs E, Hill CL, Bain G, Morris T. Suprascapular nerve block for treating adhesive capsulitis: a randomized, double-masked placebo-controlled trial. RMD Open. 2022;8(2):e002648. https://doi.org/10.1136/rmdopen-2022-002648.
12. Chang L-R, Anand P, Varacallo M. Anatomy, shoulder and upper limb, glenohumeral joint. In: StatPearls. StatPearls Publishing; 2024. http://www.ncbi.nlm.nih.gov/books/NBK537018/.
13. Raeissadat SA, Ghazi Hosseini P, Bahrami MH, Salman Roghani R, Fathi M, Gharooee Ahangar A, Darvish M. The comparison effects of intra-articular injection of platelet rich plasma (PRP), plasma rich in growth factor (PRGF), hyaluronic acid (HA), and ozone in knee osteoarthritis; a one-year randomized clinical trial. BMC Musculoskelet Disord. 2021;22(1):134. https://doi.org/10.1186/s12891-021-04017-x.
14. Rossi LA, Piuzzi NS, Shapiro SA. Glenohumeral osteoarthritis: the role for orthobiologic therapies. JBJS Rev. 2020;8(2):–e0075. https://doi.org/10.2106/JBJS.RVW.19.00075.

Elbow and Forearm

3

Sina Davari Farid, Reza Salman Roghani,
Brian Palacios, Mohammad R. Nezamabadi,
and Naffiseh Jafarian

3.1 Introduction

The elbow, a complex hinge joint, plays a crucial role in upper limb function by facilitating flexion, extension, and rotational movements. Due to its intricate biomechanics and vulnerability to musculoskeletal disorders, ultrasound has become an essential imaging technique for evaluating elbow anatomy, diagnosing soft tissue injuries, and guiding interventions. This chapter delves into the sonographic assessment of the elbow joint, focusing on its three primary articulations: the humeroulnar, humeroradial, and proximal radioulnar joints. Moreover, it elucidates the ligamentous structures, such as the ulnar and radial collateral ligaments and the annular ligament, which are vital for joint stability. The muscular and tendinous structures surrounding the elbow, including the flexor-pronator and extensor-supinator groups, are also examined for common pathologies like epicondylitis and tendinopathy. Ultrasound-guided interventions have transformed the management of elbow pain and dysfunction, providing precision for therapeutic injections. This chapter offers detailed instructions on performing ultrasound-guided injections for lateral epicondylitis (tennis elbow) and medial epicondylitis (golfer's elbow), focusing on pathological tendon changes treated with corticosteroids, platelet-rich plasma (PRP), or other regenerative therapies. Additionally, the chapter discusses the role of ultrasound in guiding botulinum toxin injections for spasticity and dystonia impacting elbow-related muscles, thereby enhancing treatment efficacy and minimizing complications. Musculoskeletal ultrasound permits dynamic, high-resolution evaluations of these structures, enabling early diagnosis and intervention for conditions such as ligament injuries, tendon degeneration, and nerve entrapments. This chapter presents a comprehensive approach to elbow ultrasound imaging, emphasizing both diagnostic applications and interventional techniques to optimize patient care.

Supplementary Information The online version contains supplementary material available at https://doi.org/10.1007/978-3-031-81037-4_3.

S. D. Farid
Division of Pain Medicine, Department of Anesthesiology and Critical Care Medicine, George Washington University, Washington, DC, USA
e-mail: sdavari@mfa.gwu.edu

R. S. Roghani (✉) · B. Palacios
Department of Physical Medicine and Rehabilitation, Larkin Community Hospital, Nova Southeastern University, Miami, FL, USA

M. R. Nezamabadi
Neshat Pain Clinic, Fardis, Karaj, Iran

N. Jafarian
Department of Physical Medicine and Rehabilitation, Shohada Hospital, Shahid Beheshti University of Medical Science, Tajrish, Tehran, Iran

R. S. Roghani, J. J. Diaz (eds.), *Video Atlas of Neuromusculoskeletal Ultrasound*,
https://doi.org/10.1007/978-3-031-81037-4_3

3.1.1 Elbow Scan Protocol

Anterior

- Short Axis
  - Elbow: Brachial vasculatures, nerves, and muscles, and elbow joint
  - Forearm: Muscles, nerves, and tendons
- Long Axis
  - Anterolateral: Humeroradial joint
  - Anteromedial: Humeroulnar joint
  - Oblique: Distal biceps tendon

Lateral

- Long Axis
  - Common extensor tendon and radio capitellar joint
- Short Axis
  - Radial nerve

Medial

- Long Axis
  - Common flexor tendon and humeroulnar joint
- Short Axis

- Ulnar nerve

Posterior

- Long Axis
  - Triceps tendon, olecranon process bursa, posterior humeroulnar joint
- Short Axis
  - Posteromedial: Ulnar nerve

3.2 Anatomy

3.2.1 Elbow

The cross-sectional anatomy of the elbow at the antebrachial fossa offers a comprehensive examination of vital musculoskeletal and neurovascular components essential for effective diagnostic and interventional ultrasound practices. Within this anatomical context, the brachial artery is centrally located, serving as a significant landmark for vascular access and identifying surrounding nerves. The median nerve is positioned medially to the brachial artery, traversing in close association with it while running superficially to the brachialis muscle, which underpins the anterior region of the elbow. Laterally, the brachioradialis muscle is prominent, delineating the lateral boundary of the antebrachial fossa and playing a functional role in the flexion of the forearm. The radial nerve courses laterally between the brachialis and brachioradialis muscles, bifurcating into superficial and deep branches. The deep branch proceeds into the posterior compartment of the forearm, navigating through the supinator muscle, while the superficial branch advances along a more superficial path toward the wrist. The pulsatile brachial artery is a pivotal vascular landmark essential for ultrasound-guided procedures involving vascular access and nerve blocks. Beneath this neurovascular ensemble lies the humeral portion of the elbow joint, which is encased in articular cartilage, promoting smooth movement. The medial epicondyle stands out as a notable bony landmark, serving as the point of attachment for various common flexor tendons. Conversely, the lateral epicondyle is critical as it provides the origin for the extensor tendons, which are significant in extending the forearm and wrist. The ulnar nerve traverses posteromedially behind the medial epicondyle, often situated near the medial head of the triceps muscle, thereby rendering it vulnerable to compression or irritation. At the posterior aspect of the elbow, the olecranon of the ulna articulates with the humerus, playing an essential role in maintaining elbow stability and function. This bony projection serves as the insertion site for the triceps tendon, which is involved in forearm extension. A thorough understanding of the detailed anatomy of these structures through the lens of ultrasound not only enhances diagnostic accuracy but also improves the precision of interventional techniques, such as ultrasound-guided injections for medial and lateral epicondylitis (commonly known as golfer's and tennis elbow) and botulinum toxin injections aimed at treating muscle spasticity and dystonia (Fig. 3.1).

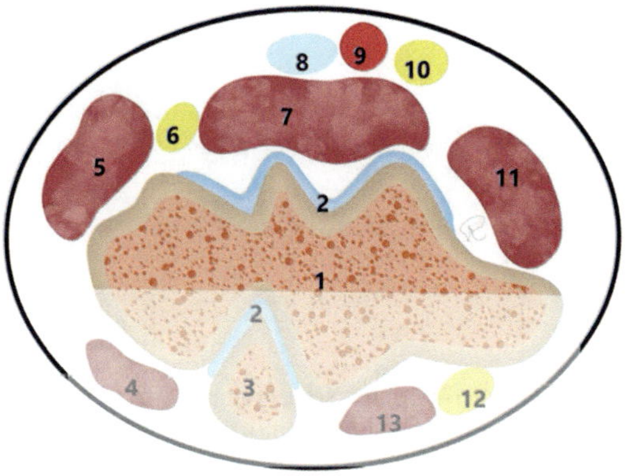

Fig. 3.1 Elbow cross-sectional anatomy. A schematic illustration of the antebrachial fossa is centered around key bony structures, serving as a clear anatomical reference. The posterior region is depicted with reduced clarity to highlight the more clinically relevant landmarks in the anterior aspect. The brachial artery, an essential vascular structure, is marked with a distinct round red circle in the anterior portion of the fossa. Each anatomical component is systematically labeled from 1 to 13, facilitating precise identification of muscles, tendons, nerves, and vascular structures. (1) Distal humerus, (2) joint space, (3) Ulnar olecranon, (4) Triceps lateral head, (5) Brachioradialis, (6) Radial nerve, (7) Brachialis, (8) Biceps tendon, (9) Brachial artery, (10) Median nerve, (11) Flexor carpi ulnaris, (12) The ulnar nerve, (13) Triceps medial head. (© Reza Roghani 2024. All Rights Reserved)

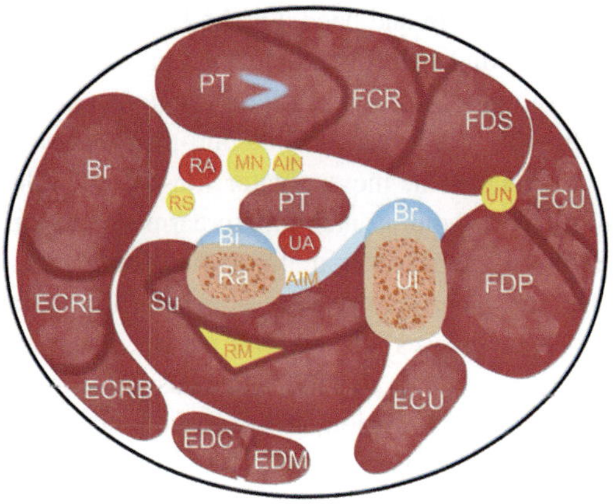

Fig. 3.2 Forearm cross-sectional area. A cross-sectional diagram of the forearm showing various muscles, nerves, and arteries. The structures are color-coded, with nerves in yellow circles, arteries in red, tendons in blue and muscles in pink. The diagram highlights the spatial relationships between these anatomical features. The image is labeled with abbreviations as *Ra* radius, *Su* supinator, *Br* brachioradialis, *PT* pronator teres, *CT* central tendon, *FCR* flexor carpi radialis, *PL* palmaris longus, *FDS* flexor digitorum superficialis, *FCU* flexor carpi ulnaris, *Ul* ulna, *Br* brachialis tendon, *IM* interosseous membrane, *UA* ulnar artery, *Bi* biceps tendon, *AIN* anterior interosseous nerve, *MN* median nerve, *RA* radial artery, *SPN* superficial radial nerve, *UN* the ulnar nerve, *RM* radial nerve motor branch. (© Reza Roghani 2024. All Rights Reserved)

3.2.2 Forearm

The anatomy of the proximal forearm, when examined in cross-section, reveals a sophisticated interplay of muscular, neural, and vascular components vital for its functional performance. The radius and ulna serve as the principal bony structures, with associated muscles delineating specific compartments. The anterior compartment is characterized by the flexor-pronator group, while the posterior compartment includes the extensor-supinator muscles. Vascular supply is provided by the brachial artery, which bifurcates into the radial and ulnar arteries, supporting both the forearm and hand. About 2 inches distal to the anterior elbow, the flexor muscles become increasingly pronounced, shaping the muscular framework of the proximal forearm. In the center of this cross-section lies the pronator teres muscle, identifiable by its central tendon that forms a "V" shape. This muscle is essential for forearm pronation and serves as a critical anatomical marker. (see Fig. 3.2). The median nerve traverses between the dual heads of the pronator teres, from which it gives rise to the anterior interosseous nerve. This nerve branch runs posterior to the main trunk but remains anterior to the interosseous membrane, providing motor innervation to the deep flexor muscles. Medially adjacent to the pronator teres is the flexor carpi radialis, notable for its resemblance to a large, open fish mouth. Continuing further medially, one observes the palmaris longus, followed by the flexor digitorum superficialis and the flexor carpi ulnaris. The ulnar nerve is located just beneath the flexor carpi ulnaris and travels alongside the ulnar artery towards the wrist, offering both motor innervation to intrinsic hand muscles and sensory innervation to the medial forearm and hand. On the lateral side, the brachioradialis runs parallel to the pronator teres and primarily facilitates elbow flexion, particularly when the forearm is in a mid-pronated position. Beneath it, the supinator muscle encircles the proximal radius, aiding in forearm supination. Between the brachioradialis and supinator muscles, the superficial sensory branch of the radial nerve progresses distally, ultimately emerging subcutaneously to provide cutaneous sensation to the dorsolateral region of the hand. This cross-sectional analysis elucidates the intricate spatial relationships among these fundamental neurovascular and muscular structures, which are crucial for clinical evaluations and ultrasound-guided procedures in the proximal forearm [1–3].

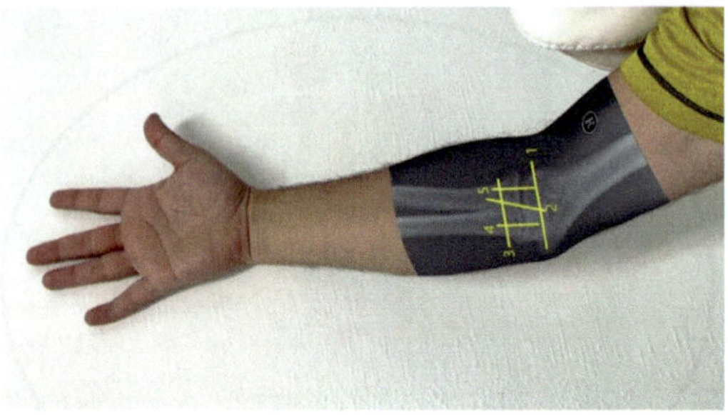

Fig. 3.3 Anterior elbow scan protocol. The illustration depicts a forearm in supination, overlaid with an X-ray image that highlights the underlying bone structures. Five yellow lines, each labeled with numbers 1 through 5, indicate key scanning positions for the anterior elbow and forearm ultrasound protocol. These positions include: (1) the anterior elbow in the short axis for an initial assessment of superficial structures, (2) an oblique view for a comprehensive evaluation of the distal biceps tendon, (3) a short-axis scan of the anterior forearm to enhance visualization of the forearm muscles, (4) the anteromedial long-axis view to assess the humeroulnar joint and associated tendons, and (5) the anterolateral long-axis view for examining the humeroradial joint and its tendons. (© Reza Roghani 2024. All Rights Reserved)

3.3 Anterior Elbow and Forearm

3.3.1 Scan

The five-step anterior elbow ultrasound scan protocol is meticulously designed to offer a comprehensive evaluation of the elbow joint and its surrounding structures. The process begins with imaging the anterior elbow and forearm in the short axis to assess superficial elements such as the brachial artery, flexor muscles and tendons, and nerve pathways. Next, an anterolateral long axis scan is conducted, concentrating on critical structures like the humeroradial joint and annular ligament. Following this, the anteromedial long axis view is performed to highlight the humeroulnar Joint , facilitating the assessment of conditions such as humeroulnar arthritis or tendinitis. An oblique view is then obtained to evaluate distal bicipital tendinitis (Fig. 3.3).

3.3.1.1 Elbow Short Axis (Video 3.1)

Patient position: During an anterior elbow scan, the patient is positioned supine with the arm fully extended and relaxed on a flat surface, with the palm facing upward to enhance visualization of the anterior structures. The elbow crease serves as a landmark for the home base position, enabling a systematic examination of the anterior elbow and forearm. Proper positioning is essential for obtaining consistent images and aids in the identification of important anatomical structures, including tendons, muscles, nerves, and vascular components.

Probe position: To effectively position the linear transducer on the elbow crease, align it with the imaginary line that connects the medial and lateral epicondyles. This alignment provides an optimal short-axis view of the anterior elbow structures. Making slight adjustments to the angle and applying gentle pressure can further enhance the visualization of tendons, muscles, nerves, and vascular structures in the anterior elbow region (Fig. 3.4a, b).

Scanning: The short-axis ultrasound image of the anterior elbow reveals distinct anatomical structures with impressive clarity. The humerus bone appears as the brightest hyperechoic line at the depths of the image, serving as a landmark. The brachialis muscle is visualized just above the humerus, creating a soft tissue layer between the bone and the neurovascular structures. Above the brachialis, the pulsatile brachial artery is clearly identifiable, positioned adjacent to the median nerve, which displays a characteristic

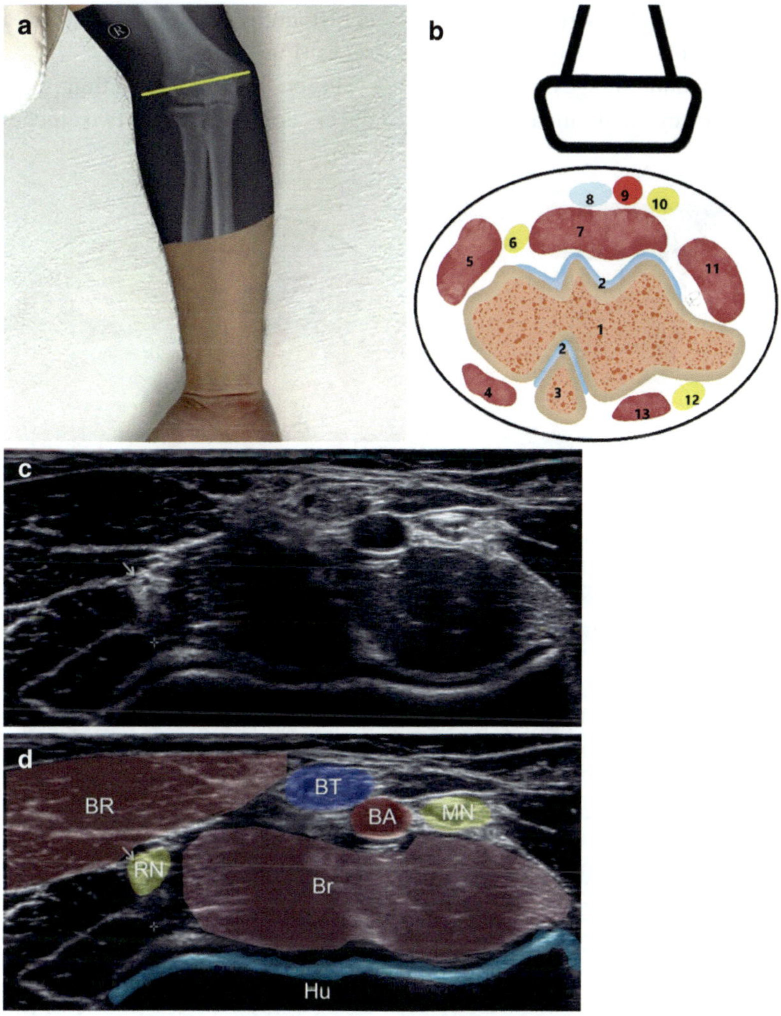

Fig. 3.4 Short axis anterior elbow US scan. This four-panel illustration offers a comprehensive overview of the anatomy and ultrasound imaging of the arm. Panel (**a**) depicts the forearm in a supinated position, featuring an X-ray image that highlights the underlying bony structures and a reference line between the medial and lateral epicondyles to ensure accurate probe placement. Panel (**b**) includes a labeled cross-sectional diagram of the elbow, indicating essential anatomical structures: (1) distal humerus, (2) joint space, (3) ulnar olecranon, (4) lateral head of the triceps, (5) brachioradialis, (6) radial nerve, (7) brachialis, (8) biceps tendon, (9) brachial artery, (10) median nerve, (11) flexor carpi ulnaris, (12) ulnar nerve, and (13) medial head of the triceps. Panel (**c**) presents an ultrasound image of the elbow, allowing for real-time visualization of internal structures. Panel (**d**) enhances this ultrasound view with a color-coded overlay, clearly identifying critical muscles and nerves, such as the brachioradialis (BR), biceps tendon (BT), radial nerve (RN), brachial artery (BA), median nerve (MN), brachialis (Br)and humerus (Hu). This detailed representation supports anatomical correlation and aids in the precision of ultrasound-guided procedures. (© Reza Roghani 2024. All Rights Reserved)

honeycomb appearance. Laterally, the fibrillar biceps tendon runs parallel to the brachial artery. Superficially, the brachioradialis muscle is located lateral to the brachialis, with the radial nerve emerging as a distinct honeycomb structure nestled between these two muscles (Fig. 3.4c, d).

3.3.1.2 Anterior Forearm Short Axis (Video 3.2)

Patient position: For anterior forearm scans, the patient should be positioned supine with the elbow fully extended and the forearm in supination, resting comfortably on the examination table. This positioning guarantees optimal exposure of the anterior elbow region, facilitating accurate probe placement and producing high-quality ultrasound images. The elbow crease serves as a key anatomical landmark, contributing to consistent and reproducible scans (Fig. 3.5a).

Probe position: Position the linear transducer approximately two inches below the

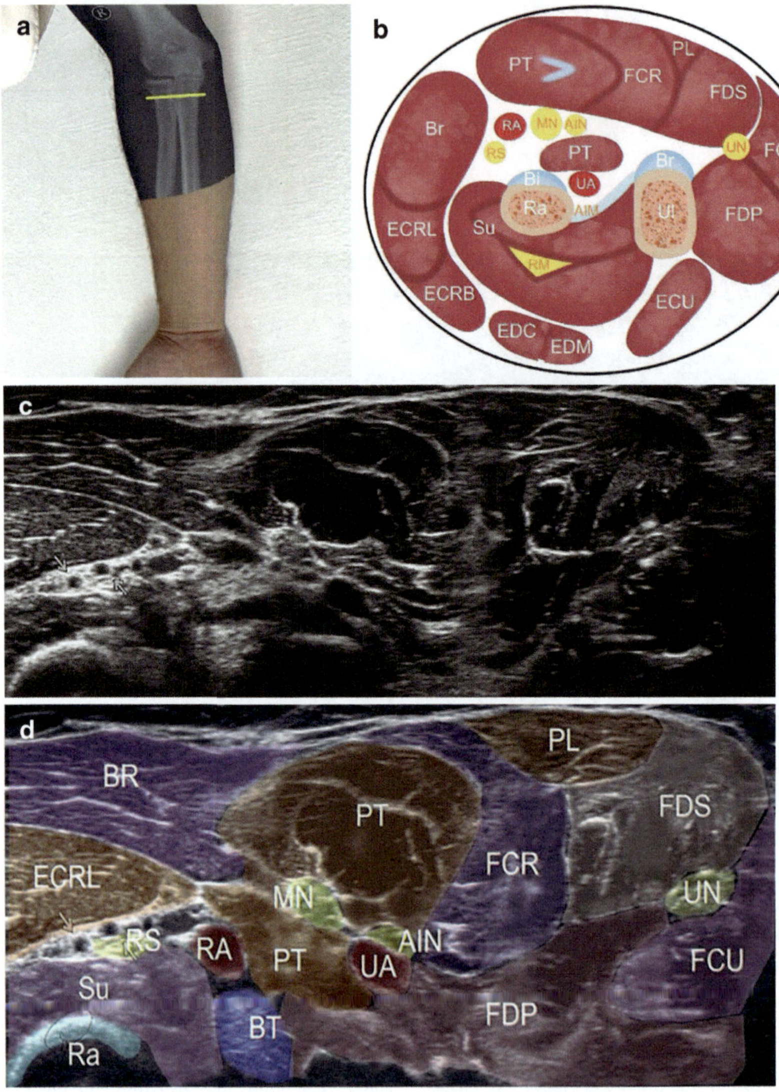

Fig. 3.5 Short axis anterior forearm. The image is composed of four panels that illustrate the anatomy and ultrasound imaging of the forearm. Panel (**a**) features a forearm with a highlighted yellow line indicating the optimal positioning of the ultrasound probe. Panel (**b**) provides a cross-sectional diagram of the forearm, labeling key muscles, nerves, and vascular structures. These include the brachioradialis (Br), pronator teres (PT), palmaris longus (PL), flexor carpi ulnaris (FCU), ulnar nerve (UN), flexor digitorum superficialis (FDS), flexor carpi radialis (FCR), anterior interosseous nerve (AIN), ulnar artery (UA), flexor digitorum profundus (FDP), biceps tendon (BT), radial artery (RA), superficial radial nerve (RS), radius (Ra), ulna (Ul), supinator (Su), extensor carpi radialis longus (ECRL), extensor carpi radialis brevis (ECRB), extensor digitorum communis (EDC), and extensor digiti minimi (EDM). Panel (**c**) showcases a panaromic ultrasound image of the anterior forearm, capturing these anatomical structures in a real-time scan. Lastly, Panel (**d**) overlays anatomical labels onto the ultrasound image, clearly identifying the same structures as shown in the anterior portion of Panel (**b**) to enhance the correlation between the diagrammatic representation and imaging findings. (© Reza Roghani 2024. All Rights Reserved)

elbow crease, ensuring that it remains parallel to the crease. This placement optimizes the visualization of the underlying structures, including the pronator teres muscle, median nerve, and biceps tendon. By maintaining a steady hand and applying appropriate pressure, you can enhance image clarity, allowing for a more accurate assessment of the anterior forearm anatomy (Fig. 3.5a, b).

Scanning: Utilizing the median nerve and pronator teres (PT) muscle as key landmarks, the ulnar artery can be located medially and deep to the median nerve. Moving medially from the PT, the flexor carpi radialis (FCR), palmaris longus (PL), flexor digitorum superficialis (FDS), and flexor carpi ulnaris (FCU) muscles appear sequentially. Lateral to the PT, the brachioradialis (BR) muscle is positioned superficially, while the supinator muscle lies deep, encircling the radius. The radial nerve and radial artery are visible between these muscle groups. Anterior to the interosseous membrane, the anterior interosseous nerve (AIN) and flexor digitorum profundus (FDP) can be found. The ulnar nerve, resembling a honeycomb structure, is situated between the FDP, FDS, and FCU muscles. In patients with a larger body habitus, it may be challenging to visualize all these structures in a single scan, necessitating medial and lateral probe sliding and an increased scanning depth for optimal imaging (Fig. 3.5c, d).

3.3.1.3 Anterolateral Long Axis: Humeroradial Joint (Video 3.3)

Patient position: For an anterolateral elbow ultrasound exam, the patient should be positioned lying supine with the arm extended and the palm facing upward. This position allows for optimal probe placement and visualization of key anatomical structures along the anterolateral forearm (Fig. 3.6a).

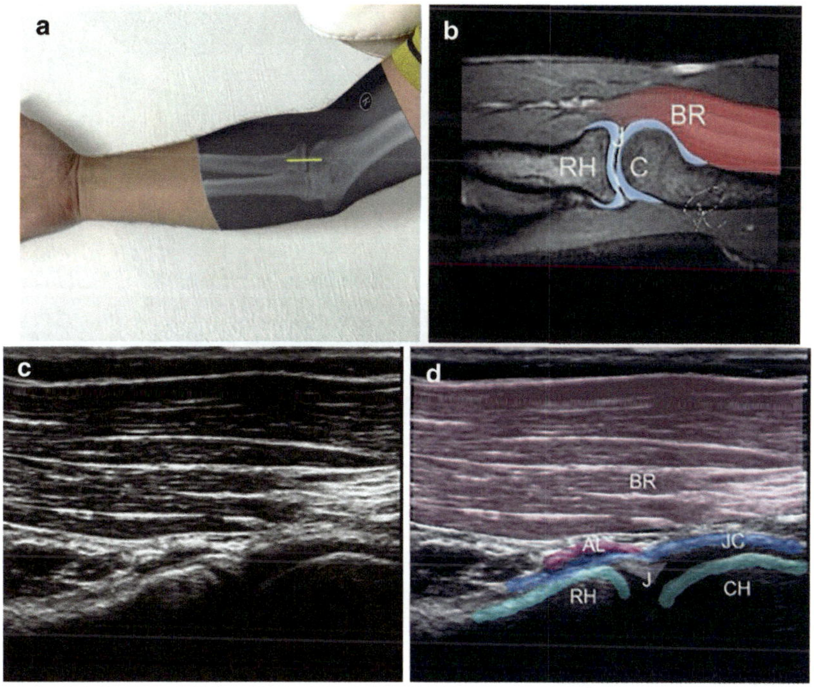

Fig. 3.6 Anterolateral elbow long axis: The image comprises a composite featuring four panels, each illustrating various views and imaging techniques of the elbow region. Panel (**a**) presents an elbow x-ray superimposed on a photograph of the elbow, highlighting the radial head and capitellum of the humerus, with a yellow line indicating the probe's position. Panel (**b**) showcases a labeled MRI scan that highlights the brachioradialis (BR) muscle, radial head (RH), and capitellum (C). Panel (**c**) illustrates an ultrasound image of the anterolateral elbow, primarily focusing on the surrounding soft tissue structures. Finally, panel (**d**) includes a color-enhanced ultrasound image, complete with labels for the brachioradialis (BR), radial head (RH), capitellum of the humerus (CH), annular ligament (AL), and joint capsule (JC), providing a comprehensive overview of the joint's anatomy.

Probe position: To perform an anterolateral elbow ultrasound examination, position the probe longitudinally along the lateral border of the humerus, centering it at the elbow flexor crease. Gradually slide the probe distally while sweeping it medially until you can visualize a gap between two bony structures deep within the image. Ensure that proper centering is maintained for optimal visualization throughout the process (Fig. 3.6c, d).

Scanning: This positioning facilitates a clear visualization of the key anatomical landmarks of the humeroradial joint, including the radial head, the capitellum of the humerus, and the V-shaped gap between them, which signifies the articulation of these structures. Additionally, the humeral fossa, which accommodates the radial head during flexion, can be identified, offering insight into joint congruency and alignment (Fig. 3.6c, d). With careful adjustments of the probe, the articular cartilage of the humeroradial joint can also be evaluated, appearing as a thin, anechoic layer covering the bony surfaces. Furthermore, the adjacent soft tissues, including the annular ligament surrounding the radial head, can be examined for signs of inflammation or pathology. Proper angulation and depth adjustments of the probe ensure optimal image clarity, allowing for a thorough assessment of the anterolateral elbow structures.

3.3.1.4 Anteromedial Long Axis: Humeroulnar Joint (Video 3.4)

Patient position: To perform an ultrasound exam of the anteromedial elbow, the patient needs to lie on their back with their arm extended and palm facing up. This positioning facilitates the best placement of the probe and the visualization of important anatomical structures along the anteromedial forearm (Fig. 3.7a).

Probe position: To perform an anteromedial elbow ultrasound examination, position the probe

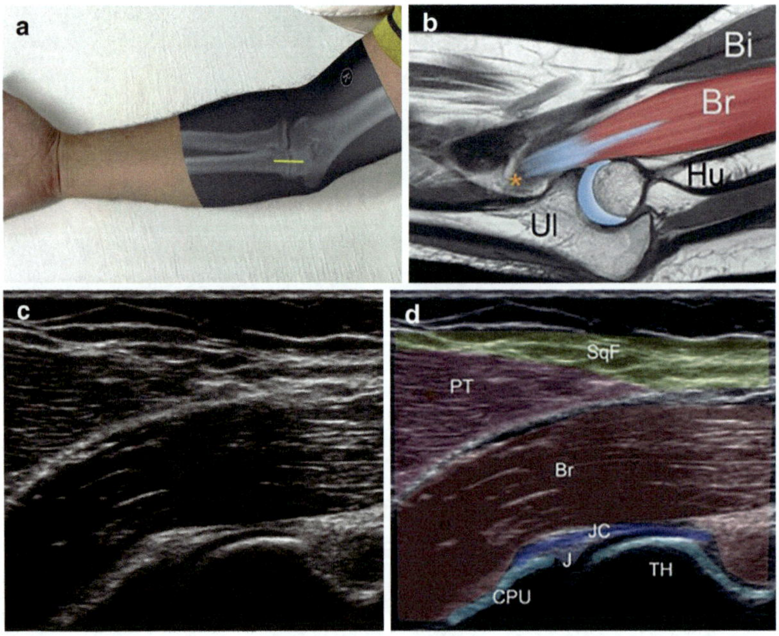

Fig. 3.7 Anteromedial elbow long axis: A composite image of four panels illustrates the anteromedial elbow's anatomy and imaging. Panel (**a**) shows an elbow with a highlighted region marked by a yellow line, indicating the correct probe position for an ultrasound examination. Panel (**b**) features a labeled sagittal MRI slice, identifying key anatomical structures, including the biceps (Bi), brachialis (Br), humerus (Hu), and ulna (Ul). Panel (**c**) presents a grayscale ultrasound image capturing the anteromedial elbow in the long axis, revealing soft tissue and bony landmarks. Panel (**d**) enhances the ultrasound image with color-coded overlays, clearly labeling critical structures such as the subcutaneous fat (SqF), pronator teres (PT), brachialis (Br), joint capsule (JC), capitellum of ulna (CPU) and trochlea of the humerus (TH), providing a more detailed and intuitive visualization of the region. (© Reza Roghani 2024. All Rights Reserved)

longitudinally along the medial edge of the humerus, directing it toward the crease of the elbow flexion. Gradually slide the probe distally while sweeping it laterally until a space between the two bony structures becomes visible deep within the image. Ensure proper alignment is maintained throughout the procedure for optimal visualization (Fig. 3.7a).

Scanning: During the scanning process, it is important to observe the interaction between the humeral trochlea and the ulna, which together form a V-shaped joint. The trochlea is a spool-shaped structure located on the distal humerus and articulates with the trochlear notch of the ulna, facilitating smooth flexion and extension of the elbow. Proper positioning of the probe will allow for clear visualization of the joint space, which should appear as a hypoechoic (dark) gap between the bony surfaces, indicating the presence of articular cartilage. The contours of both the trochlea and the ulna should be well-defined, showing no signs of irregularities or osteophytes that might suggest degenerative changes. Additionally, the medial and lateral joint recesses should be assessed for any signs of synovial thickening or fluid accumulation, as these may indicate inflammatory or degenerative joint conditions (Fig. 3.7c, d).

3.3.1.5 Anterior Oblique Long Axis: Biceps Tendon (Video 3.5)

Patient position: In the context of conducting an anterior oblique elbow ultrasound scan, the patient should be placed in a supine position, with the elbow fully extended and the forearm in a supinated position. This alignment facilitates better access and clarity during the ultrasound examination (Fig. 3.8a).

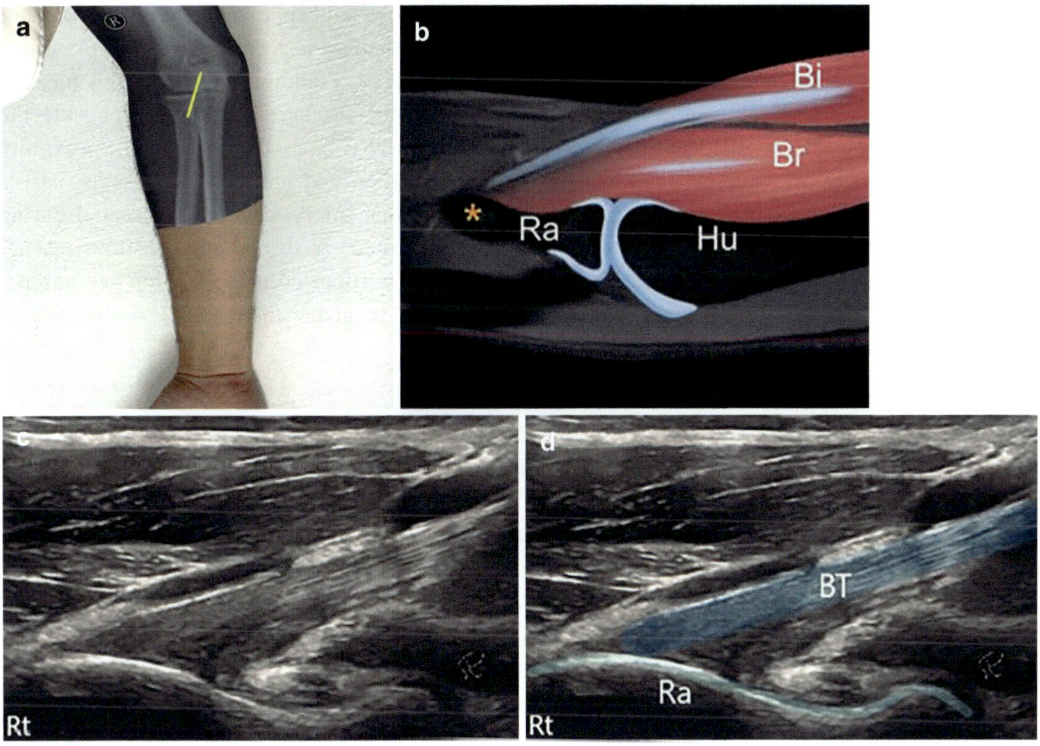

Fig. 3.8 Anterior oblique long axis scan: The illustration comprises four panels that showcase anatomical and ultrasound views of the elbow. Panel (**a**) depicts a human elbow, with a yellow line indicating the optimal placement for the ultrasound probe to achieve the best imaging results. Panel (**b**) features a detailed anatomical diagram that highlights the distal biceps tendon, labeling critical structures such as the biceps (Bi), brachialis (Br), radius bone (Ra), and humerus (Hu). Panel (**c**) presents a grayscale ultrasound image that captures the relevant structures of the biceps tendon during the anterior oblique elbow ultrasound scan. Lastly, panel (**d**) is an annotated version of the ultrasound image, incorporating blue-tone highlights to distinguish the biceps tendon (BT) and its insertion on the radial tuberosity (Ra), thereby enhancing the visualization of anatomical relationships.

Probe position: To enhance the visualization of the biceps tendon in the anterior elbow, begin by positioning the ultrasound probe in a short-axis view at the elbow. Identify and center the biceps tendon within the image. Once the probe is correctly aligned, gradually rotate it along the course of the tendon towards the radius bone, ensuring continuous visualization of its structure and its relationship with the surrounding anatomical landmarks (Fig. 3.8a).

Scanning: As you perform the scan, pay close attention to the fibrillar echotexture of the biceps tendon, ensuring that it remains properly aligned with the orientation of the probe. The tendon should appear as a continuous, hyperechoic structure extending toward its insertion on the radial tuberosity. If the visualization is unclear, consider adjusting the depth and gain settings to enhance image clarity. Increasing the depth can help reveal deeper structures, while optimizing the gain improves contrast, allowing for better differentiation between the tendon and surrounding tissues. Additionally, making constant adjustments to probe placement—such as slight tilting, fanning, or having the patient contract the biceps—can significantly improve visualization of the tendon's attachment to the radial tuberosity. This technique is particularly effective for identifying subtle anatomical variations or pathological changes, including tendinosis, partial tears, or enthesopathy (Fig. 3.8c, d).

3.3.2 Injections

3.3.2.1 Distal Biceps Tendon Injection (Video 3.6)

Scan the biceps tendon as described above. Under continuous ultrasound guidance, carefully insert a needle into the biceps tendon sheath from distal to proximal. Adjust the needle tip if you encounter significant resistance, ensuring the injectate spreads around the tendon from distal to proximal (Fig. 3.9) [4]. A therapeutic injection typically includes corticosteroid medication and a local anesthetic.

3.3.2.2 PT Syndrome and Injection (Video 3.7)

Perform a scan of the anterior forearm in a short axis, following the instructions above. Locate both the pronator teres and median nerve. Adopt a medial-to-lateral approach towards the pronator teres and median nerve, ensuring that the injection is precisely administered between the two heads of the pronator teres and alongside the median nerve (Fig. 3.10) [5]. Given the proximity of the median and anterior interosseous nerves and the ulnar artery, caution is essential during this procedure. A therapeutic injection usually involves a corticosteroid medication in combination with a local anesthetic.

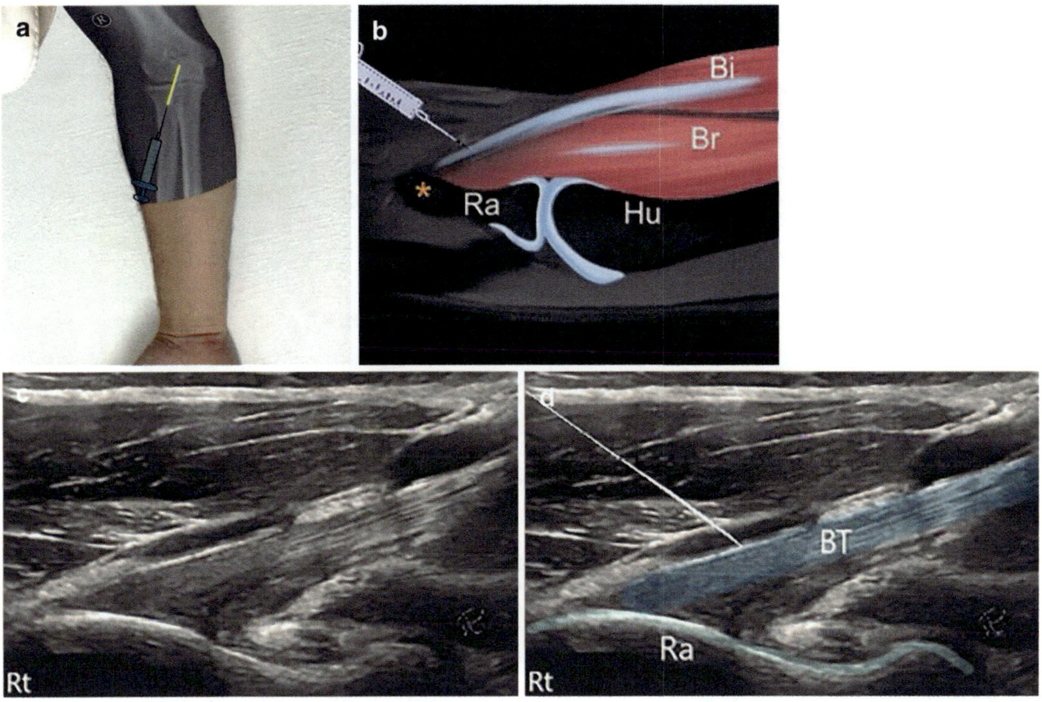

Fig. 3.9 Distal biceps tendon injection. The illustration is comprised of four panels that present both anatomical and ultrasound perspectives of the elbow. Panel (**a**) depicts a human elbow, featuring a yellow line that marks the ideal position for the ultrasound probe to ensure optimal imaging results. It also indicates the site for syringe and needle insertion. Panel (**b**) presents a detailed anatomical diagram that highlights the distal biceps tendon and labels key structures, including the biceps (Bi), brachialis (Br), radius (Ra), and humerus (Hu), as well as the needle trajectory and target point. Panel (**c**) showcases a grayscale ultrasound image that illustrates the relevant components of the biceps tendon during an anterior oblique elbow ultrasound examination. Lastly, panel (**d**) provides an annotated version of the ultrasound image, incorporating blue-tone highlights to distinguish the biceps tendon (BT) and its attachment to the radial tuberosity (Ra), along with the needle trajectory and the needle tip, which pierces the tendon sheath without penetrating the tendon itself. (© Reza Roghani 2024. All Rights Reserved)

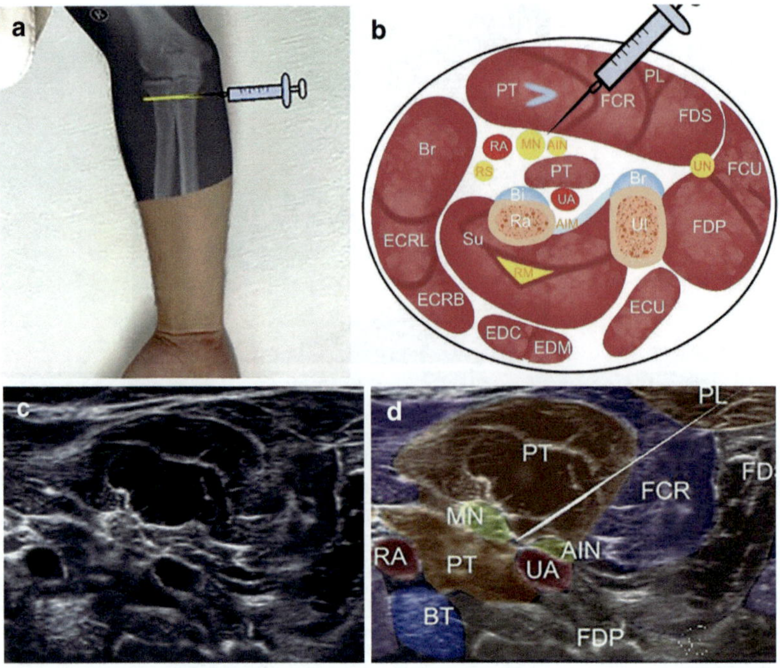

Fig. 3.10 Pronator teres syndrome injection.The image is a composite composed of four panels that illustrate a medical procedure related to the forearm. Panel (**a**) displays the forearm with a yellow line indicating the placement of the ultrasound probe, alongside a syringe to mark the intended needle in plane insertion site. Panel (**b**) features a cross-sectional anatomical diagram of the forearm, labeling key muscles, nerves, and vascular structures, including the pronator teres (PT), flexor carpi radialis (FCR), median nerve (MN), anterior interosseous nerve (AIN), and ulnar artery (UA). This panel also demonstrates the planned needle trajectory and target point. Panel (**c**) showcases a real-time ultrasound scan of the forearm, revealing internal structures with a focus on the bifurcation of the pronator teres muscle and the median nerve located in between. Finally, panel (**d**) presents an annotated version of the ultrasound image, highlighting essential anatomical landmarks such as the brachioradialis (Br), pronator teres (PT), palmaris longus (PL), flexor carpi ulnaris (FCU), ulnar nerve (UN), flexor digitorum superficialis (FDS), flexor carpi radialis (FCR), anterior interosseous nerve (AIN), median nerve (MN), ulnar artery (UA), flexor digitorum profundus (FDP), biceps tendon (BT), and radial artery (RA). This composite image aims to enhance the understanding of the anatomical relationships involved in ultrasound-guided injections for pronator teres syndrome, ensuring precise needle placement around the median nerve.

3.4 Lateral Elbow

3.4.1 Anatomy

The lateral elbow cross-section primarily focuses on structures aligned within the midcoronal plane, underscoring essential musculoskeletal components integral to movement and stability. Key bony structures in this region include the humerus, specifically the lateral epicondyle, which serves as the origin of the common extensor tendon. The radial head forms an articulation with the capitellum of the humerus, thereby creating the humeroradial joint. The lateral collateral ligament (LCL) extends from the lateral epicondyle to the annular ligament, playing a crucial role in providing lateral stability to the elbow. The annular ligament encircles the radial head, ensuring its secure placement within the ulna's radial notch, facilitating smooth forearm rotation. Muscular structures within this area consist of the common extensor tendon that originates from the lateral epicondyle and encompasses the extensor carpi radialis brevis, extensor digitorum communis, extensor digiti minimi, and extensor carpi ulnaris muscles. The brachioradialis is located superficially and laterally in relation to these muscles. From a clinical perspective, the lateral elbow is a common site for various conditions, most notably lateral epicondylitis, often referred to as tennis elbow. This condition arises from inflammation of the common extensor tendon, particularly affecting the extensor carpi radialis brevis. Radial head fractures are frequently assessed through ultrasound, which can identify discontinuities in the cortical surface. Injuries involving the lateral collateral ligament may lead to posterolateral rotatory instability, while damage to the annular ligament can contribute to radial head subluxation, a condition commonly encountered in scenarios such as nursemaid's elbow (see Fig. 3.11a, b).

3.4.2 Scan

3.4.2.1 Long Axis: Common Extensor Tendon (Video 3.8)

Patient position: For a lateral elbow scan, position the patient in a seated posture with the elbow flexed and the forearm pronated, resting on a pillow. This setup optimizes imaging of the lateral structures (Fig. 3.11a).

Probe position: Place the probe on the lateral epicondyle of the elbow, parallel to the radius. Center the radiohumeral joint on the screen and adjust the angle as needed to visualize the charac-

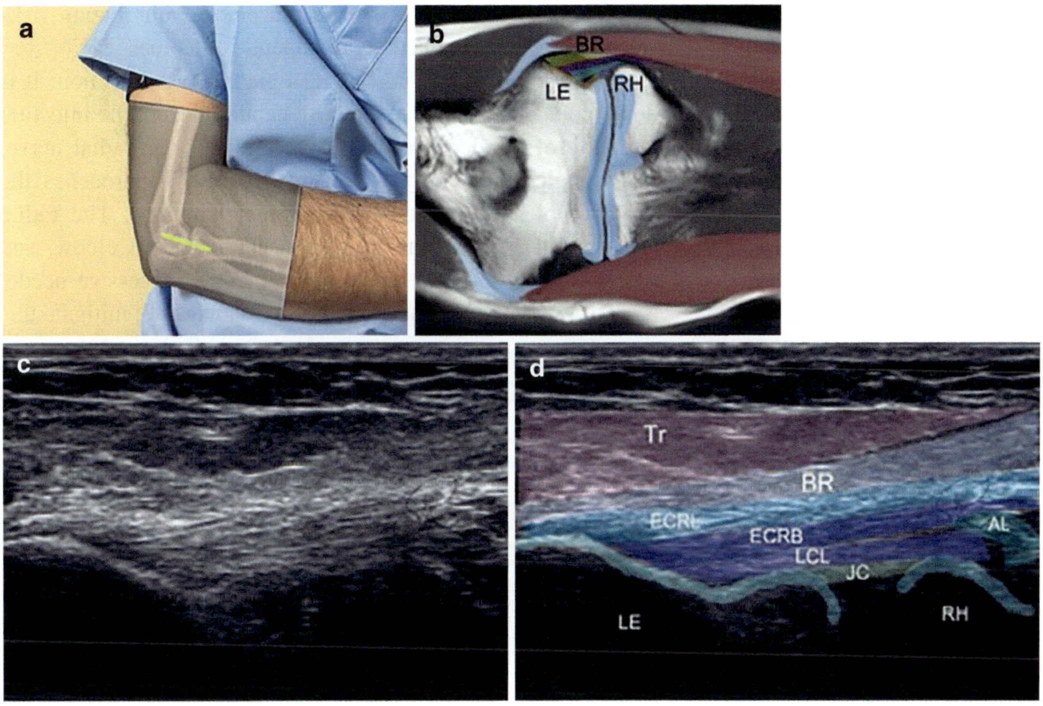

Fig. 3.11 Lateral elbow long axis scan. A composite image featuring four panels that illustrate elbow anatomy and imaging techniques. Panel (**a**) shows a flexed elbow with a pronated forearm, overlaid by an X-ray that highlights the elbow joint. A yellow line indicates the area of interest for cross-section analysis and the position for probe placement. Panel (**b**) presents a labeled anatomical diagram derived from a coronal MRI slice of the elbow, identifying key structures such as the brachioradialis (BR), lateral epicondyle (LE), and radial head (RH). Panel (**c**) displays an ultrasound image of the lateral elbow without annotations. Finally, panel (**d**) features a labeled ultrasound image that marks significant anatomical structures, including the triceps (Tr), brachioradialis (BR), extensor carpi radialis longus (ECRL), extensor carpi radialis brevis (ECRB), lateral collateral ligament (LCL), joint capsule (JC), annular ligament (AL), lateral epicondyle (LE), and radial head (RH). (© Reza Roghani 2024. All Rights Reserved)

teristic proximal "hockey stick" pattern formed by the radial head and capitellum (Fig. 3.11c).

Scanning: At the superior aspect of the joint, a thin hyperechoic line denotes the joint capsule, immediately followed by the lateral collateral ligament. The distal portion of this ligament seamlessly merges with the annular ligament, which encircles and stabilizes the radial head. Just above the lateral collateral ligament, the extensor tendons are visible, with the extensor carpi radialis brevis (ECRB) positioned centrally. More superficially, the extensor carpi radialis longus (ECRL) and brachioradialis (BR) can be observed, both contributing to lateral elbow stability and movement. As you perform the scan, pay attention to any tendon thickening, which may indicate chronic tendinopathy, as well as joint effusion or increased vascularity, which can be assessed using Doppler ultrasound. These findings could suggest lateral epicondylitis or inflammation of the radiohumeral joint. Adjusting the probe angle may be necessary to enhance the visualization of these structures and distinguish between normal and pathological findings [6, 7].

3.4.3 Injection (Video 3.9)

Lateral Epicondylitis Injection: Begin by scanning the lateral epicondyle as previously described, ensuring clear visualization of the extensor carpi radialis brevis (ECRB) tendon. Once the tendon is properly identified, administer small amounts of injectate at multiple sites along the tendon, beginning at the distal portion and progressively working proximally. This technique promotes even distribution of the medication across the tendon (Fig. 3.12).

For the treatment of lateral epicondylitis, the injectate typically consists of a combination of corticosteroid and local anesthetic, providing both anti-inflammatory effects and immediate pain relief. Alternatives such as platelet-rich plasma (PRP) and prolotherapy may be considered, particularly in refractory cases. Utilizing ultrasound guidance during this procedure allows for precise needle placement, minimizing risks and enhancing therapeutic outcomes [8].

Caution: Lateral Epicondylitis Injection: It is essential to exercise caution during the injection procedure to prevent injury to the radial nerve, especially when the needle tip approaches the more anterior or proximal regions. The radial nerve runs closely near the lateral elbow, and improper needle placement or excessive needle depth may lead to nerve damage. To mitigate this risk, ensure precise ultrasound guidance and accurate needle placement—particularly the tip of the needle—as well as proper visualization of the surrounding structures. Always proceed slowly and deliberately when injecting in proximity to sensitive areas.

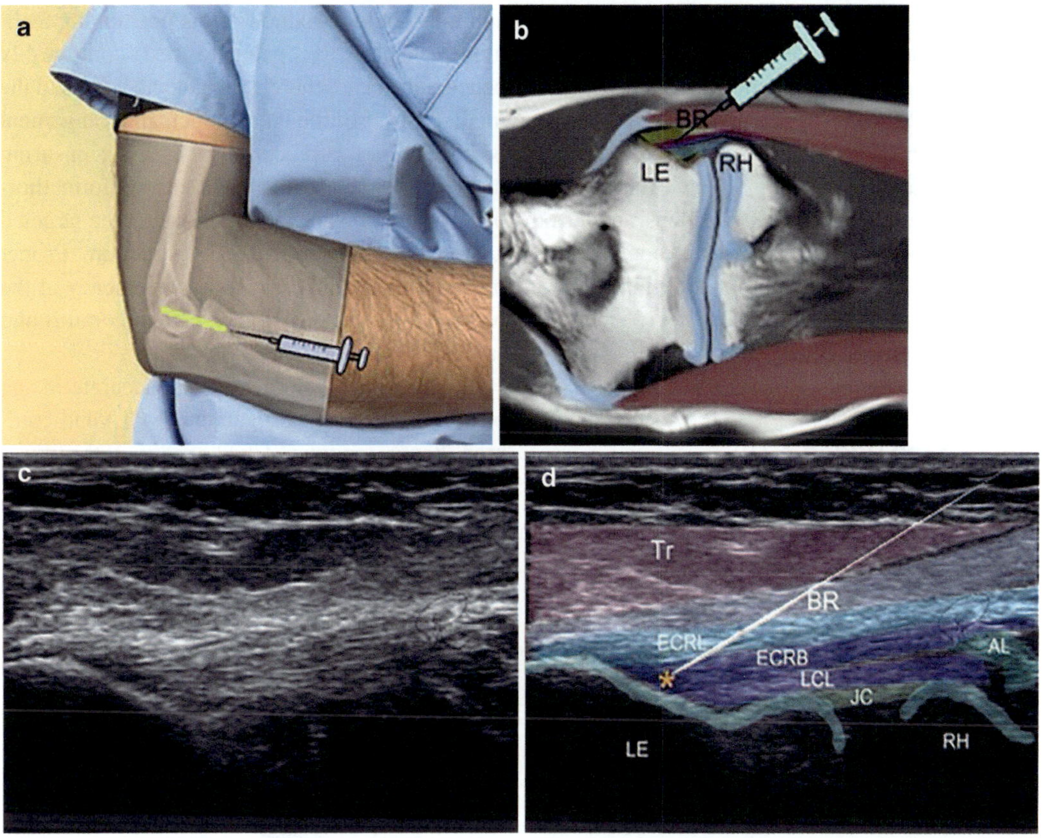

Fig. 3.12 Tennis elbow injection. The image consists of four panels illustrating the injection process for the lateral epicondyle. Panel (**a**) depicts the surface anatomy of the lateral elbow, featuring a yellow line that marks the optimal probe position alongside a syringe, indicating the needle insertion site. Panel (**b**) offers a cross-sectional diagram of the elbow, emphasizing anatomical structures such as the brachioradialis (BR), lateral epicondyle (LE), and radial head (RH). The syringe in this panel illustrates the trajectory of the needle as it passes through the extensor carpi radialis brevis (ECRB) tendon at the midpoint of the "hockey stick" handle. Panel (**c**) presents an ultrasound image of the lateral elbow, centering on the radiohumeral joint and the "hockey stick" in the middle, without annotations. Lastly, panel (**d**) displays the same ultrasound image but with structures labeled and highlighted in various colors, including the triceps (Tr), extensor carpi radialis longus (ECRL), extensor carpi radialis brevis (ECRB), lateral collateral ligament (LCL), and joint capsule (JC). This panel also presents a needle trajectory and a star mark for the ideal injection site for treating tennis elbow. (© Reza Roghani 2024. All Rights Reserved)

3.5 Medial Elbow

3.5.1 Anatomy

The area of focus in the inner elbow aligns with the midcoronal plane, which serves as a reference for understanding the anatomical structures in this region. Within this plane, one can locate the medial epicondyle of the humerus, a prominent bony feature on the inner side of the elbow. Adjacent to the medial epicondyle is the trochlea of the ulna, which is a component of the elbow's hinge joint. The humeral trochlea articulates with the ulna, and between these two structures lies a layer of cartilage that cushions the elbow joint. Above the joint, the joint capsule—a fibrous structure—encloses and stabilizes the elbow joint, containing synovial fluid that lubricates the joint for smooth movement. Superficially to the joint capsule, the medial collateral ligament (MCL) provides stability to the inner aspect of the elbow by resisting valgus stress or outward forces, which could otherwise compromise the structures in this area. Just medial and superficial to the MCL are the common flexor tendons of the forearm muscles, including those from the flexor digitorum superficialis (FDS) and flexor carpi radialis (FCR). The flexor carpi ulnaris muscle and part of its tendon cover up the deeper layers. This arrangement of structures—the medial epicondyle, trochlea of the ulna, joint capsule, medial collateral ligament, common flexor tendons, and flexor carpi ulnaris—constitutes an essential complex that ensures the stability and mobility of the inner elbow and forearm, facilitating a wide range of motions vital for daily activities (Fig. 3.13b) [9].

3.5.2 Scan (Video 3.10)

Patient position: The patient lies in a supine position, which allows for optimal alignment of the body's major structures. With the elbow flexed and the shoulder abducted, this positioning technique enables the palm to rest comfortably beneath the head, thereby enhancing access to the medial aspect of the elbow. Such an arrangement is beneficial for precise assessments, ensuring that healthcare professionals can perform thorough evaluations or interventions on the targeted anatomical region without obstruction. Proper positioning not only improves the efficacy of the procedure but also enhances patient comfort and safety (Fig. 3.13a).

Probe position: To achieve an accurate image of the ulnar collateral ligament (UCL) and common flexor tendons (CFT), position the ultrasound probe longitudinally along the medial aspect of the elbow, directly over the medial epicondyle and toward the path of the flexor carpi ulnaris (FCU) muscle. Ensure the probe is aligned

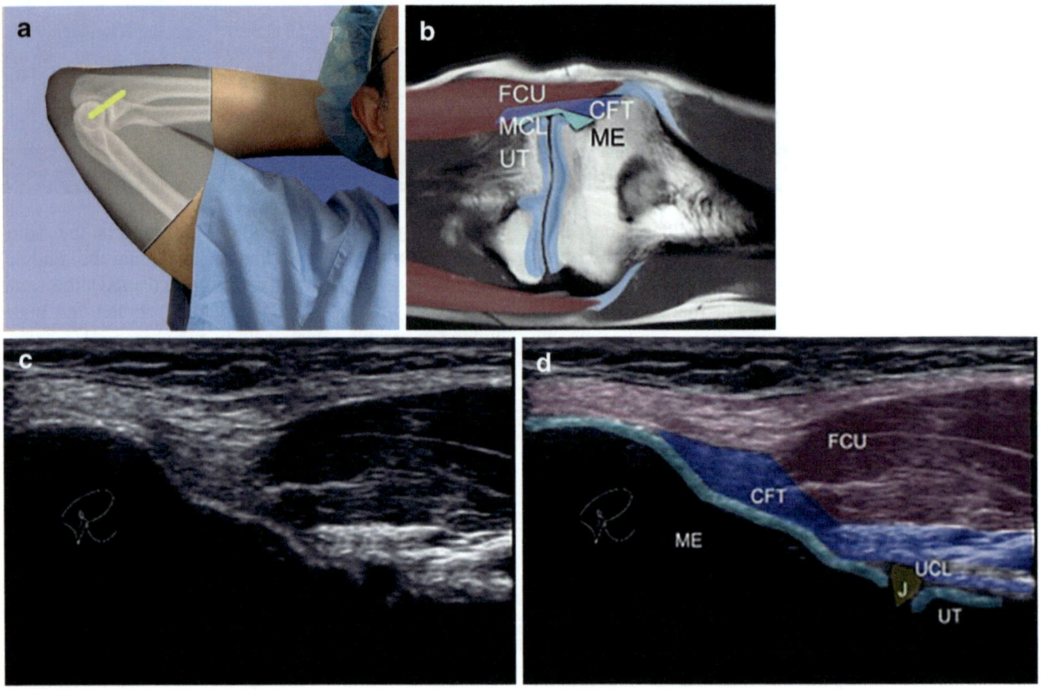

Fig. 3.13 Medial elbow scanning. The image comprises four panels that depict the anatomy and ultrasound imaging of the medial elbow. Panel (a) features a photograph of a flexed elbow superimposed with an X-ray image. A yellow line indicates the optimal position for the ultrasound probe, ensuring precise visualization of the anatomical structures. Panel (b) presents a labeled cross-sectional MRI scan of the elbow in the coronal plane, highlighting key structures such as the flexor carpi ulnaris (FCU), common flexor tendon (CFT), ulnar trochlear (UT), and the medial epicondyle (ME). Panel (c) showcases an ultrasound image of the medial elbow without annotations, concentrating on the humeroulnar joint and surrounding tissues. Panel (d) overlays the ultrasound image with color-coded anatomical labels, identifying the flexor carpi ulnaris (FCU), medial collateral ligament (MCL), ulnar trochlear (UT), common flexor tendon (CFT), medial epicondyle (ME), joint space (J), and the ulnar collateral ligament (UCL).

parallel to the forearm to facilitate clear visualization of the MCL, common flexor tendons, and adjacent structures. Adjust the angle as necessary to obtain optimal imaging of these important anatomical features (Fig. 3.13a).

Scanning: Start the scanning process by adjusting the probe to center the humeroulnar joint within the image. In this position, the ulnar collateral ligament (UCL) will be visible just above the joint. The common flexor tendons will appear more proximal and superficial to the joint. Notably, the flexor carpi ulnaris (FCU)—the most superficial layer—will be easily identifiable, with its tendon terminating at the medial condyle ridge. Make sure to fine-tune the probe's position and angle to ensure these structures are well visualized with minimal anisotropy (Fig. 3.13c, d) [10].

3.5.3 Injection (Video 3.11)

Medial Epicondylitis injection: To properly treat medial epicondylitis, begin by following the scanning process described above and approach in-plane from distal to proximal (Fig. 3.14). Administer the injectate in small quantities at various points along the common

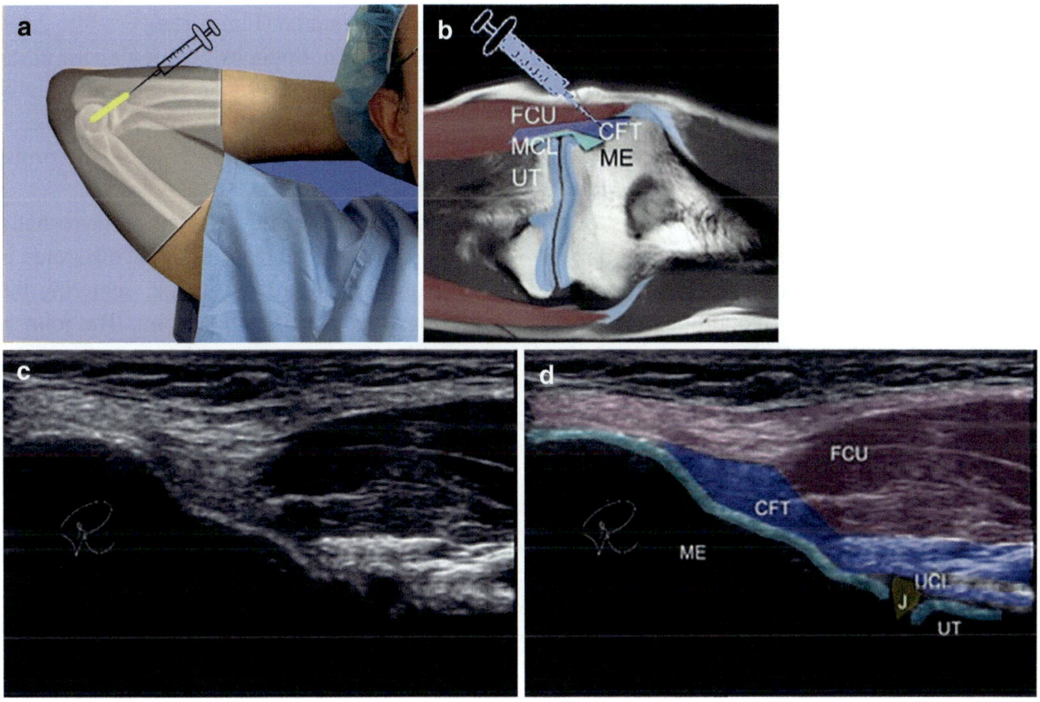

Fig. 3.14 Medial Epicondylitis injection. The image comprises four panels that depict the anatomy and ultrasound imaging of the medial elbow. Panel (**a**) The surface anatomy of the medial elbow is depicted, featuring a yellow line that marks the optimal probe position next to a syringe, which indicates the needle insertion site. Panel (**b**) presents a labeled cross-sectional MRI scan of the elbow in the coronal plane, highlighting key structures such as the flexor carpi ulnaris (FCU), common flexor tendon (CFT), ulnar trochlear (UT), and the medial epicondyle (ME). The syringe depicted in this panel illustrates the trajectory of the needle as it navigates through the midpoint of the common flexor tendon (CFT) insertion located on the medial epicondyle. Understanding this trajectory is essential for minimizing complications during injections or interventions in this anatomical region. Panel (**c**) showcases an ultrasound image of the medial elbow without annotations, concentrating on the humeroulnar joint and surrounding tissues. Panel (**d**) overlays the ultrasound image with color-coded anatomical labels, identifying the flexor carpi ulnaris (FCU), medial collateral ligament (MCL), ulnar trochlear (UT), common flexor tendon (CFT), medial epicondyle (ME), joint space (J), and the ulnar collateral ligament (UCL).

flexor tendons (CFT) [11]. The injectate typically consists of corticosteroids and local anesthetics, which can provide anti-inflammatory effects and immediate pain relief [12]. However, it is crucial to exercise caution and ensure that the entire needle remains visible under ultrasound guidance, as any movement too posterior or proximal could result in accidental penetration of the ulnar nerve.

3.6 Posterior Elbow

3.6.1 Anatomy

The posterior region of the elbow can be anatomically divided into three distinct areas: the medial, central, and lateral regions. Each of these areas plays a unique role in elbow functionality and holds varying degrees of clinical significance. The central region is particularly important, as it encompasses critical structures such as the triceps tendon and the olecranon process of the ulna. These structures are often assessed through neuromusculoskeletal ultrasound of the elbow due to their relevance in conditions like tendinopathies, bursitis, and other musculoskeletal disorders. The triceps tendon, specifically, is vital for elbow extension, and any abnormalities or pathologies in this area can significantly affect the patient's functionality. Conversely, the lateral region of the elbow generally holds minimal clinical relevance regarding musculoskeletal pathologies, injuries, or disorders. The medial region, however, is of considerable importance as it serves as the pathway for the ulnar nerve. This nerve runs along the medial aspect of the elbow, making it vulnerable to compression or irritation, especially in conditions such as cubital tunnel syndrome. Understanding the anatomy of this region is crucial for diagnosing and managing disorders associated with the ulnar nerve, which can manifest as numbness, tingling, or weakness in the hand and fingers [1, 2].

3.6.2 Scan

3.6.2.1 Central Part (Video 3.12)

In the case of the central elbow, the mid-axial cross-section is of particular interest, where the layers of the triceps tendon attach to the olecranon just beneath the skin. The elbow joint itself is located proximal to the olecranon, with a fat pad situated between the triceps tendon and the humerus, which is also positioned proximal to the joint (Fig. 3.15b) [13].

Patient Position: To ensure optimal comfort and accuracy, we suggest placing the patient supine with their hand gently placed palm-up under their head. This will help ease discomfort and provide a clear, unobstructed view for a seamless examination (Fig. 3.15a).

Probe position: Begin by positioning the ultrasound probe on the olecranon process and gently sliding it proximally until the olecranon process is directly beneath the distal edge of the probe (Fig. 3.15a).

Scanning: Continue scanning proximally along the mid-sagittal plane until the olecranon is visible on one side of the image, centering the posterior aspect of the elbow joint. The joint is encased by the synovial membrane and capsule, which can be distinguished as distinct layers covering its surface. Additionally, the triceps tendon fibers will be observable as they extend distally to attach to the olecranon, while proximally they merge with the triceps muscle (Fig. 3.15). A fat pad is situated proximal to the joint, located between the humerus bone and the triceps muscle and tendon, serving as a cushioning structure that can be identified during the scanning process.

3.6.2.2 Medial Part: Cubital Tunnel (Video 3.13)

Regarding the medial aspect of posterior ulna, the relevant cross-section is a transverse view taken between the olecranon and the medial epicondyle. Here, the medial head of the triceps is located near the olecranon, while the ulnar nerve

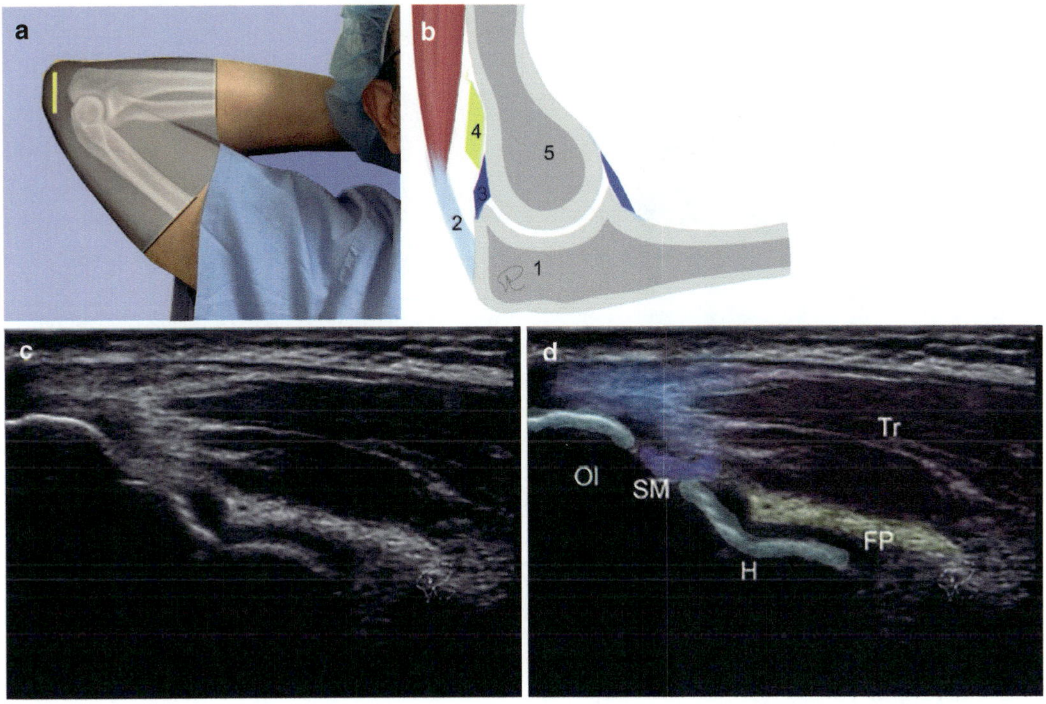

Fig. 3.15 Posterior elbow central part scan. The image features a composite of four panels that illustrate the posterocentral anatomy of the elbow along with its ultrasound imaging. Panel (**a**) depicts an individual with their elbow flexed, overlaid with an X-ray that highlights the joint and a yellow line indicating the optimal position for the ultrasound probe. Panel (**b**) includes a labeled anatomical diagram of the elbow joint, with structures numbered from 1 to 5, which are: (1) olecranon, (2) triceps tendon, (3) synovial membrane, (4) fat pad, and (5) humerus. Panels (**c**) and (**d**) present ultrasound images of the elbow, with Panel (**d**) featuring color-coded regions labeled as follows: (Ol) for olecranon, (Tr) for triceps tendon, (SM) for synovial membrane, (FP) for fat pad, and (H) for humerus.

runs adjacent to the medial epicondyle (Fig. 3.16a)

Patient position: We recommend placing the patient supine for the best possible comfort and accuracy during the examination. The patient's hand should be gently placed palm-up under their head. This will help alleviate any potential discomfort and provide a clear, unobstructed view for a smooth examination.

Probe position: Place one side of the probe on the olecranon process and the other on the medial epicondyle (Fig. 3.16a).

Scanning: The olecranon (OL) process is prominently featured on one side of the image, while the medial epicondyle (ME) is visible on the opposite side, serving as important anatomical landmarks for this scan. The floor of the image is defined by the elbow groove (G) of the medial condyle of the humerus, which acts as a pathway for the ulnar nerve. Adjacent to the medial epicondyle, the ulnar nerve (UN) stands out with its honeycomb-like structure, indicative of its fascicular architecture. This distinctive appearance arises from the hypoechoic nerve fascicles interspersed within a hyperechoic framework of connective tissue. The nerve traverses the cubital tunnel, a region known for its vulnerability to entrapment or irritation, making it critical for ultrasound evaluation. The cubital tunnel retinaculum (R), a fibrous band that stabilizes the nerve, forms the roof of this anatomical space. Near the olecranon, the medial head of the triceps (T) muscle is clearly delineated, playing a key role in elbow extension. Its fibers can be traced proximally toward the muscle belly and distally toward their insertion on the olecranon (Fig. 3.16b, d) [14]. Fanning the probe during this

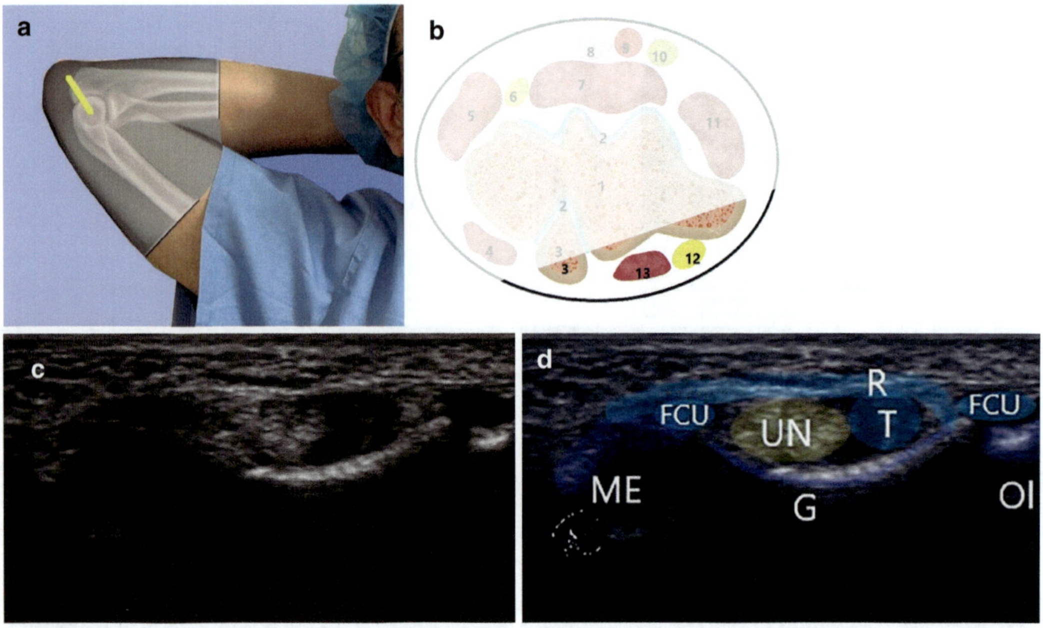

Fig. 3.16 Posterior elbow medial part scanning. The image comprises four panels that illustrate the anatomy and imaging of the elbow. Panel (**a**) depicts a person with their elbow flexed and their palm resting under their head, overshadowed by an overlaid X-ray. A yellow line indicates the optimal positioning for both patient and the ultrasound probe during the evaluation. Panel (**b**) presents a cross-sectional diagram of the posteromedial elbow, labeling key anatomical structures with numbers, including the olecranon (3), triceps (13), and ulnar nerve (12). Panel (**c**) features a grayscale ultrasound image of the posteromedial elbow, clearly showcasing the ulnar groove and its contents. Panel (**d**) provides a color-coded ultrasound image with labeled structures, including the ulnar nerve (UN), triceps (T), olecranon (Ol), ulnar groove (G), medial epicondyle (ME), flexor carpi ulnaris (FCU), and retinaculum (R).

scan is vital to ensure that the ultrasound beam remains perpendicular to the triceps myotendinous junction. Proper angulation of the probe enhances image clarity by optimizing echogenicity, reducing anisotropy, and facilitating a more precise assessment of the tendon structure in this view. This technique is essential for identifying subtle abnormalities such as partial tears, tendinopathy, or calcifications that might otherwise be missed due to inadequate insonation angles.

3.6.3 Injections

3.6.3.1 Supinator Syndrome (Video 3.14)

Supinator syndrome, also known as supinator canal syndrome, is a rare condition characterized by the compression of the deep branch of the radial nerve, the posterior interosseous nerve (PIN). This compression happens as the PIN passes through the supinator muscle in the forearm near the elbow [15].

Patient Position: The patient is lying comfortably on their back in bed with their elbow bent and their palm resting gently on their abdomen.

Probe Position: To begin the scan, place the probe about 2 inches below the elbow crease and scan the posteromedial side of the forearm in a short axis orientation.

Scanning and injection: Within the image, you will notice the bony structure of the radius surrounded by the supinator muscle. Above the supinator muscle are two honeycomb structures: a smaller one representing the sensory branch of the radial nerve and a larger, more lateral one representing the motor branch or posterior interosseous nerve (Fig. 3.17). The ECRL muscle sits on top, with the brachioradialis muscle superficial to it.

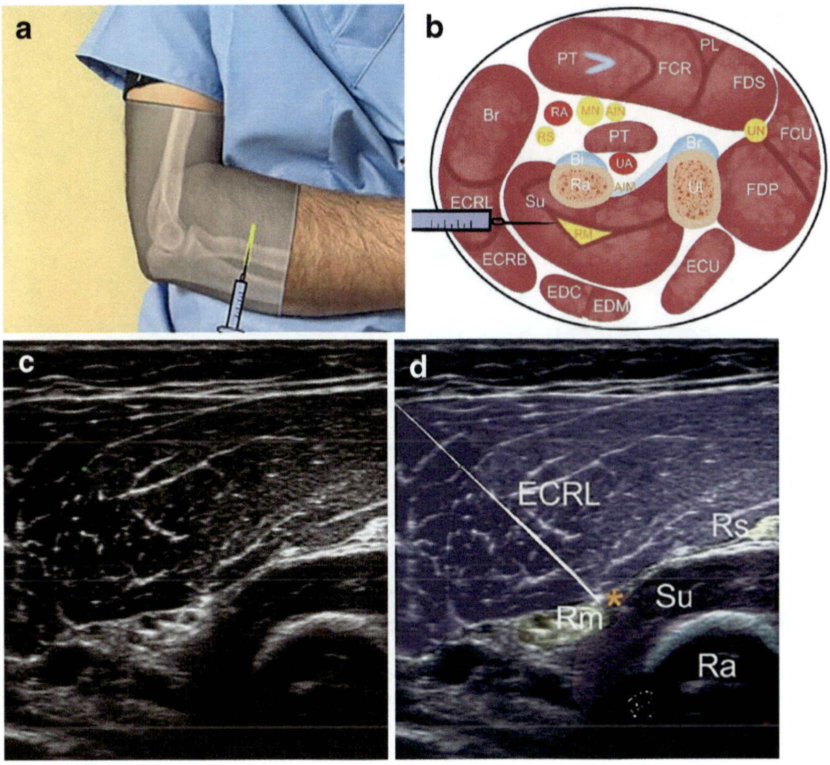

Fig. 3.17 Posterior interosseous nerve block. The image is a composite of four panels illustrating an ultrasound-guided supinator syndrome procedure on the forearm. Panel (**a**) shows a person's forearm with a transparent overlay of the underlying bone structure, depicted through an X-ray. A yellow line indicates the probe's position, while a syringe approaches in-plane, demonstrating the injection technique. Panel (**b**) presents a cross-sectional anatomical diagram of the forearm, labeling key muscles and nerves, including the extensor carpi radialis longus (ECRL), extensor carpi radialis brevis (ECRB), supinator (su), radius bone (Ra), and radial nerve motor branch (RM), providing essential anatomical context. Panel (**c**) displays an ultrasound image of the forearm, displaying the radial nerve branches and associated structures. Panel (**d**) presents the same ultrasound scan with labeled anatomical structures, including the extensor carpi radialis longus (ECRL), radial nerve motor branch (Rm), supinator muscle (Su), and radial nerve sensory branch (Rs), as well as the radial bone (Ra). A needle trajectory is illustrated from left to right, with an orange asterisk marking the target point for the nerve block. (© Reza Roghani 2024. All Rights Reserved)

3.6.3.2 Triceps Tendon (Video 3.15)

Triceps tendinitis is characterized by inflammation and irritation of the triceps tendon at its insertion on the olecranon, leading to significant pain, weakness, and functional limitations. This condition often affects individuals engaged in repetitive pushing, overhead activities, or forceful elbow extensions. It is commonly observed in athletes, weightlifters, manual laborers, and musicians who regularly exert their upper limbs under substantial mechanical load. Ultrasound-guided injections offer a precise and effective approach to managing triceps tendinitis, enabling targeted delivery of therapeutic agents while minimizing the risk of complications.

Patient position: To ensure optimal comfort and accuracy, we recommend positioning the patient supine with their hand gently resting palm-up beneath their head. This posture will alleviate discomfort and provide a clear, unobstructed view for a seamless examination (Fig. 3.18a).

Probe position: To properly position the ultrasound probe for optimal visualization of the olecranon process, place the probe directly on the olecranon process itself. From this initial position, gently slide the probe in a proximal direc-

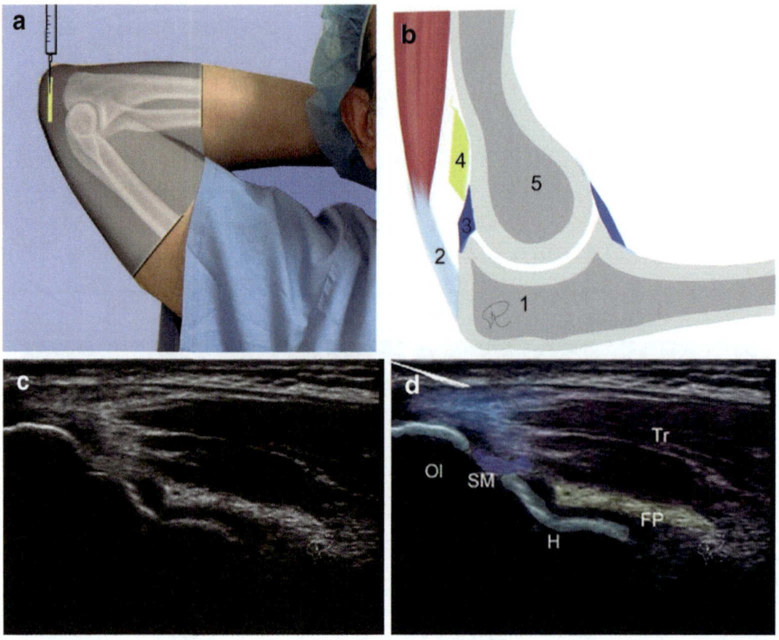

Fig. 3.18 Triceps tendon injection. The image features a composite of four panels that illustrate the posterocentral anatomy of the elbow along with its ultrasound imaging. Panel (**a**) depicts an individual with their elbow flexed, overlaid with an X-ray that highlights the joint and a yellow line indicating the optimal position for the ultrasound probe. A syringe illustrating the point of needle insertion. Panel (**b**) includes a labeled anatomical diagram of the elbow joint, with structures numbered from 1 to 5, which are: (1) olecranon, (2) triceps tendon, (3) synovial membrane, (4) fat pad, and (5) humerus. Panels (**c**) and (**d**) present ultrasound images of the elbow, with Panel (**d**) featuring color-coded regions labeled as follows: (Ol) for olecranon, (Tr) for triceps tendon, (SM) for synovial membrane, (FP) for fat pad, and (H) for humerus. A needle trajectory and a target point are shown in the upper left corner of image (**d**). (© Reza Roghani 2024. All Rights Reserved)

tion until the olecranon process is situated directly beneath the distal edge of the probe. This alignment ensures that the anatomical structure is effectively imaged for diagnostic purposes (Fig. 3.18a).

Scanning and injection: Under real-time ultrasound guidance, gently slide the probe slightly proximal until the olecranon process be visible on the distal edge of the image. Insert the needle in-plane beneath the distal end of the probe and carefully advance it toward the target site, ensuring that the tip punctures the tendon sheath (Fig. 3.18). If you encounter any significant resistance, slightly withdraw the needle and reposition it to optimize placement. A 25-gauge needle, typically ranging from 1 to 1.5 inches in length, is commonly used, while syringe volumes generally vary from 3 to 5 mL, depending on the selected injectate. The objective of the injection is to alleviate pain and inflammation by precisely delivering corticosteroids and local anesthetics, thus ensuring effective symptom relief while minimizing the risk of complications.

3.6.3.3 Cubital Tunnel (Video 3.16)

The cubital tunnel is a narrow anatomical passage located on the medial side of the elbow, bordered by the two heads of the flexor carpi ulnaris (FCU) muscle and the medial epicondyle of the humerus. This tunnel serves as a pathway for the ulnar nerve, which is responsible for both motor and sensory innervation to the forearm and hand. Factors such as repetitive elbow flexion, prolonged pressure, or mechanical strain can lead to inflammation, swelling, or fibrosis within the cubital tunnel. This can reduce the available space and increase compression on the ulnar nerve, disrupting its normal function. As a result, individuals may experience pain, numbness, tingling, and weakness, particularly in the ring and little fingers. Corticosteroid injections can help manage acute inflammation and provide symptomatic relief; however, their use should be limited to avoid potential weakening of the tendon or nerve. Another effective technique is hydrodissection, where fluid is injected around the ulnar nerve to separate it from surrounding structures, thereby reducing entrapment and enhancing mobility [16].

Probe position and scanning: To properly scan the cubital tunnel, please refer to the protocol outlined in Sect. 3.6.2.2.

Scanning and injection: Start by locating the ulnar nerve in the short axis between the medial epicondyle and olecranon, where it appears as a honeycomb-like structure within the cubital tunnel. Once identified, rotate the ultrasound probe 90° to obtain a long-axis view, ensuring continuous monitoring of the nerve's pathway. For the injection, utilize an in-plane approach from the proximal aspect, carefully advancing the needle under direct ultrasound guidance until the tip is positioned above the nerve within the tunnel (Fig. 3.19). Take great care to avoid penetrating the nerve sheath, as an inadvertent intraneural injection may result in complications. To alleviate inflammation and provide symptomatic relief, prepare the injectate by combining 3 cc of a local anesthetic with a corticosteroid, ensuring optimal dispersion within the cubital tunnel while minimizing potential irritation.

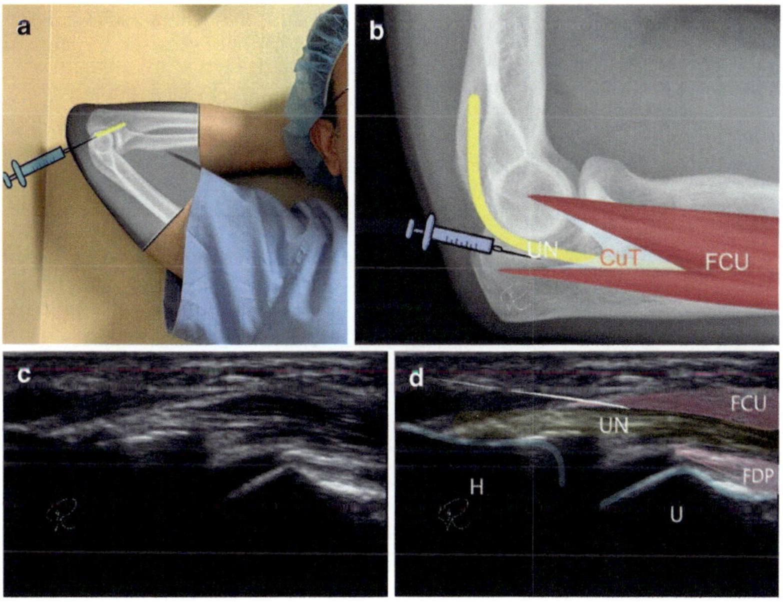

Fig. 3.19 Cubital tunnel injection. The image consists of a composite illustration divided into four panels, depicting the cubital tunnel scan and injection procedure. Panel (a) shows a patient positioned with their elbow flexed and palm resting under their head, an arrangement that optimizes the evaluation of the cubital tunnel. An overlaid X-ray provides anatomical context, while a yellow guideline indicates the ideal positioning for the ultrasound probe. Additionally, a syringe icon marks the precise point for needle insertion. Panel (b) features a detailed, annotated illustration superimposed on an X-ray of the elbow, highlighting the needle's trajectory and crucial anatomical structures, including the flexor carpi ulnaris (FCU), ulnar nerve (UN), and cubital tunnel (CuT). Panels (c) and (d) present ultrasound images of the elbow, showcasing the cubital tunnel and the injection site. Panel (d) includes labeled structures such as the flexor carpi ulnaris (FCU), flexor digitorum profundus (FDP), ulnar nerve (UN), and cubital tunnel (CuT), providing a clear depiction of the needle trajectory and target point for accurate intervention. (© Reza Roghani 2024. All Rights Reserved)

References

1. Chin K, Hussain S, Mazis G, Arya A. Clinical anatomy and biomechanics of the elbow. J Clin Orthop Trauma. 2021;20:101485. https://doi.org/10.1016/j.jcot.2021.101485.
2. Malagelada F, Dalmau-Pastor M, Vega J, Golanó P. Elbow anatomy. In: Doral MN, Karlsson J, editors. Sports injuries: prevention, diagnosis, treatment, and rehabilitation. Springer; 2014. p. 1–30. https://doi.org/10.1007/978-3-642-36801-1_38-1.
3. Boles CA, Kannam S, Cardwell AB. The forearm. Am J Roentgenol. 2000;174(1):151–9. https://doi.org/10.2214/ajr.174.1.1740151.
4. van der Vis J, Janssen SJ, Bleys RLAW, Eygendaal D, van den Bekerom MPJ. Distal biceps tendon injection. Clin Shoulder Elb. 2021;24(2):93–7. https://doi.org/10.5397/cise.2021.00010.
5. Delzell PB, Patel M. Ultrasound-guided perineural injection for pronator syndrome caused by median nerve entrapment. J Ultrasound Med. 2020;39(5):1023–9. https://doi.org/10.1002/jum.15166.
6. Hohmann E, Tetsworth K, Glatt V. Corticosteroid injections for the treatment of lateral epicondylitis are superior to platelet-rich plasma at one month, but platelet-rich plasma is more effective at six months: an updated systematic review and meta-analysis of level 1 and 2 studies. J Shoulder Elb Surg. 2023;32(9):1770–83. https://doi.org/10.1016/j.jse.2023.04.018.
7. Omoumi P, Gondim Teixeira PA, Ward SR, Trudell D, Resnick D. Practical ultrasonographic technique to precisely identify and differentiate tendons and ligaments of the elbow at the level of the humeral epicondyles: anatomical study. Skeletal Radiol. 2021;50(7):1369–77. https://doi.org/10.1007/s00256-020-03693-5.
8. Sun JQ, Stillson QA, Strelzow JA, Shi LL. Trends in corticosteroid injections for treatment of lateral epicondylitis: an analysis of 80,169 patients. JAAOS Glob Res Rev. 2021;5(9):e21.00186. https://doi.org/10.5435/JAAOSGlobal-D-21-00186.
9. Cinque ME, Schickendantz M, Frangiamore S. Review of anatomy of the medial ulnar collateral ligament complex of the elbow. Curr Rev Musculoskelet Med. 2020;13(1):96–102. https://doi.org/10.1007/s12178-020-09609-z.
10. Konarski W, Poboży T, Kotela A, Hordowicz M, Poboży K. Ultrasound in the differential diagnosis of medial epicondylalgia and medial elbow pain—imaging findings and narrative literature review. Healthcare. 2022;10(8):1529. https://doi.org/10.3390/healthcare10081529.
11. Ergönenç T. Ultrasound-guided elbow injection techniques. In: El Miedany Y, editor. Musculoskeletal ultrasound-guided regenerative medicine. Springer; 2022. p. 109–18. https://doi.org/10.1007/978-3-030-98256-0_6.
12. Zahn KV, Byerly DW. Medial epicondyle injection. In: StatPearls. StatPearls Publishing; 2024. http://www.ncbi.nlm.nih.gov/books/NBK551506/.
13. Kunc V, Benes M, Veigl D, Kachlik D. Anatomical variants are complicating the posterior approaches towards the elbow joint. Surg Radiol Anat. 2023;45(5):587–92. https://doi.org/10.1007/s00276-023-03124-9.
14. Tamborrini G, Müller-Gerbl M, Vogel N, Haeni D. Ultrasound of the elbow with emphasis on the sonoanatomy of the distal biceps tendon and its importance for the surgical treatment of tendon lesions. J Ultrason. 2020;20(81):e129–34. https://doi.org/10.15557/JoU.2020.0021.
15. Jeon A, Kim Y-G, Kwon S-O, Lee J-H. Relationship between the branching patterns of the radial nerve and supinator muscle. Biomed Res Int. 2021;2021:8691114. https://doi.org/10.1155/2021/8691114.
16. Anderson D, Woods B, Abubakar T, Koontz C, Li N, Hasoon J, Viswanath O, Kaye AD, Urits I. A comprehensive review of cubital tunnel syndrome. Orthop Rev. 2022;14(3):38239. https://doi.org/10.52965/001c.38239.

4 Wrist and Hand

Andrew M. Mendelson, Reza Salman Roghani, Megan McGuire, Jasmine Sidhu, Naffiseh Jafarian, and Ghazaleh Ebrahimi

4.1 Introduction

The wrist and hand consist of a complex network of tendons, ligaments, nerves, and small joints, making neuromusculoskeletal (NMSK) ultrasound an invaluable imaging modality for precise evaluation and guided interventions. This chapter delves into the utilization of high-resolution ultrasound for diagnosing and managing prevalent wrist and hand pathologies, including tendinopathies, ligament injuries, nerve entrapments (such as carpal tunnel syndrome), inflammatory arthropathies, and mechanical disorders like trigger finger. A comprehensive review of the sonographic anatomy of the extensor and flexor tendons is presented, with particular focus on their organization into six extensor compartments, as well as the maneuver of flexor tendons through the carpal tunnel and Guyon's canal. The chapter discusses flexor pulley system pathology, especially A1 pulley thickening related to trigger finger, alongside dynamic scanning techniques to evaluate stenosing tenosynovitis and identify abnormal tendon movement or impingement. The chapter highlights the diagnosis and severity grading of carpal tunnel syndrome (CTS) using ultrasound, emphasizing the measurement of the median nerve's cross-sectional area (CSA) at the pisiform level. Additional sonographic markers are explored, including the loss of fascicular pattern, restricted nerve mobility, and increased vascularity on Doppler imaging, which are crucial for distinguishing between mild, moderate, and severe CTS. Furthermore, the text outlines scanning protocols and diagnostic criteria for conditions such as tenosynovitis, partial and complete tendon tears, and impingement syndromes. The chapter also reviews important ultrasound-guided interventions, including corticosteroid injections, hydrodissection for nerve entrapments, and regenerative therapies (e.g., PRP injections). By integrating ultrasound imaging into clinical practice, healthcare providers can achieve real-time, dynamic assessments of wrist and hand conditions, ultimately enhancing diagnostic accuracy and treatment effectiveness.

Supplementary Information The online version contains supplementary material available at https://doi.org/10.1007/978-3-031-81037-4_4.

A. M. Mendelson
Pain Management Division, Department of Anesthesia, University of Virginia School of Medicine, Charlottesville, VA, USA
e-mail: hav4pm@uvahealth.org

R. S. Roghani (✉) · J. Sidhu · G. Ebrahimi
Department of Physical Medicine and Rehabilitation, Larkin Community Hospital, Nova Southeastern University, Miami, FL, USA

M. McGuire
Pohlman Pain Associates, Coral Springs, FL, USA

N. Jafarian
Department of Physical Medicine and Rehabilitation, Shohada Hospital, Shahid Beheshti University of Medical Science, Tajrish, Tehran, Iran

R. S. Roghani, J. J. Diaz (eds.), *Video Atlas of Neuromusculoskeletal Ultrasound*,
https://doi.org/10.1007/978-3-031-81037-4_4

4.1.1 Wrist and Hand Ultrasound Protocol

Dorsal Wrist

- **Transverse Plane (Short Axis):**
  - Evaluate the **extensor tendon compartments** in short axis.
  - Assess **radiocarpal** and **midcarpal joints** for pathology and guide **intra-articular injections**.
- **Coronal Plane:**
  - Guide injections for **de Quervain's tenosynovitis**.
  - Visualize and access the **radiocarpal** and **ulnocarpal joints** for diagnostic or therapeutic procedures.

Volar Wrist

- **Transverse Plane (Short Axis):**
  - Cross-sectional evaluation of the **carpal tunnel** and **Guyon's canal**.
  - Guide injections for **median nerve** and **ulnar nerve** entrapment syndromes.
- **Sagittal Plane (Long Axis):**
  - Longitudinal evaluation of the **median nerve** for dynamic assessment and injection guidance.

Hand

- **Short Axis:**
  - Assess the **thenar** and **hypothenar eminences** for structural abnormalities and guide focal injections.
- **Long Axis:**
  - Visualize the **flexor pulley system** for evaluation of **trigger finger** or tenosynovitis interventions.

4.2 Dorsal Wrist

4.2.1 Joints

4.2.1.1 Anatomy

The wrist is a sophisticated anatomical region comprised of eight carpal bones organized into two distinct rows, along with numerous articulations that facilitate both mobility and stability. These carpal bones and associated joints establish the fundamental framework for wrist movement, grip strength, and overall hand dexterity. The radius articulates distally with the scaphoid and lunate bones, thereby forming the radiocarpal joint, which is critical for wrist flexion and extension. In contrast, the ulna does not have direct contact with the carpal bones; it forms the ulnocarpal joint through interaction with the lunate and triquetrum, supported by the triangular fibrocartilage complex (TFCC). Above these articulations lies the distal radioulnar joint (DRUJ), where the radius and ulna function together to facilitate forearm pronation and supination. This joint is vital for wrist mobility and is reinforced by the interosseous membrane and DRUJ ligaments, which ensure smooth motion between the two bones. On the volar side of the wrist, the pisiform bone, a small sesamoid bone nestled within the tendon of the flexor carpi ulnaris (FCU), sits atop the triquetrum. This anatomical arrangement enhances the mechanical leverage of the FCU, playing a significant role in wrist flexion and ulnar deviation. The distal carpal row, arranged from radial to ulnar, is composed of the trapezium, trapezoid, capitate, and hamate bones. These bones articulate proximally with the first-row carpal bones and distally with the metacarpals, forming the carpometacarpal (CMC) joints, which are essential for hand dexterity and grip strength. The capitate serves as the largest carpal bone, acting as the central axis for wrist motion, while the trapezium is particularly important for the mobility of the thumb through the first CMC joint. Neuromusculoskeletal ultrasound has emerged as a vital tool for assessing the structures of the wrist and hand. It is particularly useful in evaluating the integrity of the radiocarpal, ulnocarpal, and DRUJ joints, while also facilitating the detection of ligamentous injuries. This imaging modality guides interventions for issues such as carpal instability, TFCC tears, and osteoarthritis. High-resolution ultrasound allows for dynamic assessment, enabling real-time visualization of joint congruency, tendon movement, and synovial pathology, thus becoming a cornerstone of contemporary musculoskeletal diagnostics [1, 2].

4.2.1.2 Scan (Video 4.1)

Patient position: The patient sits with their hand placed palm down on the examination table, with

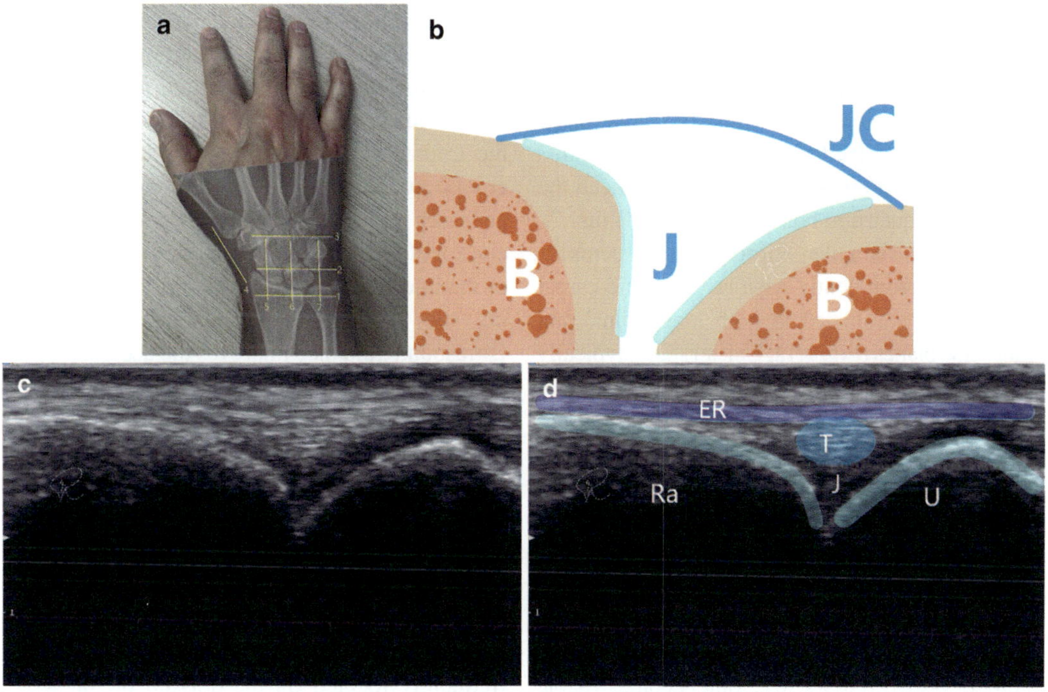

Fig. 4.1 Wrist joints. The image comprises a composite of four panels that illustrate wrist anatomy, joint positioning, and ultrasound imaging. Panel (**a**) displays a human hand with an overlaid X-ray, which distinctly highlights the wrist bones. Numbered yellow lines indicate the specific positions of the ultrasound probe used to scan various joints for a thorough evaluation. Panel (**b**) presents a detailed diagram of a joint, with labeled structures: "B" for bone, "J" for joint, and "JC" for joint capsule, providing a schematic representation of the wrist's structural components. Panel (**c**) showcases an ultrasound image of the wrist, revealing both bone and the surrounding soft tissue structures. Panel (**d**) is an annotated version of panel (**c**), featuring labels that identify key anatomical landmarks: "ER" for extensor retinaculum, "T" for tendon, "J" for joint, "Ra" for radius, and "U" for ulna. Collectively, these panels integrate anatomical, radiographic, and ultrasound perspectives, offering a comprehensive visual guide for evaluating the wrist joint.

a rolled towel under the wrist to allow for mild flexion.

Probe position: The ultrasound probe is systematically positioned at seven distinct locations on the dorsal aspect of the wrist, utilizing both longitudinal and transverse axes to facilitate a comprehensive evaluation of the underlying structures. The assessment begins at Line 1, corresponding to the transverse axis of the distal radioulnar joint (DRUJ). This initial position allows for clear visualization of the articulation between the radius and ulna, enabling an assessment of joint stability, effusion, and ligament integrity. As the probe is advanced along the dorsal wrist, adjustments are made to capture various anatomical landmarks, including the radiocarpal joint, midcarpal joint, and carpometacarpal joints. Employing both longitudinal and transverse imaging planes ensures a thorough examination of the tendons, synovial sheaths, and bony structures, which aids in diagnosing conditions such as tenosynovitis, joint effusions, and ligamentous injuries. This systematic approach enhances the accuracy of ultrasound-guided interventions and improves the overall evaluation of dorsal wrist pathology (Fig. 4.1a, line 1).

Scanning: From Position 1, the examiner slides the ultrasound probe distally by approximately 1 cm to obtain a view of the proximal intercarpal joint (Line 2). Moving an additional 1 cm distally (Line 3) reveals the distal intercarpal joints. Line 4 corresponds to the radio-scaphoid and scapho-trapezoid joints. Following this, an ulnar sliding maneuver should be performed to fully visualize the radio-scaphoid joint (Fig. 4.1a, Line 5), with further ulnar movement to assess the radio-lunate joint (Fig. 4.1a, Line 6). Continuing ulnarly, a distinct V-shaped drop becomes evident between the ulna and triquetrum bones (Fig. 4.1a, Line 7), where the triangular fibrocartilage complex (TFCC) is prominently visible. The mid-carpal joints can be evaluated in both longitudinal and transverse planes (Fig. 4.1a, Lines 1, 2, 3), typically presenting a V-shape on ultrasound. To accurately identify individual joints, the examiner should methodically assess the carpal bones and intercarpal spaces, scanning from distal to proximal and radial to ulnar while counting the proximal and distal carpal bones and analyzing their articulations. For the first carpometacarpal (CMC) joint, the ultrasound probe is aligned along the long axis of the first metacarpal bone and moved proximally until the V-shaped first CMC joint becomes visible (Fig. 4.1a, Line 4). To examine the metacarpophalangeal (MCP) joint, the scan begins at the proximal phalanx and progresses proximally until the V-shaped MCP joint is clearly displayed.

4.2.1.3 Injection (Video 4.2)

Procedures involving the wrist and hand joints are frequently performed for both therapeutic and diagnostic purposes. They address a variety of conditions, including inflammatory arthropathies such as psoriatic arthritis, rheumatoid arthritis, and gout, as well as degenerative joint diseases like osteoarthritis and post-traumatic arthritis. These interventions are essential for reducing inflammation, alleviating pain, enhancing mobility, and restoring function in the affected joints. Typically, a 25–27 gauge, 1–1.5-inch needle is employed to ensure precision while minimizing the patient's discomfort. The injectate generally comprises 1 mL of local anesthetic (such as lidocaine) combined with 0.5–1.0 mL of an injectable corticosteroid (like triamcinolone or methylprednisolone), providing both immediate and sustained symptom relief. This sterile procedure utilizes an ultrasound-guided scanning technique, which allows for accurate needle placement while avoiding neurovascular structures. The needle is advanced in-plane relative to the transducer to maintain continuous visualization (Fig. 4.2), enhancing safety and efficacy. In the case of an ulno-triquetrum joint injection, meticulous care is necessary to prevent injury to the triangular fibrocartilage complex (TFCC), a crucial stabilizing structure of the wrist. This approach requires careful angulation and depth control of the needle to ensure the precise delivery of the injectate into the joint space while preserving the integrity of surrounding soft tissues. Ultrasound guidance improves the accuracy of the procedure and enhances patient safety and comfort by reducing the risk of vascular injury, intratendinous injection, or unintentional diffusion of medication into adjacent structures. This method has become the standard of care for musculoskeletal interventions involving the wrist and hand, allowing for real-time visualization, optimized needle trajectory, and improved therapeutic outcomes.

Ganglion cysts are benign, fluid-filled sacs frequently located on the dorsum of the wrist. They are most prevalent in individuals between the ages of 30 and 50, although they can manifest at any age [3]. These cysts typically possess a tortuous lumen that establishes a connection with the underlying joint, enabling communication with synovial fluid, usually originating from the wrist joint or tendon sheath. This connection may facilitate cyst growth and result in variations in size. Clinically, the presentation of ganglion cysts ranges from asymptomatic to symptomatic, with potential discomfort arising from the cyst compressing adjacent structures such as nerves or tendons. Symptoms may include restricted wrist movement, pain, swelling, and aesthetic concerns. Ultrasound imaging serves as an effective diagnostic tool for ganglion cysts, providing clear visualization of the cyst, its anatomical relationship to the joint, and surrounding soft tissues. The use of neuromusculoskeletal ultrasound is particularly advantageous during interventions, as it offers real-time imaging that enhances both accuracy and safety. The first-line treatment for ganglion cysts typically involves ultrasound-guided aspiration, often complemented by corticosteroid injection. Aspiration entails the extraction of cyst fluid, which diminishes cyst size and alleviates symp-

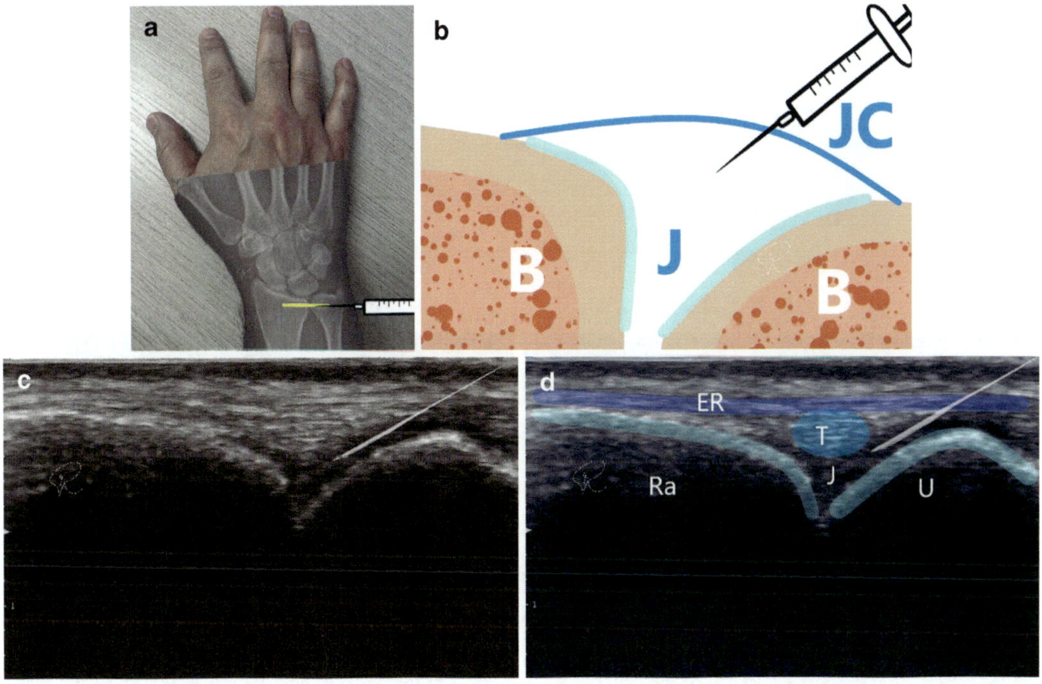

Fig. 4.2 Wrist joint injection. The text provides a detailed and structured overview of wrist joint anatomy and the ultrasound-guided injection technique, divided into four distinct panels. In Panel (**a**), a hand is depicted alongside an overlaid X-ray, which serves to highlight the wrist bones. The yellow line denotes the positioning of the ultrasound probe specifically over the distal radioulnar joint. A syringe is illustrated as it approaches the joint, indicating the target point for needle insertion. Panel (**b**) offers a cross-sectional view of the joint anatomy, where components are clearly labeled: "B" for bone, "J" for the joint, and "JC" for the joint capsule, illustrating the needle trajectory as it penetrates the joint space. Panels (**c**) and (**d**) include ultrasound images that depict the radioulnar joint. Panel (**c**) is the grayscale ultrasound image of the joint with the needle trajectory. Panel (**d**) provides a labeled anatomical reference featuring critical structures such as "ER" for extensor retinaculum, "T" for tendon, "J" for joint, "Ra" for radius, and "U" for ulna. It also elaborates on the needle trajectory and the precise target point for injection.

toms. Subsequently, a steroid injection may be administered to mitigate inflammation and reduce the likelihood of recurrence. This combined approach has demonstrated superior outcomes, especially in smaller cysts, as it can yield symptomatic relief without necessitating more invasive surgical options. Furthermore, the precision afforded by ultrasound guidance minimizes the risk of complications and promotes a higher success rate in cyst resolution [4].

A 16–18-gauge, 1.5-in. needle is commonly utilized, with 0.5 mL of local anesthetic and 0.5 mL of injectable corticosteroid. This sterile technique requires inserting the needle in-plane or out-of-plane relative to the transducer and targeting the underlying joint space (Fig. 4.3).

4.2.2 Tendons

4.2.2.1 Anatomy

4.2.2.2 Scan (Video 4.3)

Patient position: The patient should be sitting with their hand placed palm down, with their thumb held horizontally.

Probe position: To visualize the extensor tendons, position the ultrasound probe over the styloid process of the radius (Fig. 4.2a, Line 1) in the transverse plane to identify a bony prominence in the ultrasound scan.

Scanning: This bony prominence is Lister's tubercle (Fig. 4.2d). Here, the compartments of the extensor tendons can be visualized on both sides

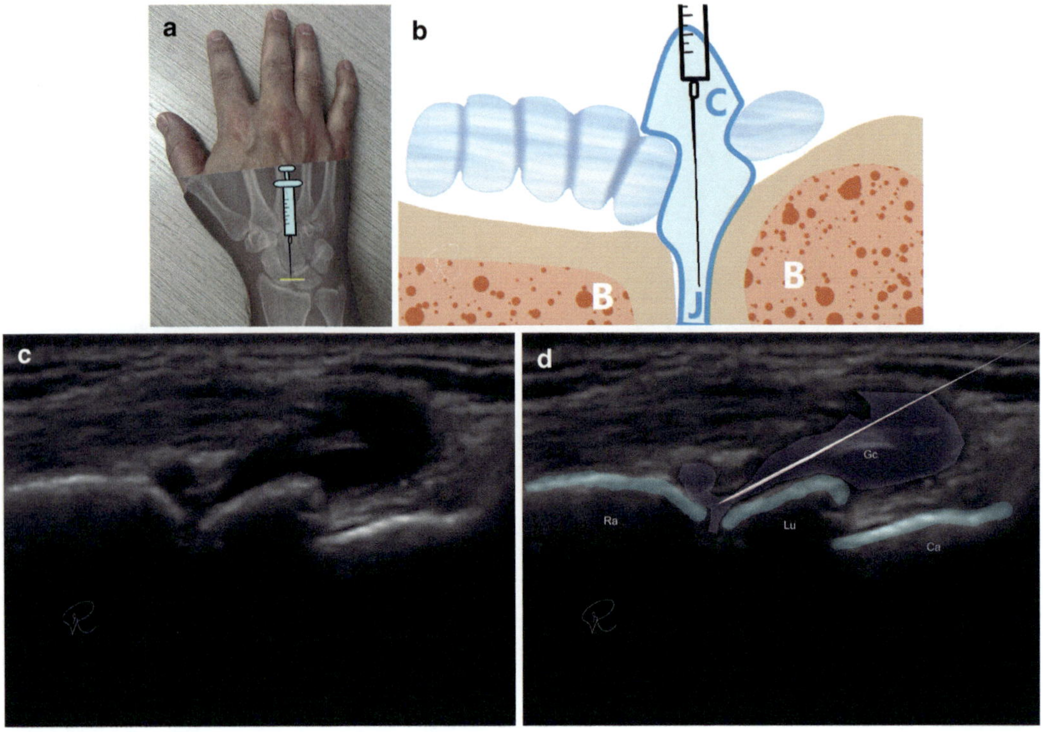

Fig. 4.3 Ganglion cyst injection. This composite image is comprised of four panels that illustrate the techniques for injecting a wrist joint and a ganglion cyst. Panel (**a**) presents a human hand with an overlaid X-ray image, demonstrating the position of a syringe for precise ganglion cyst aspiration and injection. Panel (**b**) features a diagram detailing the anatomical structures of the wrist joint, with labels "B," "C," and "J" representing bones, joints, and cyst with a multi-angle schematic structure of the ganglion cyst. Panel (**c**) showcases an ultrasound image of the wrist, emphasizing key joint structures to guide the procedure. Panel (**d**) provides the same ultrasound view with labeled anatomical landmarks, including "Ra" for radius, "Lu" for lunate, "Gc" for ganglion cyst, and "Ca" for capitate, offering a comprehensive understanding of the cyst ultrasound anatomy and injection. (© Reza Roghani 2024. All Rights Reserved)

of the tubercle. Radial to the tubercle is the second compartment containing the extensor carpi radialis longus and extensor carpi radialis brevis tendons. Further radial to the second compartment is the first compartment, with the abductor pollicis longus positioned volar to the extensor pollicis brevis tendon. Moving the probe to the ulnar side of the hand allows for visualization of the subsequent compartments. Once Lister's tubercle has been encountered, the extensor pollicis longus of the third compartment can be found on the ulnar side of it. As the probe is moved toward the ulna, the fourth compartment containing the extensor indicis proprius and extensor digitorum communis appears. Then, in the fifth compartment, extensor digiti minimi above the radio-ulnar joint can be seen. Finally, in the sixth compartment, the extensor carpi ulnaris tendons above the ulnar bone can be identified (Fig. 4.4).

4.2.2.3 Injection

Position the probe in the transverse plane to locate the first compartment, as described in the scanning section above. Insert the needle in plane until its tip reaches beneath the tendon sheath. Next, inject the steroid and anesthetic mixture beneath the sheath and above the tendon. A 25–30-gauge, 1.5-in. needle is typically used to administer 1 mL of a local anesthetic mixed with 0.5–1 mL of an injectable corticosteroid (Fig. 4.5).

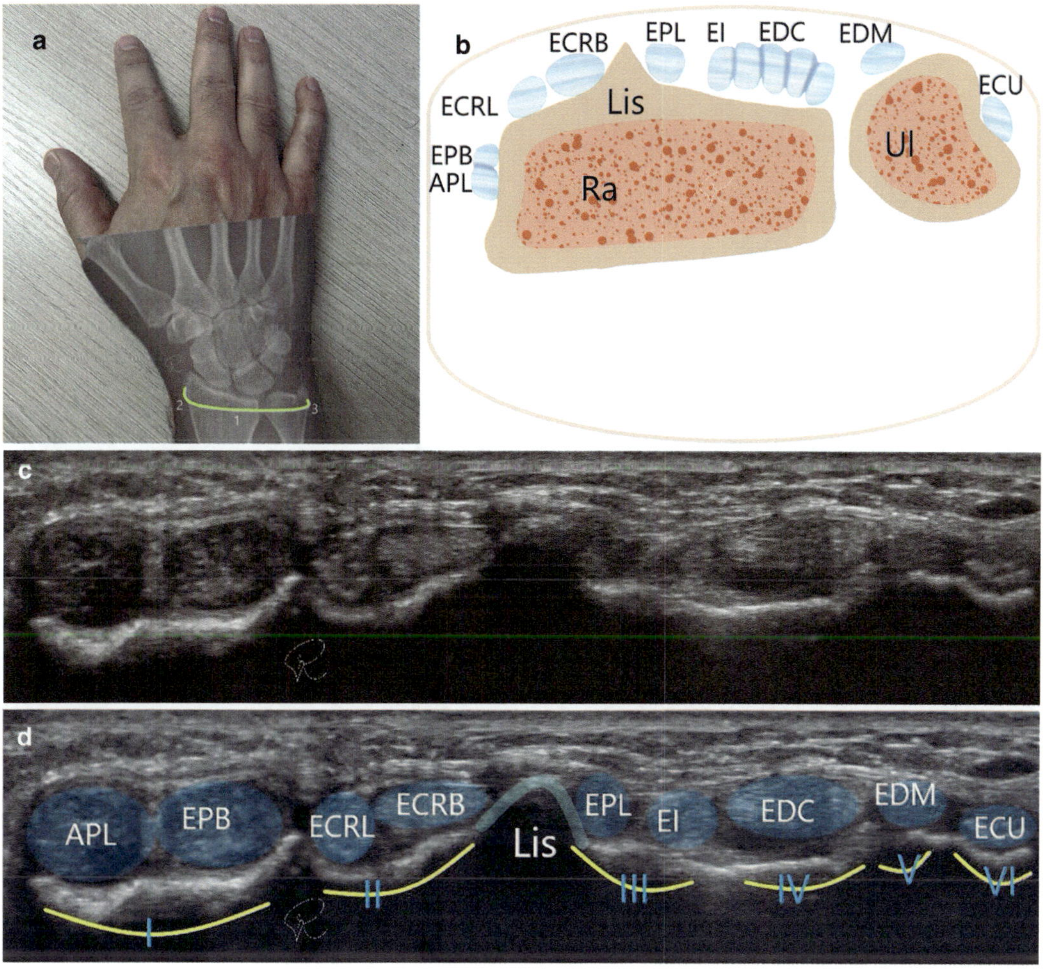

Fig. 4.4 Wrist Extensor tendons. The image comprises four panels that illustrate the anatomy and ultrasound imaging of the wrist extensor tendons. Panel (**a**) features a human hand with an overlay of the wrist bones and a green line indicating three key positions: (1) the initial probe placement for locating Lister's tubercle, (2) the position for Compartment I, and (3) the position for Compartment VI. Panel (**b**) presents a detailed anatomical diagram that labels the wrist bones and extensor tendons, including the radius (Ra), ulna (Ul), and a variety of tendons. Panel (**c**) displays a panoramic ultrasound image of the dorsal wrist, featuring multiple extensor tendons. Finally, Panel (**d**) offers an annotated ultrasound scan that highlights essential structures such as the extensor tendons and bones. The labeled structures include the abductor pollicis longus (APL), extensor pollicis brevis (EPB), extensor carpi radialis longus (ECRL), extensor carpi radialis brevis (ECRB), extensor pollicis longus (EPL), extensor indicis (EI), extensor digitorum communis (EDC), extensor digiti minimi (EDM), and extensor carpi ulnaris (ECU), with Lister's tubercle (Lis) marked as a crucial anatomical reference. Each of the six extensor compartments is systematically represented: Compartment I (APL, EPB), Compartment II (ECRL, ECRB), Compartment III (EPL), Compartment IV (EI, EDC), Compartment V (EDM), and Compartment VI (ECU). (© Reza Roghani 2024. All Rights Reserved)

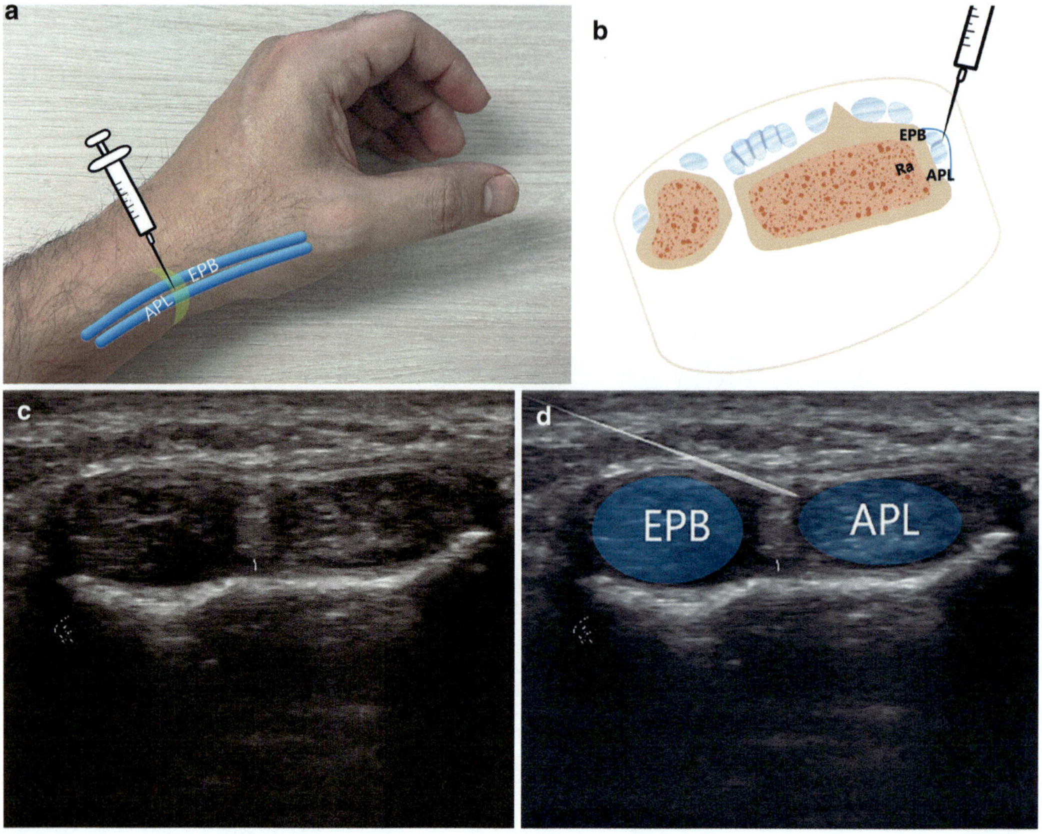

Fig. 4.5 De Quervain's tenosynovitis injection. The image consists of four panels illustrating the injection technique for de Quervain's tenosynovitis at the wrist, focusing on the needle trajectory. Panel (**a**) presents a hand with a syringe targeting the abductor pollicis longus (APL) and extensor pollicis brevis (EPB) tendons, showing the needle trajectory toward the first compartment. Panel (**b**) is a cross-sectional anatomical diagram of the wrist, indicating the injection site near the APL and EPB, along with the needle trajectory for accurate delivery of the injectate. Panels (**c**) and (**d**) display ultrasound images of the first extensor compartment of the wrist, with panel (**d**) explicitly highlighting the EPB and APL tendons, as well as the needle trajectory toward the target structures for de Quervain's tenosynovitis injection.

4.3 Volar

4.3.1 Carpal Tunnel

4.3.1.1 Anatomy

The carpal tunnel is located on the volar side of the wrist—the carpal bones and the transverse carpal ligament form it. The carpal bones, which comprise the floor and sides of the carpal tunnel, are organized into two rows. The proximal row contains the scaphoid, lunate, and triquetrum, while the distal row consists of the trapezium, trapezoid, capitate, and hamate. The roof of the carpal tunnel is constructed from the transverse carpal ligament, a robust band of fibrous tissue that spans the wrist, connecting the hook of the hamate and the pisiform bone to the tubercle of the scaphoid and the trapezium. This ligament provides support to the tendons and median nerve traversing the tunnel. The median nerve, a pivotal structure within the carpal tunnel, innervates the thumb, index, middle, and parts of the ring fingers, handling both sensory and motor functions. Nine flexor tendons pass through the carpal tunnel: four from the Flexor Digitorum Superficialis (FDS), which facilitate the bending of the middle joints of the fingers, and four from the Flexor Digitorum Profundus (FDP), which are responsible for flexing the distal joints. Additionally, the Flexor Pollicis Longus (FPL) tendon enables thumb flexion. Regarding anatomical relationships, the median nerve is centrally positioned within the carpal tunnel, flanked by the flexor tendons on either side. Carpal tunnel syndrome (CTS) occurs when the median nerve is irritated or compressed, leading to symptoms such as numbness, tingling, pain, and weakness. Contributing factors may include repetitive hand motions, wrist injuries, or anatomical variations. Diagnosis typically involves clinical examinations, nerve conduction studies, and imaging methods such as ultrasound or MRI for a detailed assessment. Ultrasound is a valuable diagnostic tool for evaluating the carpal tunnel. It allows for visualizing soft tissue structures, including tendons, ligaments, and the median nerve. It can also identify bone cortical fractures, displacements, and volar ganglion cysts. This imaging technique aids in diagnosing conditions such as carpal tunnel syndrome (CTS), assess the extent of nerve compression, and guide interventions like corticosteroid injections or surgical planning. [7].

4.3.1.2 Scan (Video 4.4)

Patient position: For a carpal tunnel ultrasound examination, the patient should be positioned with their forearm resting on a table or surface, the elbow flexed at approximately 90°, and the wrist in a neutral position, neither flexed nor extended. The hand should be relaxed with the palm facing up (supinated) to allow clear access to the carpal tunnel area. The sonographer may gently guide the wrist into slight extension to improve visualization of the carpal tunnel structures, including the median nerve, flexor tendons, and transverse carpal ligament.

Probe position: The ultrasound probe should initially be placed transversely on the volar surface of the wrist, proximal to the distal wrist crease (Fig. 4.6a, line 1).

Scanning: The scaphoid bone is located laterally, and the pisiform will be visualized medially, with the flexor retinaculum between them. Below the flexor retinaculum, the flexor digitorum superficialis (FDS) and flexor digitorum profundus (FDP) tendons can be seen (Fig. 4.6c, d). Asking the patient to flex and extend the thumb helps enhance the image of the flexor pollicis longus (FPL) tendon. The FPL tendon is located next to and deeper than the median nerve, which exhibits a honeycomb pattern and is positioned almost at the center of the tunnel below the flexor retinaculum (Fig. 4.6). Ultrasound is commonly used to diagnose carpal tunnel syndrome (CTS) and its severity [8].

The diagnostic examination for carpal tunnel syndrome (CTS) involves scanning across four distinct planes: one longitudinal and three transverse sections. The inlet area is located between the pisiform and scaphoid bones (Fig. 4.6a, Line 1). The mid-canal area is situated midway between the inlet and outlet (Fig. 4.6a, Line 2). The outlet area is positioned just beneath the distal rim of the flexor retinaculum, at the level of the hook of the hamate (Fig. 4.6a, Line 3). In the longitudinal plane, the ultrasound probe is aligned along the midline between the radius and ulna, directly centered on the median nerve (Fig. 4.6a, Line 4).

The diagnostic criteria for carpal tunnel syndrome (CTS) via ultrasound encompass several specific parameters. One of the primary indicators is the median nerve's cross-sectional area (CSA) at the carpal tunnel inlet, with values exceeding 9 mm^2 commonly suggestive of CTS. Observations may also reveal a flattening or "bowing" of the median nerve at the carpal tunnel inlet, indicative of heightened intratunnel pressure. Moreover, impaired gliding motion of the median nerve during wrist flexion and extension can be a notable finding. Decreased echogenicity of the median nerve typically points to potential inflammation or edema surrounding the nerve. Alterations in the thickness of the flexor retinaculum may exacerbate median nerve compression, and the presence of perineural edema—fluid accumulation around the median nerve—further substantiate the possibility of nerve compression. According to an established reference values, the average CSA at the wrist inlet is generally less than 9 mm^2. Classification of CTS severity is as follows: a CSA between 9 and 12 mm^2 indicates mild CTS, while moderate CTS correlates with a CSA from 12 to 17 mm^2, and severe CTS is char-

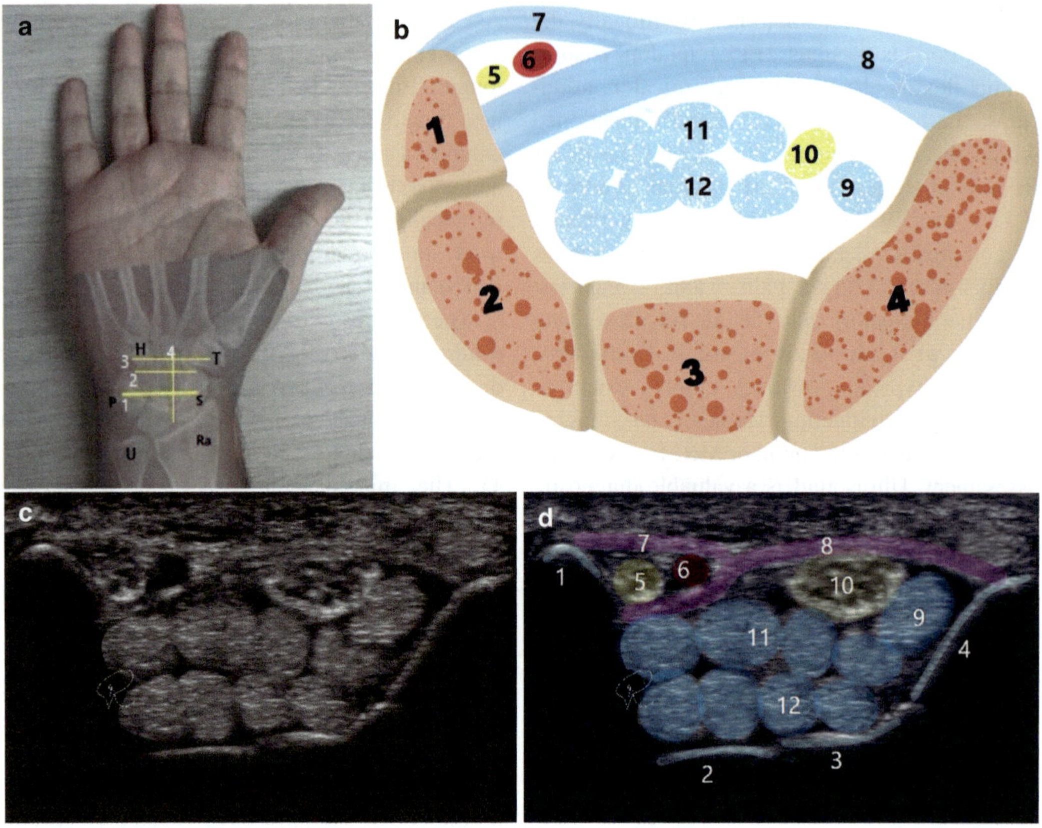

Fig. 4.6 Carpal tunnel inlet. A composite image consisting of four panels illustrating carpal tunnel anatomy and ultrasound imaging. Panel (**a**) displays a human hand with an overlay of wrist bones, labeled 'P' (Pisiform), 'S' (Scaphoid), and 'Ra' (Radius), along with a yellow line indicating the initial position of the ultrasound probe. Panel (**b**) features a detailed diagram of wrist anatomy, with sections numbered 1 to 12, as follows: (1) Pisiform bone, (2) Triquetrum, (3) Lunate, (4) Scaphoid, (5) Ulnar nerve, (6) Ulnar artery, (7 and 8) Flexor retinaculum, (9) Flexor pollicis longus, (10) Median nerve, (11) Flexor digitorum superficialis, (12) Flexor retinaculum profundus. Panel (**c**) presents a high-resolution ultrasound image of the carpal tunnel. Panel (**d**) shows the same ultrasound image with color-coding, where numbered sections correspond to the diagram in panel (b) for clear anatomical comparison.

acterized by a CSA that exceeds 17 mm². It is essential to recognize that these reference values may fluctuate in older populations due to age-related changes in nerve morphology, and geographic phenotypic variations may also impact nerve measurements. Ultimately, these ultrasound findings, when interpreted alongside clinical symptoms and supplementary diagnostic evaluations, are crucial for confirming the diagnosis and determining the severity of CTS [9].

4.3.1.3 Injection (Video 4.5)

Ultrasound-guided corticosteroid injection serves as a valuable intervention for patients diagnosed with mild to moderate carpal tunnel syndrome (CTS), particularly those who continue to experience persistent symptoms despite undergoing conservative management strategies. Empirical evidence demonstrates that corticosteroid injections can lead to significant symptom improvement within a short-term framework, typically spanning four to twelve weeks. Many patients report a significant decrease in pain and alleviation of tingling and nocturnal symptoms. A substantial number of patients sustain this symptom relief over the intermediate term, which ranges from three to six months. However, it is not uncommon for some individuals to require repeat injections should their symptoms recur. Ultrasound guidance in the injection process markedly enhances the precision of medication delivery around the median nerve and minimizes the likelihood of complications associated with the procedure. Compared to traditional landmark-guided methods, ultrasound-guided techniques yield higher rates of symptom relief, accompanied by a reduction in side effects and a lower risk of intraneural injection. While it is critical to note that corticosteroid injection does not serve as a definitive cure for CTS, it plays a pivotal role in symptom management. This intervention provides temporary relief and can postpone or lessen the need for surgical intervention in appropriately selected patients [9,10,11].

Patient Position: For a carpal tunnel syndrome (CTS) injection, the patient is typically positioned as follows: The most common setup involves the patient either sitting or lying supine, with their arm resting on an examination table or armrest. The wrist should be placed in slight dorsiflexion (approximately 20–30 degrees), with the palm facing upward. It's often beneficial to support the wrist with a rolled towel or small cushion to optimize access to the carpal tunnel.

Probe Position: The ultrasound probe is positioned transversely over the carpal tunnel inlet to visualize the flexor retinaculum, the cross-section of the median nerve, the flexor tendons, and surrounding vascular structures before needle insertion. Ensuring that the patient is relaxed and minimizing hand movement is essential for a successful injection, regardless of the chosen position.

Scanning and injection: The ulnar-side ultrasound-guided approach for injecting corticosteroids in carpal tunnel syndrome (CTS) offers a precise and minimally invasive method for alleviating median nerve compression. Using a 22–25-gauge needle, the injection is performed from the ulnar side, aligned in-plane with the ultrasound probe, and carefully advanced toward the median nerve. (Fig. 4.7a), Attention to the needle's trajectory is crucial to avoid the ulnar artery and nerve. Hydrodissection is achieved by injecting a solution that typically consists of 1 mL of local anesthetic (such as 2% lidocaine) and 2 mL of corticosteroid (such as triamcinolone). To enhance anti-inflammatory effects and promote symptom relief, we recommend using 2 cc of corticosteroid. The injectate is precisely deposited just above and around the median nerve, effectively creating additional space between the nerve and surrounding structures while reducing inflammation. (Fig. 4.7c, d). The combination of hydrodissection and flexor retinaculum fenestration has shown to provide better outcomes in symptom relief and functional recovery compared to traditional injection methods, making it a promising treatment option for patients with carpal tunnel syndrome (CTS)[10,11]. We recommend that the real-time ultrasound-guided procedure follows a structured four-step approach to ensure precision and optimal therapeutic results. The first step is identifying the mid-canal transverse line (Fig. 4.7a) to mark the medial needle insertion point. In the second step, the needle is advanced toward the lower pole of the median nerve, carefully avoiding the ulnar artery, ulnar nerve, and median nerve, while injecting the first one-third of the injectate. The third step involves repositioning the needle over the upper pole of the median nerve to inject the second one-third. Finally, in the fourth step, the needle is repositioned at the flexor retinaculum to administer the remaining injectate(Fig. 4.7c, d) [9–11].

Careful attention is necessary to prevent any accidental injury to nearby arteries. Color flow (CF) Doppler feature is employed to minimize the risk of injury to nearby vascular structures and to ensure proper visualization of the injected fluid (Fig. 4.7).

4.3.2 Guyon's Canal

4.3.2.1 Anatomy

Guyon's canal, also referred to as the ulnar tunnel, is an anatomical structure located on the palmar side of the wrist. It serves as a conduit for the ulnar nerve and artery as they travel into the hand. This canal is situated between the pisiform bone and the hook of the hamate, creating a fibro-osseous tunnel. The roof is constructed from the palmar carpal ligament, which is a continuation of the flexor retinaculum, while the floor consists

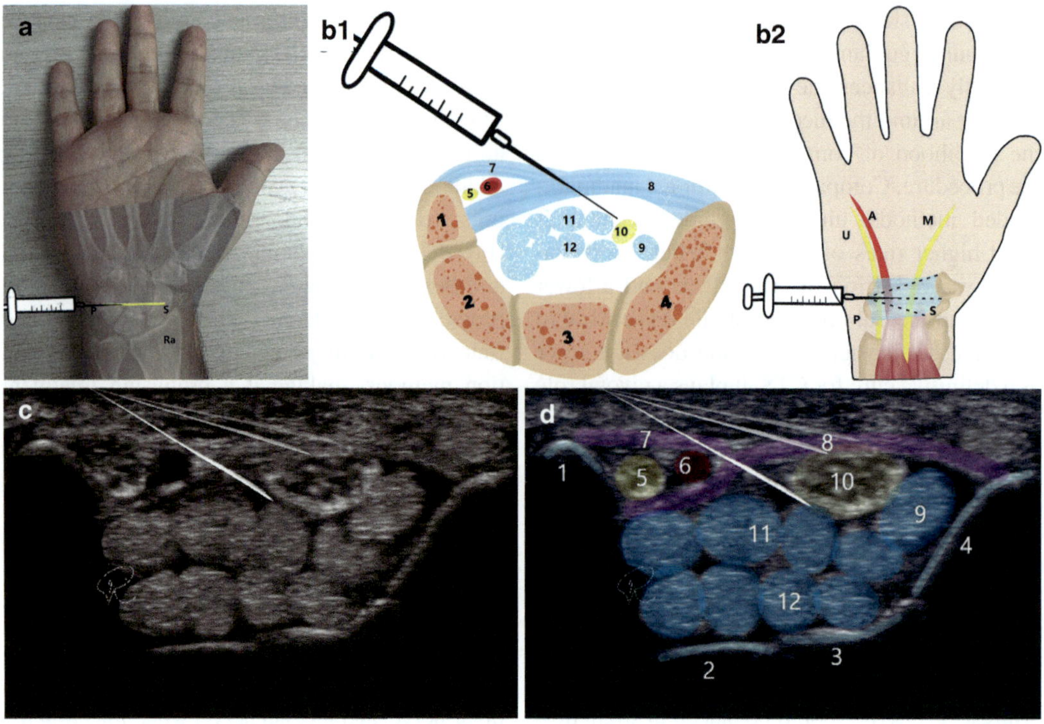

Fig. 4.7 Carpal tunnel injection. This image serves as a comprehensive guide to ultrasound-guided carpal tunnel injection, organized across four distinct panels. Panel (**a**) depicts a hand overlaid with a transparent representation of wrist anatomy, highlighting the position of the ultrasound probe and the needle insertion site. Panels (**b1** and **b2**) provide a cross-sectional schematic of the wrist, detailing key anatomical structures with numbered labels. A syringe is illustrated to indicate the precise entry point and trajectory of the injection needle within the carpal tunnel. Panel (**c**) showcases an actual ultrasound image of the carpal tunnel, revealing the internal structures and the needle's three trajectories as it approaches the lower and upper poles of the median nerve and the flexor retinaculum. Finally, panel (**d**) enhances the ultrasound image with color overlays and corresponding numbered labels for clear anatomical identification. The labeled structures include (1) the pisiform bone (P), (2) the triquetrum, (3) the lunate, (4) the scaphoid (S), (5) the ulnar nerve (U), (6) the ulnar artery (A), (7 and 8) the flexor retinaculum, (9) the flexor pollicis longus, (10) the median nerve (M), (11) the flexor digitorum superficialis, and (12) the deep flexor retinaculum. (© Reza Roghani 2024. All Rights Reserved)

of the transverse carpal ligament and the pisohamate ligament. Medially, it is bordered by the pisiform bone, and laterally by the hook of the hamate. Within the canal, the ulnar nerve divides into two branches: the superficial sensory branch, which supplies sensation to the ulnar aspect of the hand, and the deep motor branch, responsible for innervating the intrinsic muscles of the hand. Guyon's Canal Syndrome arises from the entrapment of the ulnar nerve at the wrist. In contrast to cubital tunnel syndrome, this condition does not affect sensation on the dorsal hand, as the dorsal cutaneous branch of the ulnar nerve exits proximal to the canal. The syndrome is commonly associated with repetitive trauma, particularly in individuals who engage in activities that involve sustained wrist compression, such as cyclists and weightlifters. Other contributing factors include the presence of ganglion cysts, which are the prevalent space-occupying lesions in the canal, fractures of the hamate or pisiform that may narrow the tunnel, ulnar artery thrombosis that compresses the nerve, and in rare cases, tumors or lipomas. Diagnosis of Guyon's Canal Syndrome hinges on clinical examination, which may uncover sensory deficits, muscle weakness, Froment's sign, and Wartenberg's sign, characterized by the sustained abduction of the little finger. Electromyography (EMG) and nerve conduction studies (NCS) are instrumental in confirming the presence and extent of ulnar nerve compression. Additionally, imaging modalities such as ultrasound or MRI are valuable in identifying compressive lesions, fractures, or vascular anomalies. Management strategies for Guyon's Canal Syndrome depend on the severity of the condition. Conservative approaches include modification of activities to minimize prolonged wrist compression, the application of wrist splints in a neutral position, and the administration of anti-inflammatory medications or ultrasound guided corticosteroid injections. These measures aim to alleviate symptoms and prevent further nerve damage [12].

4.3.2.2 Scan (Video 4.6)

Patient position: The patient should sit on the examination table with their hand placed on their thigh in a supinated position. Alternatively, the individual rests supine on a table with the forearm supinated and positioned on an armrest.

Probe position: The ultrasound probe should initially be placed transversely on the volar surface of the wrist, proximal to the distal wrist crease.

Scanning: To begin scanning the ulnar nerve in Guyon's canal, position the ultrasound probe transversely at the proximal wrist, using the pisiform bone as a key landmark. From there, move the probe distally to scan the entire canal, tracing the ulnar nerve as it courses between the pisiform bone and the hook of the hamate. The ulnar nerve appears as a hyperechoic, honeycomb-like structure, consisting of multiple small fascicles surrounded by a hypoechoic perineurium. The ulnar artery, identifiable by its characteristic pulsation on Doppler imaging, lies adjacent to the nerve. As you advance the probe distally, you can visualize the bifurcation of the ulnar nerve into its superficial sensory and deep motor branches. The deep motor branch moves radially and dorsally toward the intrinsic muscles of the hand, while the superficial branch continues along the palm to provide sensory innervation. It is crucial to identify potential compressive structures, such as ganglion cysts, fibrotic bands, or vascular anomalies, during the scanning process. Additionally, performing a dynamic ultrasound assessment, including wrist flexion and extension, can help evaluate nerve mobility and detect any positional compression (Fig. 4.8).

4.3.2.3 Injection (Video 4.7)

Guyon's canal syndrome frequently coexists with carpal tunnel syndrome (CTS), and treatment for CTS often alleviates symptoms. However, in cases where Guyon canal syndrome presents as a standalone issue, ultrasound-guided injections can provide valuable assistance and relief. The standard ulnar nerve block or Guyon's canal injection approach is a short-axis, in-plane ulnar-side approach. The positioning is like the one described above, except lying down is preferred. The equipment required for performing injections in cases of Guyon Canal syndrome includes a needle ranging from 23 to 25 gauge and a nerve block injectate consisting of 1 mL of local anesthetic, optionally complemented by 1 mL of injectable corticosteroids (Fig. 4.9).

4.4 Hand

4.4.1 Thenar

4.4.1.1 Anatomy

The cross-sectional anatomy of the thenar prominence reveals a complex arrangement of muscles, nerves, tendons, and vascular structures vital for thumb movement and function. Superficially, the skin and subcutaneous tissue envelop the thenar eminence, followed by the palmar fascia, which provides structural support. Beneath this fascia lie the three primary thenar muscles: the abductor pollicis brevis, flexor pollicis brevis, and opponens pollicis. These muscles originate from the flexor retinaculum and adjacent carpal bones, creating a distinct compartment within the hand. The opponens pollicis, the deepest of the three muscles, attaches to the first metacarpal, while the abductor pollicis brevis and flexor pollicis brevis are situated more superficially. Deep to the thenar muscles, the adductor pollicis muscle, composed of transverse and oblique heads, is located medially and contributes to thumb adduction. This muscle is innervated by the ulnar nerve

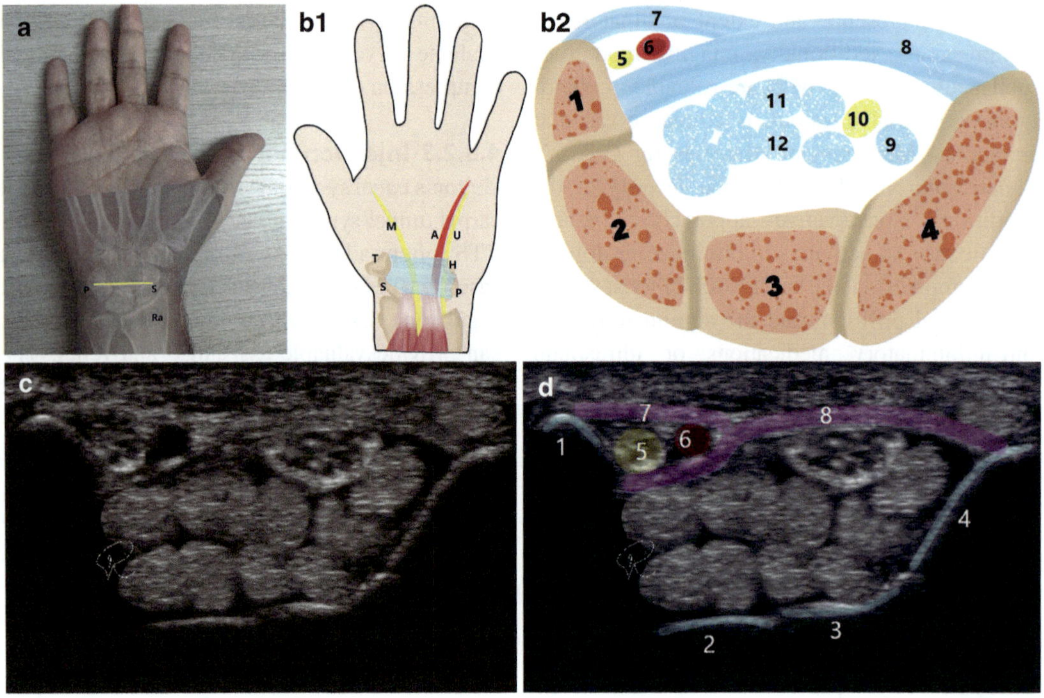

Fig. 4.8 Guyon's canal. This composite image offers anatomical and ultrasound perspectives of the wrist, delivering a comprehensive overview of the carpal tunnel and Guyon's canal. Panel (**a**) showcases a human hand with an overlay of wrist bones, emphasizing key structures labeled "P" for pisiform, "Ra" for the radius, "S" for scaphoid and a yellow line indicating the probe placement. Panel (**b1**) features a hand diagram with detailed anatomical labels, while panel (**b2**) presents a cross-sectional view of the wrist, highlighting structures 1 through 12, including bones, nerves, and tendons. Panel (**c**) displays an ultrasound image that captures the internal anatomy of the wrist, featuring the carpal tunnel and Guyon's canal. In panel (**d**), this ultrasound image is enhanced with colored overlays and numbered labels for greater clarity. The labeled structures include (1) the pisiform bone, (2) the triquetrum, (3) the lunate, (4) the scaphoid, (5) the ulnar nerve, (6) the ulnar artery, (7 and 8) the flexor retinaculum, (9) the flexor pollicis longus, (10) the median nerve, (11) the flexor digitorum superficialis, and (12) the flexor digitorum profundus. The trapezium (T), median nerve (M), hamate (H), scaphoid (S), pisiform (P), the ulnar nerve (U) and the ulnar artery (A) are also identified, providing a complete anatomical reference for clinical and diagnostic purposes. ()

and is positioned adjacent to the first dorsal interosseous muscle. Additionally, the tendons of the flexor pollicis longus traverse the thenar region, surrounded by synovial sheaths that minimize friction during thumb flexion. The interaction between these tendons and the thenar muscles enables the precise movements required for grasping and manipulating objects [2].

4.4.1.2 Scanning

Patient position: The patient is supine on the examination table, with the hand supinated on the armrest.

Probe position: The ultrasound probe is positioned in a transverse plane over the thenar prominence (Fig. 4.10 a).

Scanning: To ensure optimal imaging, adjust the probe tilt so that its plane is perpendicular to the area of interest, enhancing the visibility of the muscles and tendons in the thenar region while minimizing anisotropy. In this image, the first metacarpal bone is prominently displayed, generating a distinct hyperechoic (bright) echo deep within the scan. Surrounding the bone are the adjacent muscles—the opponens pollicis, abductor pollicis brevis, and flexor pollicis brevis

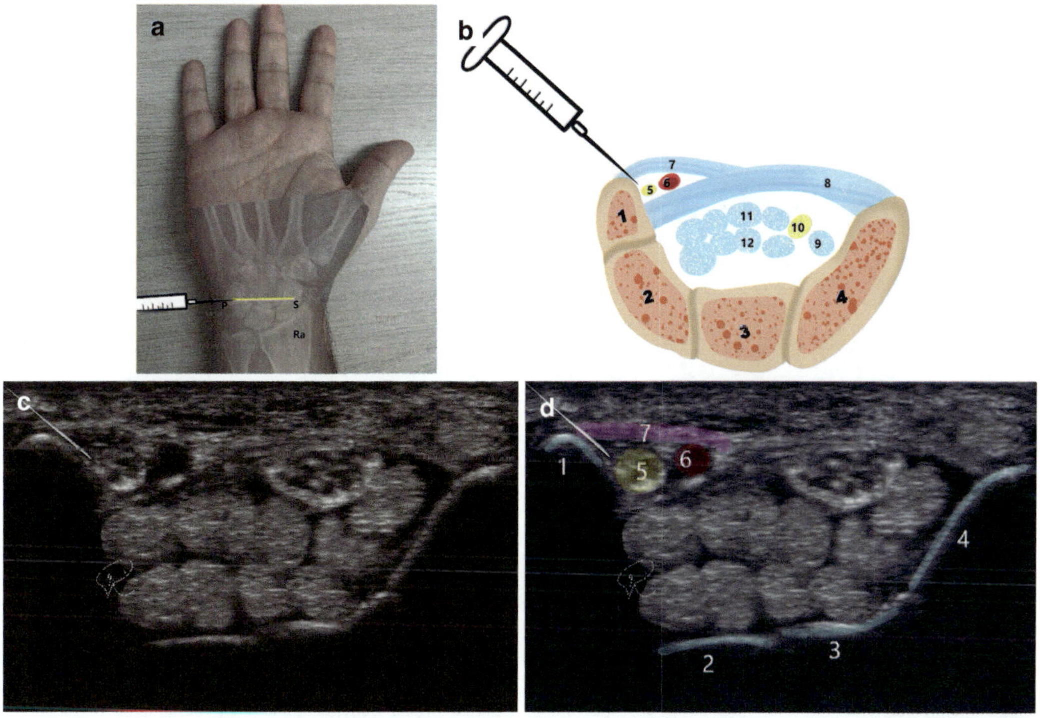

Fig. 4.9 Guyon's canal injection. A composite image that illustrates the anatomy of Guyon's canal and its injection techniques is divided into four distinct panels. Panel (**a**) depicts a human hand overlaid with wrist bones, detailing the positioning of the patient and probe, along with a syringe directed towards the wrist, demonstrating the needle insertion point and labeled "P" for pisiform, "Ra" for the radius, and "S" for scaphoid. Panel (**b**) features a cross-sectional diagram of the wrist with a syringe, highlighting numerous anatomical structures numbered 1 to 12. Panel (**c**) presents an ultrasound image of the wrist, showcasing the needle trajectory. Panel (**d**) offers the same ultrasound image color-coded with labeled anatomical structures numbered 1 to 7. The identified structures include (1) the pisiform bone, (2) the triquetrum, (3) the lunate, (4) the scaphoid, (5) the ulnar nerve, (6) the ulnar artery, (7 and 8) the flexor retinaculum, (9) the flexor pollicis longus, (10) the median nerve, (11) the flexor digitorum superficialis, and (12) the flexor digitorum profundus.

(FPB)—which are readily identifiable as hypoechoic (darker) areas. The flexor pollicis longus (FPL) tendon, responsible for thumb flexion, is also visible as a well-defined, hyperechoic structure within its synovial sheath. This imaging technique allows for a thorough assessment of these muscles and tendons, providing critical insights for diagnosing conditions such as tendinopathy, muscle imbalances, or nerve compression in the hand. (Fig. 4.10).

4.4.2 Hypothenar

4.4.2.1 Anatomy

The hypothenar region of the hand is a muscular prominence located on the ulnar side of the palm, playing a crucial role in the movements of the little finger. It consists of four muscles: the abductor digiti minimi, which facilitates the abduction of the little finger; the flexor digiti minimi brevis, which flexes the proximal phalanx; the opponens digiti minimi, which enables

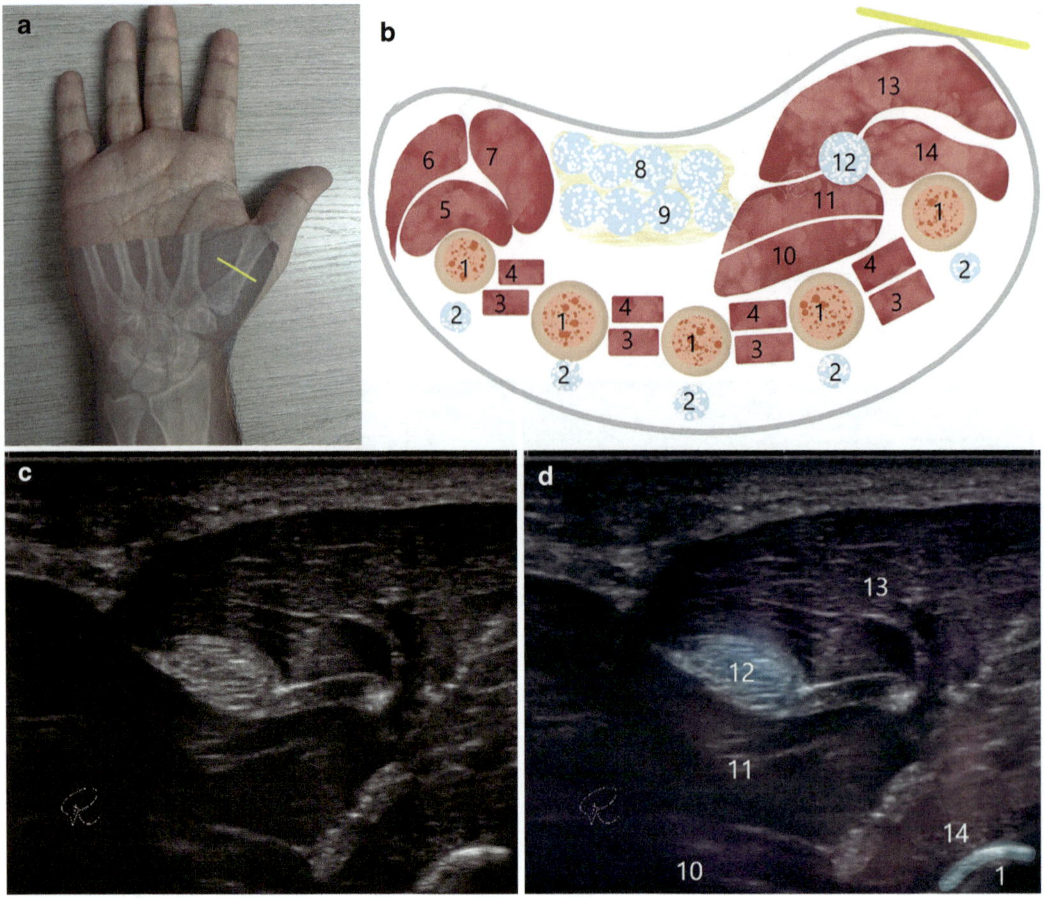

Fig. 4.10 Thenar eminence scan. The image consists of four panels, each providing a detailed view of the anatomical and ultrasound structures of the thenar area. Panel (**a**) presents a human hand overlaid with an X-ray image, highlighting the wrist and hand bones and a yellow line indicating the probe position. Panel (**b**) offers a diagrammatic cross-section of the hand, labeling key anatomical structures with corresponding numbers. Panels (**c**) and (**d**) display ultrasound images of the thenar area, with panel (**d**) color-coded and annotated with numbers 1 and 10 through 14. The structures labeled are: (1) Metacarpal bone, (2) Extensor tendon, (3) Dorsal interosseous muscle, (4) Palmar interosseous muscle, (5) Opponens digiti minimi, (6) Abductor digiti minimi, (7) Flexor digiti minimi, (8) Flexor digitorum superficialis tendons, (9) Flexor digitorum profundus tendons, (10) Adductor pollicis brevis, (11) Flexor pollicis brevis, (12) Flexor pollicis longus tendon, (13) Abductor pollicis brevis, and (14) Opponens pollicis.

opposition by rotating the fifth metacarpal; and the palmaris brevis, a superficial muscle that tightens the skin of the hypothenar eminence. These muscles are primarily innervated by the deep branch of the ulnar nerve, while the superficial branch innervates the palmaris brevis, which also provides sensory input to the medial palm and little finger. The ulnar artery supplies blood to the hypothenar region via its deep palmar branch. Clinically, ulnar nerve compression at the wrist, such as in Guyon's canal syndrome, can result in weakness of the hypothenar muscles and sensory deficits in the ulnar distribution. Additionally, repetitive trauma to the ulnar artery in this area may lead to hypothenar hammer syndrome, causing ischemic issues in the digits [2].

4.4.2.2 Scanning

Patient position: The patient lies supine on the examination table, with their hand supinated.

Probe position: The ultrasound probe is positioned in a transverse plane over the hypothenar prominence (Fig. 4.11a).

Scanning: With this probe placement, the fifth metacarpal bone appears as a hyperechoic line in the deep portion of the image. Overlying and surrounding this bone is the opponens digiti minimi (ODM). The abductor digiti minimi is visible more superficially and medially, while the most superficial and slightly lateral structure is the flexor digiti minimi. Sliding the probe cephalad reveals the superficial palmaris brevis muscle, completing the ultrasound assessment of the hypothenar region (Fig. 4.11).

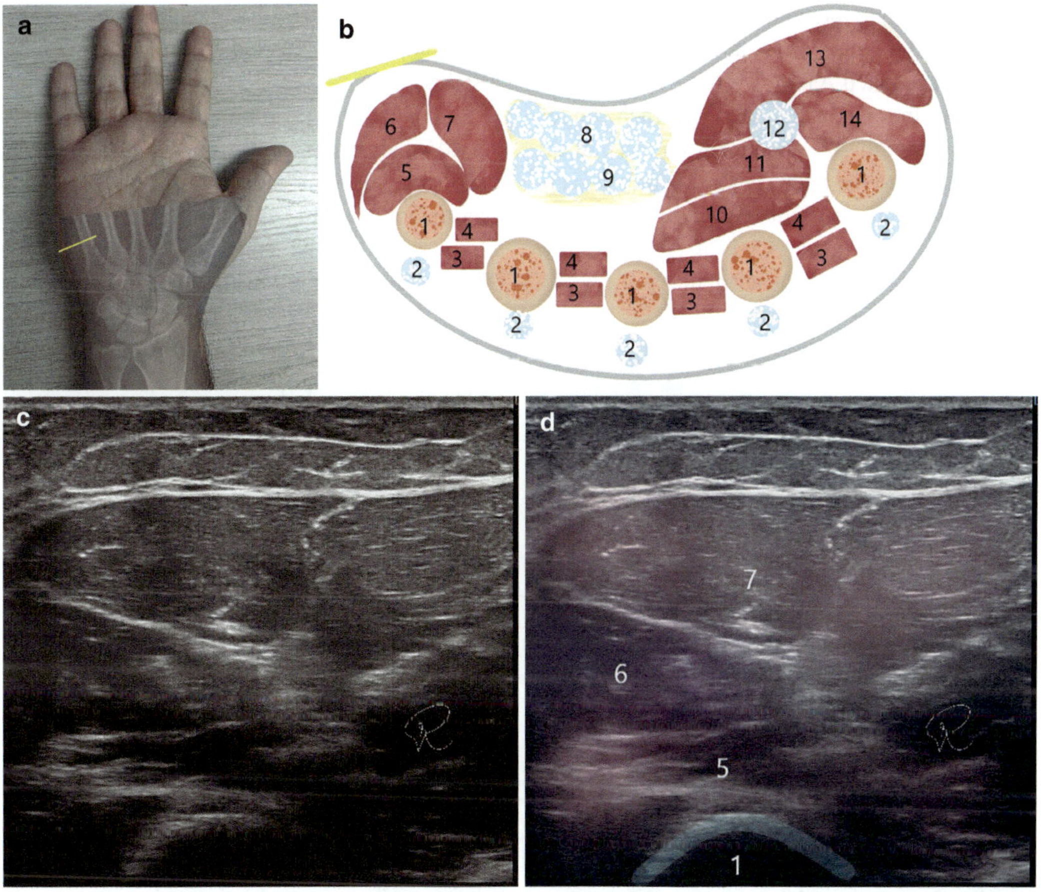

Fig. 4.11 Hypothenar muscles scan. The image consists of four panels, each providing a detailed view of the anatomical and ultrasound structures of the hypothenar area. Panel (**a**) presents an external view of the hand with a yellow line, indicating the probe position. Panel (**b**) is a detailed anatomical cross-section of the wrist, illustrating muscles, tendons, and nerves labeled with numbers for identification. Panels (**c**) and (**d**) display ultrasound images of the hypothenar region, with panel (**d**) featuring numbered annotations (1, 5, 6, and 7) corresponding to structures in the anatomical illustration. The labeled structures include (1) Metacarpal bone, (2) Extensor tendon, (3) Dorsal interosseous muscle, (4) Palmar interosseous muscle, (5) Opponens digiti minimi, (6) Abductor digiti minimi, (7) Flexor digiti minimi, (8) Flexor digitorum superficialis tendons, (9) Flexor digitorum profundus tendons, (10) Adductor pollicis brevis, (11) Flexor pollicis brevis, (12) Flexor pollicis longus tendon, (13) Abductor pollicis brevis, and (14) Opponens pollicis. (© Reza Roghani 2024. All Rights Reserved)

4.5 Palm

4.5.1 Flexor Tendon Pulley System

4.5.1.1 Anatomy

The flexor tendon pulley system comprises structures vital for finger and thumb flexion and extension, ensuring tendon alignment [13]. These structures include the annular pulleys, cruciform pulleys, and palmar aponeurosis. The annular pulleys, designated A1 to A5, form fibrous rings encircling the flexor tendons in each finger, except the thumb. A1, situated at the base of the finger closest to the palm, is particularly susceptible to inflammation-induced entrapment, leading to a trigger finger. A5 is located near the finger's distal portion. These annular pulleys prevent bowstringing of the tendons and maintain their alignment [2].

4.5.1.2 Scanning

Patient position: The patient should sit relaxed on the examination table with the hand being held supine.

Probe position: Position the ultrasound probe longitudinally over the metacarpophalangeal (MCP) joint to visualize the flexor tendon pulley system.

Scanning: This positioning allows for displaying a V-shaped joint in the middle of the screen, the distinct fibrillar pattern of the flexor tendon over the joint, and a hyperechoic cross-section of the pulley located superior to the tendon (Fig. 4.12). Dynamic scanning is beneficial in

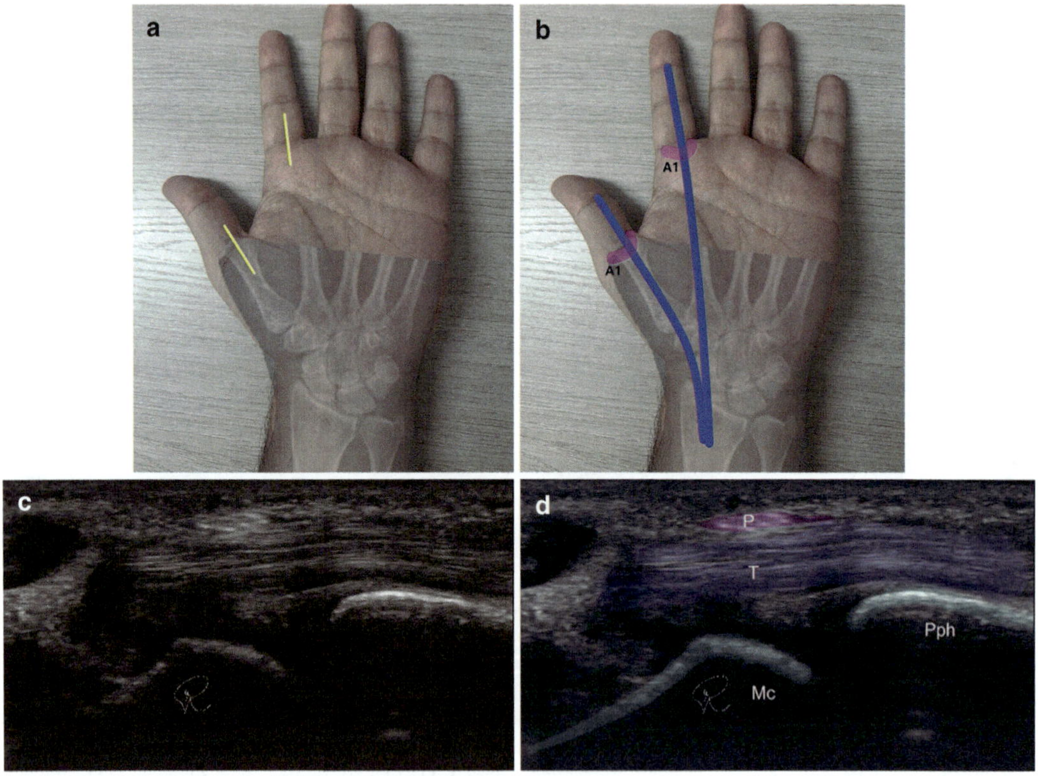

Fig. 4.12 A1 pulley scan. The image under discussion comprises four distinct panels that collectively illustrate the hand's anatomical and ultrasound perspectives, emphasizing the flexor pulley system's significance. Panel (**a**) presents a human hand accompanied by an overlaid X-ray image, which highlights the skeletal structure, alongside a yellow line that denotes the probe's position. Panel (**b**) mirrors this view, incorporating blue lines that depict the flexor tendons and violet arches labeled A1 that specify the locations of the pulleys. Panels (**c**) and (**d**) transition to ultrasound images, with panel (**c**) providing a long-axis view that clearly captures the pulley and its nearby anatomical structures. Meanwhile, panel (**d**) enhances the visual representation with a colored overlay, labeling essential anatomical components: A1 identifies the A1 pulley system, P represents the pulley itself, T corresponds to the tendons, Mc signifies the metacarpal bone, and Pph denotes the proximal phalanx.

this context as it enables the visualization of pathologies such as trigger fingers. During dynamic scanning, instruct the patient to flex their finger under ultrasound view, allowing the examiner to observe the gliding of the flexor tendon under the pulley and over the joint.

4.5.1.3 Injection (Video 4.8)

The flexor tendon pulley system can be targeted for intervention to treat stenosing tenosynovitis, commonly known as trigger finger. This condition is characterized by inflammation and subsequent tightening and narrowing of the A1 pulley. The procedure begins with scanning as described above, and the needle is approached in-plane from distal to proximal. The injection technique involves a 25–30-gauge needle to deliver 0.5 mL of local anesthetic and 0.5 mL of injectable corticosteroid into the sheath surrounding the tendon below the pulley (Fig. 4.13).

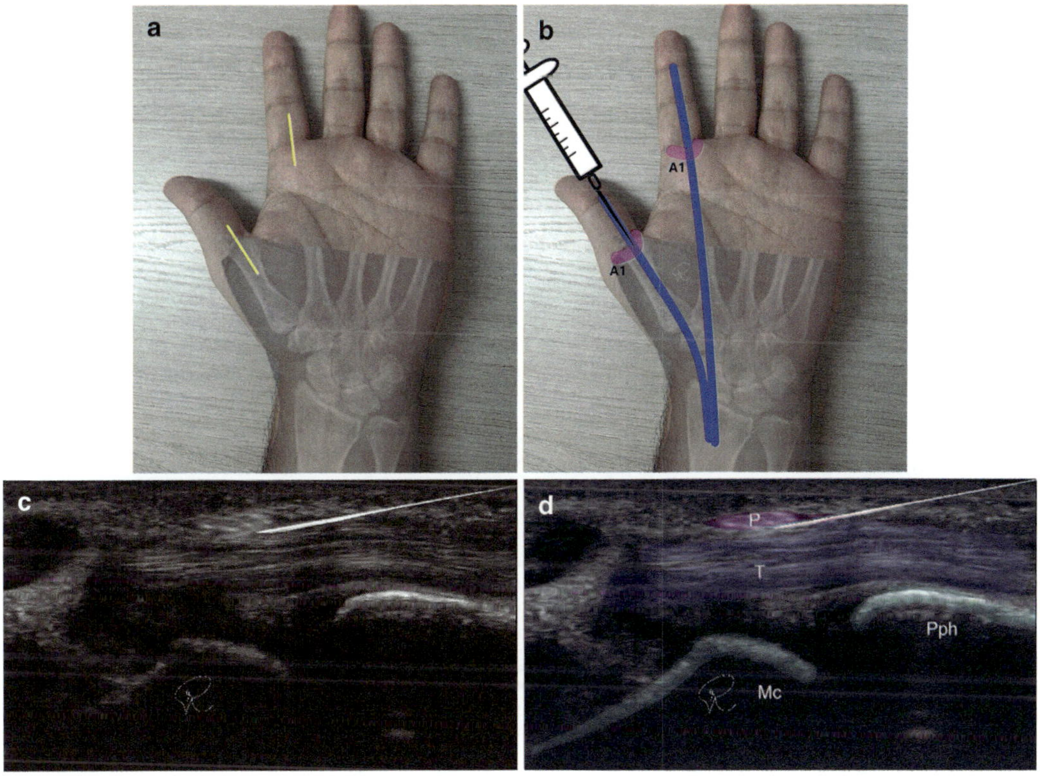

Fig. 4.13 A1 pulley injection. The image under discussion comprises four panels that collectively illustrate the hand's anatomical and ultrasound perspectives, emphasizing the flexor A1 pulley injection. Panel (**a**) presents a human hand accompanied by an overlaid X-ray image, which highlights the skeletal structure, alongside a yellow line that denotes the probe's position. Panel (**b**) mirrors this view, incorporating blue lines depicting the flexor tendons, violet arches labeled A1 that specify the locations of the pulleys and a syringe, and a needle demonstrating the needle insertion point and in-plane approach. Panels (**c**) and (**d**) transition to ultrasound images, with panel (**c**) providing a long-axis view that captures the pulley and the needle trajectory with the needle tip below the pully piercing the tendon sheet. Meanwhile, panel (**d**) enhances the visual representation with a colored overlay, labeling essential anatomical components: A1 identifies the A1 pulley system, P represents the pulley itself, T corresponds to the tendons, Mc signifies the metacarpal bone, and Pph denotes the proximal phalanx. (© Reza Roghani 2024. All Rights Reserved)

References

1. Eschweiler J, Li J, Quack V, Rath B, Baroncini A, Hildebrand F, Migliorini F. Anatomy, biomechanics, and loads of the wrist joint. Life. 2022;12(2):188. https://doi.org/10.3390/life12020188.
2. Hand and wrist anatomy and biomechanics | 9783132053410 | Thieme Webshop. Thieme USA. https://shop.thieme.com/Hand-and-Wrist-Anatomy-and-Biomechanics/9783132053410. Accessed 24 Mar 24 2024.
3. Gude W, Morelli V. Ganglion cysts of the wrist: pathophysiology, clinical picture, and management. Curr Rev Musculoskelet Med. 2008;1(3–4):205–11. https://doi.org/10.1007/s12178-008-9033-4.
4. Sinha MK, Mishra P, Mishra TS, Barman A. Aspiration and steroid injection in ganglion cysts: an ultrasound-guided response evaluation. J Clin Orthop Trauma. 2019;10(Suppl 1):S252–7. https://doi.org/10.1016/j.jcot.2019.03.004.
5. Maaref, K. (2014). Anatomy and biomechanics of the extensor tendons of the hand.
6. Fakoya AO, Tarzian M, Sabater EL, Burgos DM, Maldonado Marty GI. De Quervain's disease: a discourse on etiology, diagnosis, and treatment. Cureus. 2023;15(4):e38079. https://doi.org/10.7759/cureus.38079.
7. Presazzi A, Bortolotto C, Zacchino M, Madonia L, Draghi F. Carpal tunnel: normal anatomy, anatomical variants, and ultrasound technique. J Ultrasound. 2011;14(1):40–6. https://doi.org/10.1016/j.jus.2011.01.006.
8. Salman Roghani R, Hashemi SE, Holisaz MT, Gohari F, Delbari A, Lokk J. The diagnostic accuracy of median nerve ultrasonography in elderly patients with carpal tunnel syndrome: sensitivity and specificity assessment. Clin Interv Aging. 2018;13:1953–62. https://doi.org/10.2147/CIA.S177307.
9. Salman Roghani R, Holisaz MT, Sahami Norouzi AA, Delbari A, Gohari F, Lokk J, Boon AJ. Sensitivity of high-resolution ultrasonography in clinically diagnosed carpal tunnel syndrome patients with hand pain and normal nerve conduction studies. J Pain Res. 2018;11:1319–25. https://doi.org/10.2147/JPR.S164004.
10. Roghani RS, Kara S, Taheri MJ, Gohari F, Sadrneshin S, Thant HL, Diaz JJ, Lokk J. Intra-flexor retinaculum steroid injection in elderly patients with carpal tunnel syndrome: a randomized clinical trial. Interv Pain Med. 2022;1(3):100106. https://doi.org/10.1016/j.inpm.2022.100106.
11. Salman Roghani R, Holisaz MT, Tarkashvand M, Delbari A, Gohari F, Boon AJ, Lokk J. Different doses of steroid injection in elderly patients with carpal tunnel syndrome: a triple-blind, randomized, controlled trial. Clin Interv Aging. 2018;13:117–24. https://doi.org/10.2147/CIA.S151290.
12. Aleksenko D, Varacallo M. Guyon canal syndrome. In: StatPearls. StatPearls Publishing; 2024. http://www.ncbi.nlm.nih.gov/books/NBK431063/.
13. Zafonte B, Rendulic D, Szabo RM. Flexor pulley system: anatomy, injury, and management. J Hand Surg Am. 2014;39(12):2525–32; quiz 2533. https://doi.org/10.1016/j.jhsa.2014.06.005.

Hip

5

Reza Salman Roghani, Jorge E. Garcia-Negron, Natasha Mehta, Nicole Schneider, and Padideh Baran

5.1 Introduction

Neuromusculoskeletal (NMSK) ultrasound of the hip provides a real-time, high-resolution evaluation of essential anatomical structures, offering valuable insights for both diagnostic and interventional purposes. This imaging technique facilitates a thorough assessment of the hip joint and acetabulum, allowing for the detection of joint effusions, synovitis, and degenerative changes. The iliopsoas tendon can be analyzed for conditions such as tendinopathy, bursitis, or snapping hip syndrome. Additionally, the femoral nerve and artery serve as critical landmarks for regional anesthesia and interventional procedures. The lateral femoral cutaneous nerve, often associated with meralgia paresthetica, can also be visualized to identify potential entrapment or compression issues. Evaluating the greater trochanter and iliotibial band is essential in diagnosing greater trochanteric pain syndrome, which encompasses conditions like trochanteric bursitis and gluteal tendinopathy. Furthermore, the posterior aspects should include an assessment of the sciatic nerve and piriformis muscle, particularly concerning piriformis syndrome or sciatic neuropathy. Ultrasound also allows for precise injection into the sacroiliac joint, aiding in the treatment of inflammatory arthritis. With its real-time capabilities and high sensitivity, NMSK ultrasound of the hip is an invaluable tool for guiding clinical decision-making and interventions.

5.1.1 Hip Ultrasound Protocol

Anterior

- Axial Oblique:
  - Below the ASIS Level: Lateral femoral cutaneous nerve

Supplementary Information The online version contains supplementary material available at https://doi.org/10.1007/978-3-031-81037-4_5.

R. S. Roghani (✉)
Department of Physical Medicine and Rehabilitation, Larkin Community Hospital, Nova Southeastern University, Miami, FL, USA

J. E. Garcia-Negron
Department of Physical Medicine and Rehabilitation/Pain Medicine, West Palm Beach VA Healthcare System, U.S. Department of Veterans Affairs, West Palm Beach, FL, USA
e-mail: jorge.garcia-negron2@va.gov

N. Mehta
Division of Pain Medicine, Department of Anesthesia, Larkin Community Hospital, Nova Southeastern University, South Miami, FL, USA

N. Schneider
Dr. Kiran C. Patel College of Osteopathic Medicine, Nova Southeastern University, Fort Lauderdale, FL, USA

P. Baran
Imaging Department, University of Miami, Miami, FL, USA
e-mail: Pxb646@miami.edu

R. S. Roghani, J. J. Diaz (eds.), *Video Atlas of Neuromusculoskeletal Ultrasound*,
https://doi.org/10.1007/978-3-031-81037-4_5

- At the Level of the Hip Joint: Hip joint, femoral artery, vein, and nerve
- Sagittal Oblique:
  - Iliopsoas tendon injection
  - Hip joint injection

Lateral
- Short Axis at the Level of the Greater Trochanter: Trochanteric bursitis and gluteus medius and minimums tendinitis
- Long Axis: Long Axis at the Level of Hip Joint and Femoral Neck: Hip joint injection

Posterior
- Short Axis at the Level of Sacroiliac (SI) Joint: SI joint injection
- Axial Oblique at the Level of the Sciatic Nerve: Piriformis injection

5.2 Anterior Hip

5.2.1 Anatomy

The evaluation of the anterior hip region through musculoskeletal ultrasound involves a careful consideration of principal imaging planes, notably the axial, axial oblique, and sagittal oblique planes. Each plane provides distinct insights into key anatomical structures relevant to diagnosis and intervention. In the axial short-axis view at the level of the anterior superior iliac spine (ASIS), attention is drawn to pivotal soft tissue structures, including the serratus anterior muscle, lateral femoral cutaneous nerve, tensor fascia lata, and rectus femoris muscle (Fig. 5.1a) [1]. This perspective proves particularly beneficial for identifying entrapment syndromes, soft tissue anomalies, and nerve pathologies such as meralgia paresthetica, characterized by the involvement of the lateral femoral cutaneous nerve. As the imaging probe is advanced distally to capture the hip joint, the transition into the axial short-axis plane reveals deeper osseous and vascular components. Here, the pubic bone and acetabulum serve as significant bony landmarks, with the femoral head visible in its articulation within the acetabulum. The superficial layer displays the femoral vein, artery, and nerve arranged in a medial-to-lateral orientation. Notably, the pectineus and iliacus muscles are prominently visualized lateral to the femoral nerve, facilitating the assessment of hip flexor pathologies and possible nerve compression syndromes (Fig. 5.1b) [2]. The sagittal oblique plane, when focused on the iliopsoas tendon, allows for a thorough examination of the acetabulum, femoral head and neck, joint labrum, capsule, and iliopsoas tendon (Fig. 5.1c). This viewpoint is critical for identifying iliopsoas tendinopathy, snapping hip syndrome, and various intra-articular pathologies, including labral tears and synovial inflammation. At the level of the hip joint, the sagittal oblique plane affords unparalleled visualization of the femoral neck, excelling in delineating cortical integrity and identifying fractures or stress injuries (Fig. 5.1d). This plane also proves instrumental in assessing the joint capsule and detecting effusions, rendering it an essential modality for evaluating inflammatory and degenerative joint conditions.

5.2.2 Scan

5.2.2.1 Axial Oblique below the Level of ASIS (Video 5.1)

Patient Position: Lying down on the bed in the supine position.

Probe Position: Place the probe on the ASIS parallel to the inguinal ligament (a line between ASIS and pubis) and slide distally until the ASIS cortex has disappeared (Fig. 5.2a) [3].

Scanning: For optimal visualization of the lateral femoral cutaneous nerve (LFCN), a high-frequency linear transducer is recommended. In this ultrasound image, the deep, semi-oval hypoechoic structure with well-defined edges corresponds to the iliac bone cortex. Superficial to this landmark is the relatively hypoechoic rectus femoris muscle. Above this, two distinct hypoechoic muscular structures can be observed: the sartorius muscle medially and the tensor fascia lata laterally. Between these muscles, there is a small, honeycomb-like hyperechoic structure that represents the LFCN as it progresses toward the thigh. The fascia lata, a thin echogenic band, lies above these structures and serves as a crucial anatomical landmark. To accurately identify the LFCN and distinguish it from the sartorius tendon, it is essential to slide the probe both proximally and distally. Unlike tendons, nerves retain their characteristic honeycomb appearance along

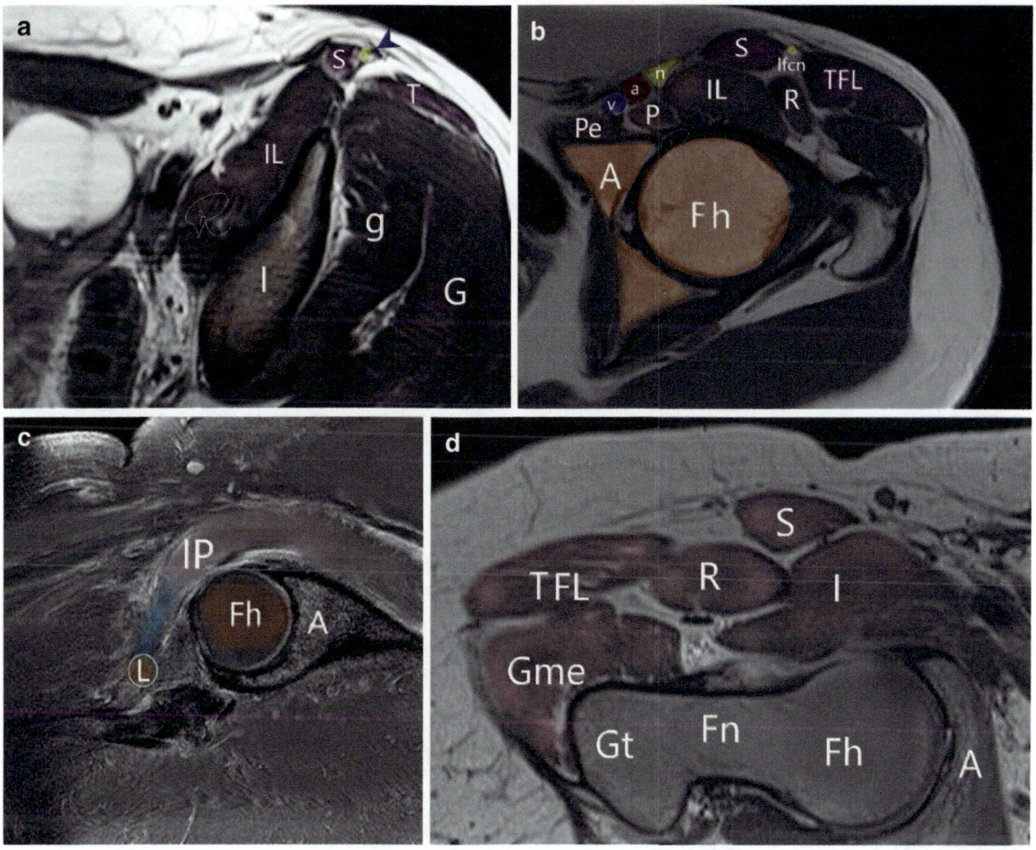

Fig. 5.1 Anterior hip anatomy: The image consists of four labeled and color-enhanced MRI scans of the hip region, each highlighting key anatomical structures and muscles in different planes. Image (**a**): This axial cross-section located just below the anterior superior iliac spine (ASIS) highlights key muscles, including the iliacus, gluteus maximus, and sartorius. The visualization of the lateral femoral cutaneous nerve emphasizes its potential involvement in conditions such as meralgia paresthetica. Image (**b**): At the level of the hip joint, this axial cross-section reveals critical components like the femoral head and acetabulum, along with the tensor fasciae latae and psoas muscles. The clear depiction of the femoral neurovascular bundle—encompassing the artery, vein, and nerve—facilitates assessments regarding joint congruency and soft tissue integrity. Image (**c**): This sagittal oblique section accentuates the iliopsoas tendon along with the femoral head and acetabulum. This perspective is crucial for diagnosing iliopsoas-related issues, such as bursitis and snapping hip syndrome. Image (**d**): Another sagittal oblique view at the hip joint level showcases the gluteus medius and minimus, as well as the femoral neck. This image aids in evaluating the integrity of the femoral neck, detecting stress fractures, and examining gluteal muscle pathologies. Additionally, the visibility of the greater trochanter and iliotibial band supports the diagnosis of greater trochanteric pain syndrome. Abbreviations for Reference: S (Sartorius), TFL (Tensor fascia lata), I (Iliac bone), IL (Iliacus), G (Gluteus maximus), Gme (Gluteus medius), Gmi (Gluteus minimus), lfcn (Lateral femoral cutaneous nerve), R (Rectus femoris), P (Psoas), Pe (Pectineus), v (Femoral vein), a (Femoral artery), n (Femoral nerve), IP (Iliopsoas), L (Lesser trochanter), Fn (Femoral neck), Gt (Greater trochanter). (© Reza Roghani 2024. All Rights Reserved)

their course. Furthermore, gentle tilting of the transducer can improve the contrast between the nerve and the surrounding tissues. (Fig. 5.2d). For a lateral femoral cutaneous nerve (LFCN) block, the recommended injection site is generally positioned near the inguinal ligament, where the LFCN runs superficially between the sartorius and tensor fascia lata muscles. The authors advocate using an in-plane technique from the lateral side. This approach provides a clear view of the needle's trajectory, ensuring accurate positioning and a safe entry point, which facilitates effective anesthetic deposition while minimizing the risk of injury to the LFCN and surrounding structures, such as blood vessels or the sartorius tendon. (Fig. 5.2e, f) (Video 5.1).

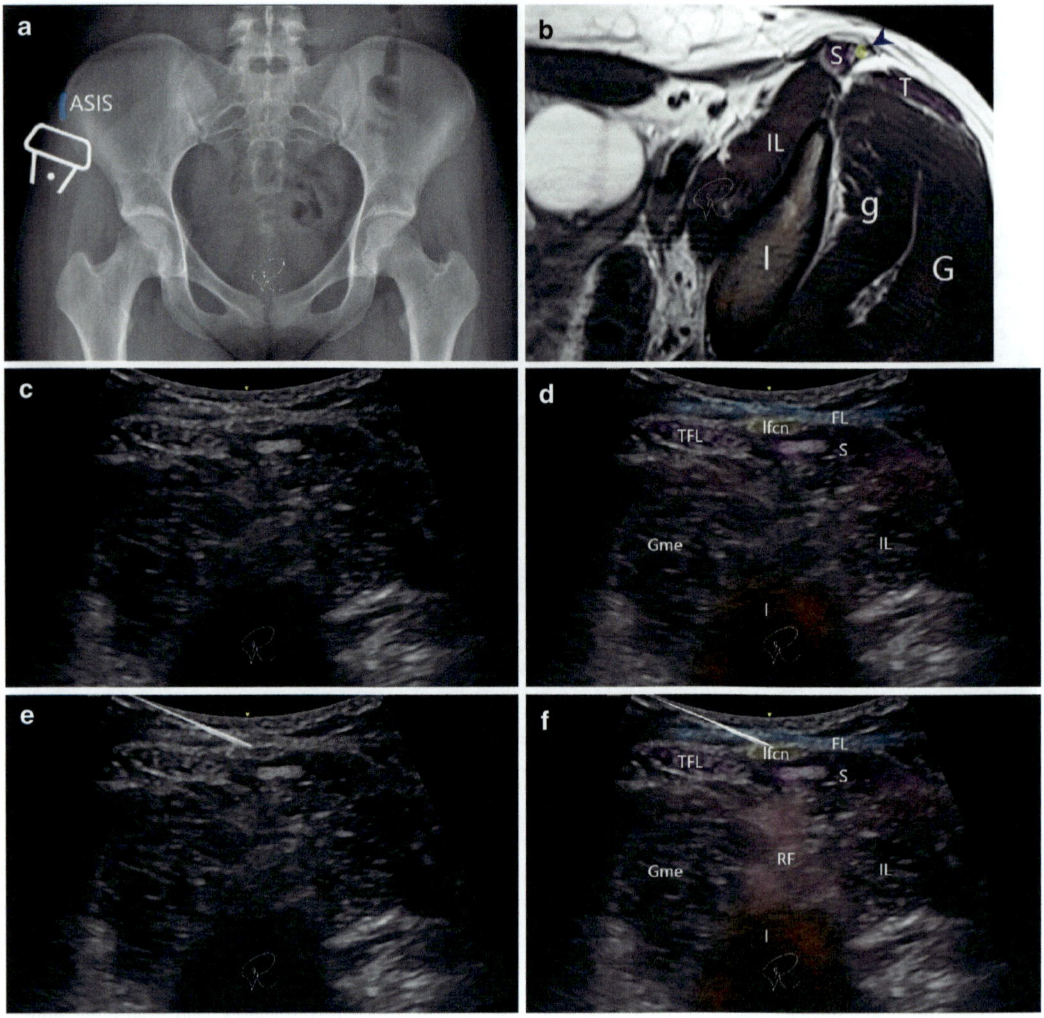

Fig. 5.2 Axial oblique below ASIS level. The image presented is a composite of six medical imaging scans focused on the lateral femoral cutaneous nerve region. Image (**a**) is an X-ray depicting the anterior superior iliac spine (ASIS), with a highlighted area and a probe illustrating an axial oblique position parallel to the inguinal ligament. Image (**b**) is an MRI scan featuring labeled structures, including S (Sartorius), T (Tensor fascia lata), IL (Iliacus), g (Gluteus medius), I (Iliacus), and G (Gluteus maximus), which represent various muscles, along with a solid arrowhead indicating the lateral femoral cutaneous nerve. Images (**c**) and (**d**) are ultrasound scans that visualize the lateral femoral cutaneous nerve, with image (**d**) being color-enhanced, labeled, and annotated to identify specific muscles and nerves, such as TFL (Tensor fascia lata), lfcn (Lateral femoral cutaneous nerve), FL (Fascia lata), S (Sartorius), Gme (Gluteus medius), IL (Iliacus), and RF (Rectus femoris). Images (**e**) and (**f**) correspond to images (c) and (d), respectively, but emphasize the needle trajectory for the lateral femoral cutaneous nerve block.

5.2.2.2 Axial Oblique at the Level of the Hip Joint (Video 5.2)

Patient Position: Lying down on the bed in the supine position.

Probe Position: Use the femoral pulse as a landmark and place the probe in a sagittal oblique plane parallel to the inguinal ligament (Fig. 5.3a) [4].

Scanning: The key vascular and neural structures—the femoral vein, femoral artery, and femoral nerve—should appear in a medial-to-lateral alignment. Once these landmarks are identified, gradually slide the transducer laterally while maintaining a perpendicular angle to the skin. This maneuver will bring the femoral head, a convex hyperechoic structure, into the center of the screen. In the deepest layer of the ultrasound image, the acetabular cortex will appear as a bright, linear structure, followed by the labrum, which may be visualized as a hyperechoic triangular or rounded structure at the acetabular rim. Adjacent to this, the femoral head cortex can be seen as another bright, well-defined contour. Superficial to these bony landmarks, the joint capsule is visible as a thin, hyperechoic line covering the femoral head and acetabulum. Above the capsule, the iliopsoas tendon can be distinguished as a fibrillar structure, and further superficial to it, the iliopsoas muscle appears as a hypoechoic, striated mass. Tilting the transducer slightly or using a dynamic scanning technique, such as external-internal rotation of the hip, can enhance differentiation of the structures and improve diagnostic accuracy. For procedural applications, color Doppler imaging can help identify adjacent vascular structures, ensuring safe needle placement during interventions such as joint injections or iliopsoas tendon evaluations. (Fig. 5.3c, d).

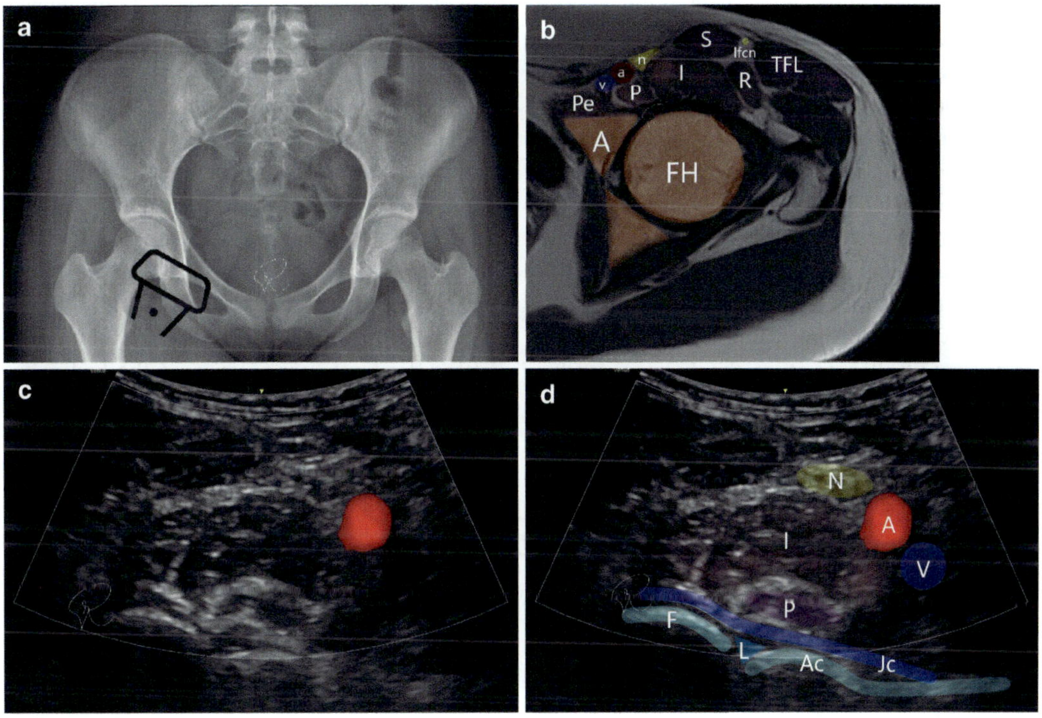

Fig. 5.3 Axial oblique at the level of the hip joint. The image consists of a composite of four medical scans illustrating an axial oblique view of the hip joint. Panel (**a**) displays an X-ray of the pelvis, with a highlighted area indicating the position of the probe. Panel (**b**) features an MRI cross-section of the hip, annotated with various anatomical structures, including Sartorius (S), Tensor Fascia Lata (TFL), Iliac Bone (I), Iliacus (IL), Gluteus Maximus (G), Gluteus Medius (g), Lateral Femoral Cutaneous Nerve (lfcn, marked by an arrowhead), Rectus Femoris (R), Psoas (P), Pectineus (Pe), Femoral Vein (v), Femoral Artery (a), Femoral Nerve (n), Iliopsoas (IP), Lesser Trochanter (L), Femoral Neck (Fn), Greater Trochanter (Gt), Gluteus Medius (Gme), and Fascia Lata (FL). Panel (**c**) presents an ultrasound image captured in color Doppler mode, emphasizing vascular structures. Panel (d) is the same ultrasound image as shown in (**c**), but it includes multiple color-coded labels that identify key anatomical features: "A" for Femoral Artery, "V" for Femoral Vein, "N" for Femoral Nerve, "P" for Psoas , "I" for Iliacus, "F" for Femur, "Jc" for Joint Capsule, "L" for Labrum, and "AC" for Acetabulum. (© Reza Roghani 2024. All Rights Reserved)

5.2.2.3 Sagittal Oblique Iliopsoas Tendon (Video 5.3)

Patient Position: Lying down on the bed in the supine position.

Probe Position: Begin by locating the femoral pulse as your initial landmark. Position the ultrasound probe in a sagittal oblique plane, ensuring it is aligned parallel to the inguinal ligament. Once the probe is properly positioned, identify the iliopsoas tendon and center it within the image for optimal visualization. After achieving this alignment, gently rotate the probe 90° around its central axis to obtain a long axis view. (Fig. 5.4a) [5].

Scanning: In the deepest layer of the neuromusculoskeletal ultrasound image of the anterior hip, the acetabular cortex should be clearly visible as a well-defined hyperechoic line. Adjacent to the acetabulum, the labrum appears as a triangular-shaped structure, while the convex hyperechoic contour of the femoral head cortex is also discernible. Notably, the transition at the femoral head-neck junction exhibits a concave shape. Superficially to these osseous and cartilaginous formations, the joint capsule presents as a thin, hyperechoic layer. Further outward, with its distinct fibrillar structure, the iliopsoas tendon courses distally, frequently accompanied by the iliopsoas bursa beneath it. This bursa may be visible in cases of effusion or inflammation. The overlying musculature, including the rectus femoris muscle, lies more superficially, demonstrating its hypoechoic muscle belly and hyperechoic fascial planes. Proper transducer positioning and optimal gain settings are essential for clearly differentiating these structures and minimizing anisotropy of the iliopsoas tendon (Fig. 5.4c, d). As you advance the transducer distally, trace the iliopsoas tendon as it courses distally and medially toward its insertion on the lesser trochanter of the femur. Upon reaching the lesser trochanter, the tendon insertion appears as a well-defined, hyperechoic structure adjacent to the cortical surface. Dynamic scanning can be conducted by asking the patient to flex and extend the hip slightly, which may aid in distinguishing the tendon from surrounding structures and in assessing for any abnormal movement, thickening, or bursitis. Furthermore, scanning in this area enables the evaluation of the iliopsoas bursa, situated between the tendon and the hip joint capsule. In cases of bursitis, fluid accumulation may present as an anechoic or hypoechoic region adjacent to the tendon. (Fig. 5.4e, f). This location serves as the ideal site for injecting the iliopsoas tendon sheath, facilitating accurate localization and effective delivery of the injectate, while minimizing the risk of injury to surrounding structures. The authors prefer utilizing an in-plane ultrasound-guided approach from the distal aspect, which allows for continuous visualization of the needle throughout its trajectory, thereby enhancing both accuracy and safety. Under real-time ultrasound guidance, a 25- to 22-gauge needle that is 2.5 inches or longer is positioned to approach the target. Once the needle tip is confirmed to be within the tendon sheath, an injectate that includes a local anesthetic and corticosteroid, or other therapeutic agents, is administered, ensuring proper dispersion around the tendon.

5.2.2.4 Sagittal Oblique Hip Joint Injection (Video 5.4)

Patient Position: Lying down on the bed in the supine position with the leg on external rotation.

Probe Position: Begin with the sequence described in Sect. 5.2.2.2. Utilize the femoral pulse as a reliable landmark to guide probe placement. Position the transducer in a sagittal oblique plane, aligned parallel to the inguinal ligament to ensure optimal alignment with key anatomical structures. In this view, the femoral vein, femoral artery, and femoral nerve should be distinctly arranged from medial to lateral. Once these landmarks are clearly visualized, gently slide the transducer laterally while maintaining a perpendicular angle to the skin. This maneuver will shift the field of view laterally, positioning the femoral head at the center of the image for optimal visualization. With the femoral head now centered, carefully rotate the probe 90° around its midpoint. This rotation will transition the image from an axial view to a longitudinal perspective, providing a clear view of the hip joint and femoral neck in the long axis. (Fig. 5.5a).

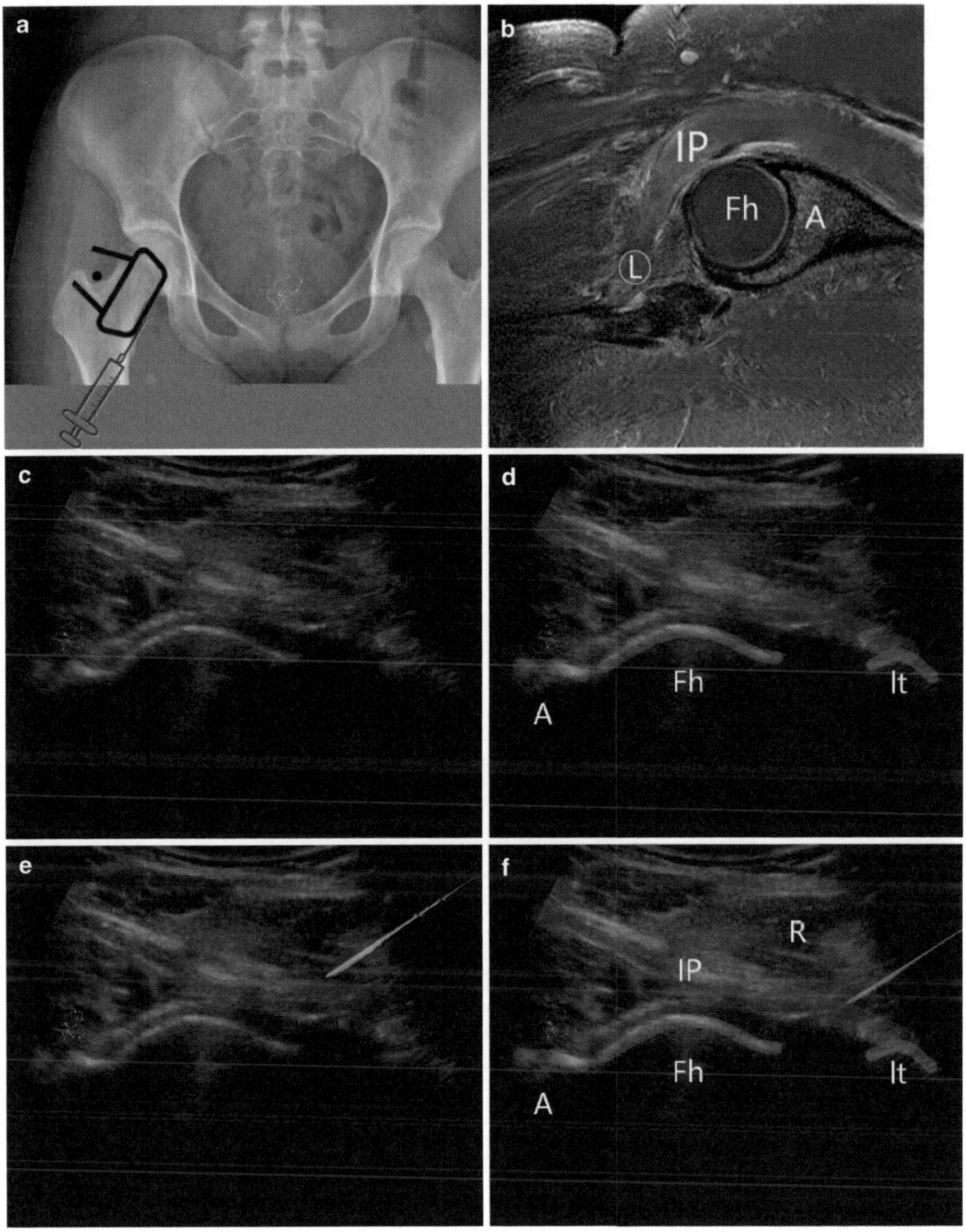

Fig. 5.4 Sagittal oblique Iliopsoas tendon. The image comprises six panels illustrating the anatomy, scanning techniques, and injection procedure for the iliopsoas tendon. Panel (**a**) presents an X-ray of the pelvis, featuring a schematic representation of a probe and syringe, which indicates the probe's positioning and the needle insertion point for the iliopsoas tendon injection. Panel (**b**) showcases a high-resolution MRI scan that highlights essential anatomical structures, including the femoral head (Fh), acetabulum (A), iliopsoas (IP), and lesser tubercle (L). Panels (**c**) and (d) display ultrasound images of the iliopsoas tendon, with panel (**d**) incorporating color overlays to identify structures such as the femoral head (Fh), acetabulum (A), iliopsoas (IP), and lesser tubercle (Lt). Panels (**e**) and (**f**) are enhanced versions of panels (**c**) and (**d**), respectively, providing additional emphasis on the needle trajectory for accurate iliopsoas tendon sheath injection. Panel (**f**) also labels the rectus femoris muscle as R.

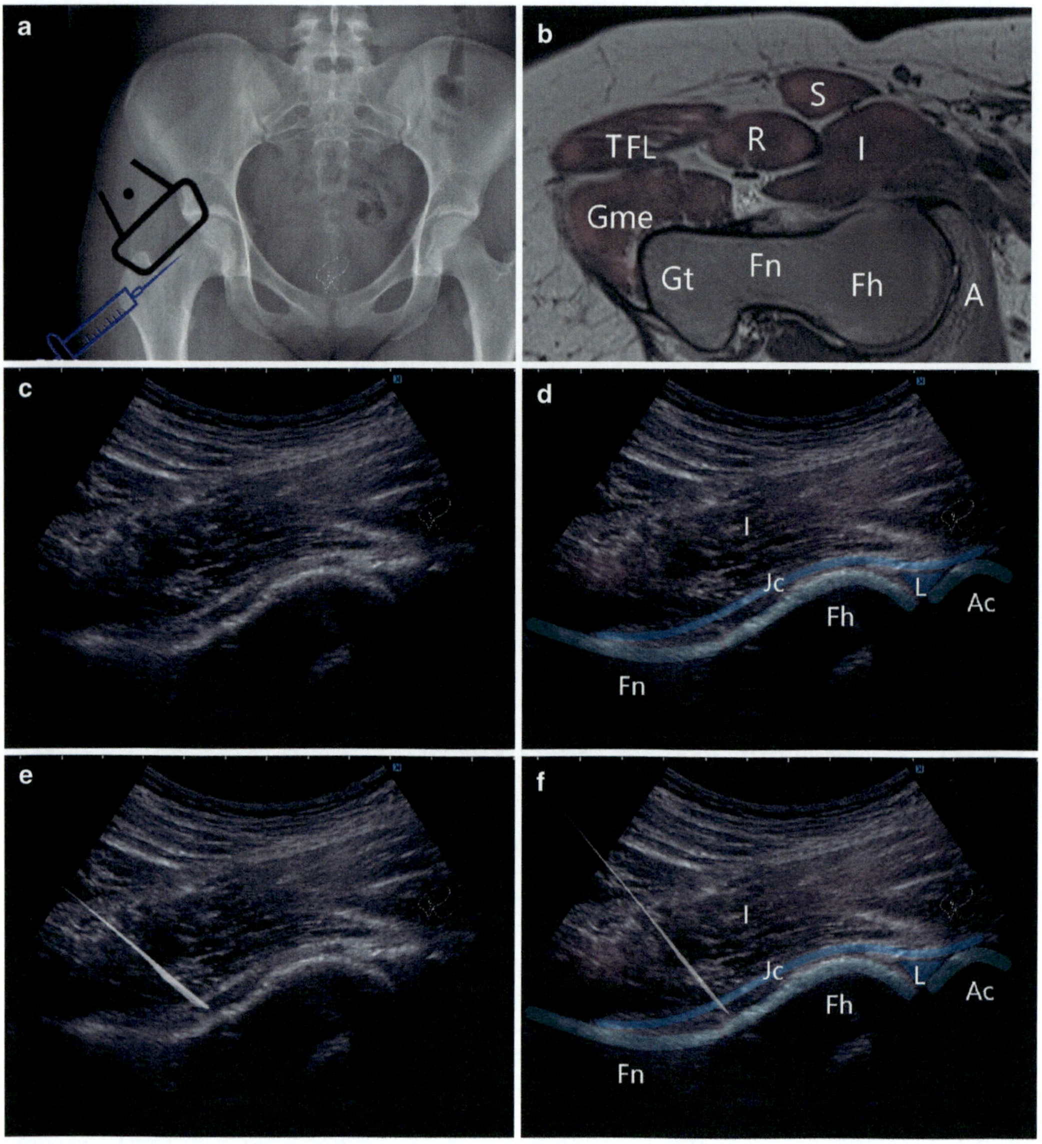

Fig. 5.5 Sagittal oblique hip joint injection. This composite image offers an in-depth exploration of hip joint anatomy through various medical imaging modalities, enhancing the understanding of both diagnostic procedures and interventional techniques. Panel (**a**) showcases an X-ray of the pelvis, supplemented by an overlay diagram illustrating the appropriate probe placement and needle insertion technique for ultrasound-guided hip joint injections. This diagram delineates the optimal needle insertion point and in-plane approach In Panel (**b**), a labeled MRI cross-section of the hip is presented, clearly identifying crucial anatomical features such as the Tensor Fasciae Latae (TFL), Gluteus Medius (Gme), Greater Trochanter (Gt), Femoral Neck (Fn), Femoral Head (Fh), Rectus Femoris (R), Sartorius (S), Ilium (I), and Acetabulum (A). Panels (**c**) and (**d**) offer ultrasound images of the hip joint, with d being colored and labeled to illustrate the femoral head (Fh) and neck (Fn), the ilium (I), the joint capsule (Jc), the labrum (L), and the acetabulum (Ac). Panels (**e**) and (**f**) expand upon the ultrasound images from (**c**) and (**d**), showcasing the needle's trajectory as it approaches the hip joint. These six panels deliver a thorough and comprehensive view of hip joint imaging, significantly aiding both the diagnostic assessment and procedural guidance in clinical practice.

Scanning: Adjust the rotation angle of the probe until the femoral neck cortex is fully visible in the deepest layer of the image. In this layer, you should be able to visualize the acetabular cortex, labrum, the convex structure of the femoral head cortex, the concave structure of the femoral head and neck junction, the femoral neck, and finally, the inter-trochanteric ridge. Positioned above these structures are the joint capsule, and the iliopsoas muscle (Fig. 5.5c, d). This image illustrates the ideal ultrasound view for conducting an anterior hip joint injection, offering a clear perspective on the relevant anatomical structures. To perform the injection, position the needle in-plane from the distal end of the probe, carefully advancing it under ultrasound guidance toward the concave junction of the femoral head and neck. This area represents the anterior joint recess, where the joint capsule is most accessible, facilitating effective distribution of the injectate. Utilizing real-time ultrasound guidance is essential to avoid nearby neurovascular structures, particularly the femoral artery and vein, which are located medially. Once the needle tip is confirmed within the joint space, proceed to administer the injectate, usually a blend of local anesthetic and corticosteroid, while monitoring for appropriate dispersion within the joint capsule. If needed, hydrodissection can be employed to enhance the spread of the injectate and reduce any potential adhesions [6].

5.3 Lateral Hip

5.3.1 Anatomy

The lateral hip is best assessed using two primary imaging planes: the axial and coronal planes. These planes provide comprehensive visualization of the anatomical structures surrounding the greater trochanter, which plays a crucial role in hip stability and movement. In the short-axis (axial) view, the key structures of interest include the greater trochanter itself, along with the tendinous insertions of the gluteus medius, gluteus minimus, and piriformis muscles. These tendons are essential for hip abduction, external rotation, and stabilization during weight-bearing activities. The trochanteric bursa, which lies between the gluteal tendons and the iliotibial band, is also a critical structure in this plane, as it is a common site of inflammation and pain in trochanteric bursitis. The iliotibial band, which extends over the lateral hip and down the thigh, is another notable feature that can be assessed for signs of thickening or friction-related pathology (Fig. 5.6a) [7]. When transitioning to the long-axis (coronal) view, more structures become apparent. This perspective allows for a detailed assessment of the gluteus medius tendon at its insertion on the greater trochanter, providing insights into potential tendinopathy or tears. The femoral head and acetabulum are also visible, facilitating an evaluation of hip joint congruency and potential degenerative changes. This view is particularly valuable for identifying intra-articular pathologies, such as hip osteoarthritis or labral abnormalities, which may contribute to lateral hip pain. (Fig. 5.6b) [8].

5.3.2 Scan

5.3.2.1 Short Axis at the Level of the Greater Trochanter (Video 5.5)

Patient Position: The patient should be positioned in a lateral decubitus position on the examination table, with the affected side facing upward and fully exposed for optimal access and visualization. (Fig. 5.7a).

Probe position: The probe should be placed in a short-axis orientation directly over the apex of the greater trochanter, ensuring optimal visualization of the underlying bony landmarks, tendinous insertions, and surrounding soft tissues [8].

Scanning Technique: When conducting an ultrasound scan of the lateral hip region, the transducer must be positioned in a short-axis orientation directly over the apex of the greater trochanter. The resulting ultrasound image should clearly depict a relatively triangular hyperechoic line indicative of the cortical surface of the greater trochanter, centrally situated within the field of view.

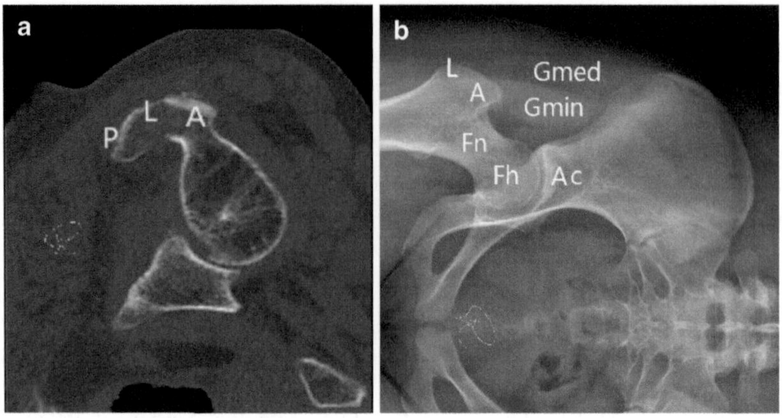

Fig. 5.6 Lateral hip anatomy: This two-part medical imaging provides a detailed anatomical assessment of the lateral hip using different imaging modalities. Image (**a**) presents a labeled CT scan of the hip joint, offering a high-resolution, cross-sectional view of bony structures. Key regions are marked, including P (Posterior facet of the greater trochanter), L (Lateral facet of the greater trochanter), and A (Anterior facet of the greater trochanter). This image represents different parts of the greater trochanter. Image (**b**) features a labeled X-ray of the hip joint, colored and highlighting key anatomical landmarks commonly assessed in lateral hip anatomy. This image includes L (Lateral facet of the greater trochanter), A (Anterior facet of the greater trochanter), Fn (Femoral Neck), Gmed (Gluteus Medius), Gmin (Gluteus Minimus), and Ac (Acetabulum).

It is crucial to meticulously evaluate the tendinous insertions of relevant musculature during the examination. The gluteus minimus tendon, which inserts onto the anterior facet of the greater trochanter, can be recognized as a well-defined fibrillar structure. Observations of any thickening, hypoechogenicity, or irregularities in this area may be indicative of tendinopathy or partial tearing. Similarly, the gluteus medius tendon inserts onto the lateral facet of the greater trochanter and is typically visualized as a distinct hyperechoic structure exhibiting a well-organized fibrillar pattern. Degenerative alterations, including tendinosis or tears, may manifest as regions of hypoechogenicity, disorganization of normal structure, or fluid accumulation surrounding the tendon. To optimize image resolution and clarity, it is imperative to adjust transducer pressure and angulation throughout the assessment, particularly while evaluating tendon integrity. (Fig. 5.7c, d).

5.3.2.2 Long Axis at the Level of Hip Joint and Femoral Neck (Video 5.6)

Patient Position: In preparing for the examination, the patient must be positioned in a lateral decubitus position on the examination table. The affected side should be oriented upward, ensuring complete exposure of the area of interest. This positioning facilitates optimal access and visualization, which is crucial for an accurate assessment and intervention. (Fig. 5.8a).

Probe Placement: The probe should be aligned along the long axis of the greater trochanter to obtain a longitudinal view of the cortical surface and the insertion points of the gluteus medius and minimus tendons. This positioning facilitates optimal visualization of tendon integrity, potential pathological changes, and the surrounding soft tissues, such as the trochanteric bursa and the iliotibial band. Proper transducer placement is essential for accurate assessment and guidance for interventional procedures (Fig. 5.8a).

Scanning Technique: During the ultrasonographic examination of the hip, it is essential to identify a triangular-shaped hyperechoic line situated centrally within the image. This line denotes the cortical surface of the greater trochanter and is a crucial landmark for evaluating the adjacent tendons and soft tissues. Attention should be directed to the insertion points of the gluteus medius tendon, specifically located on the superoanterior and lateral

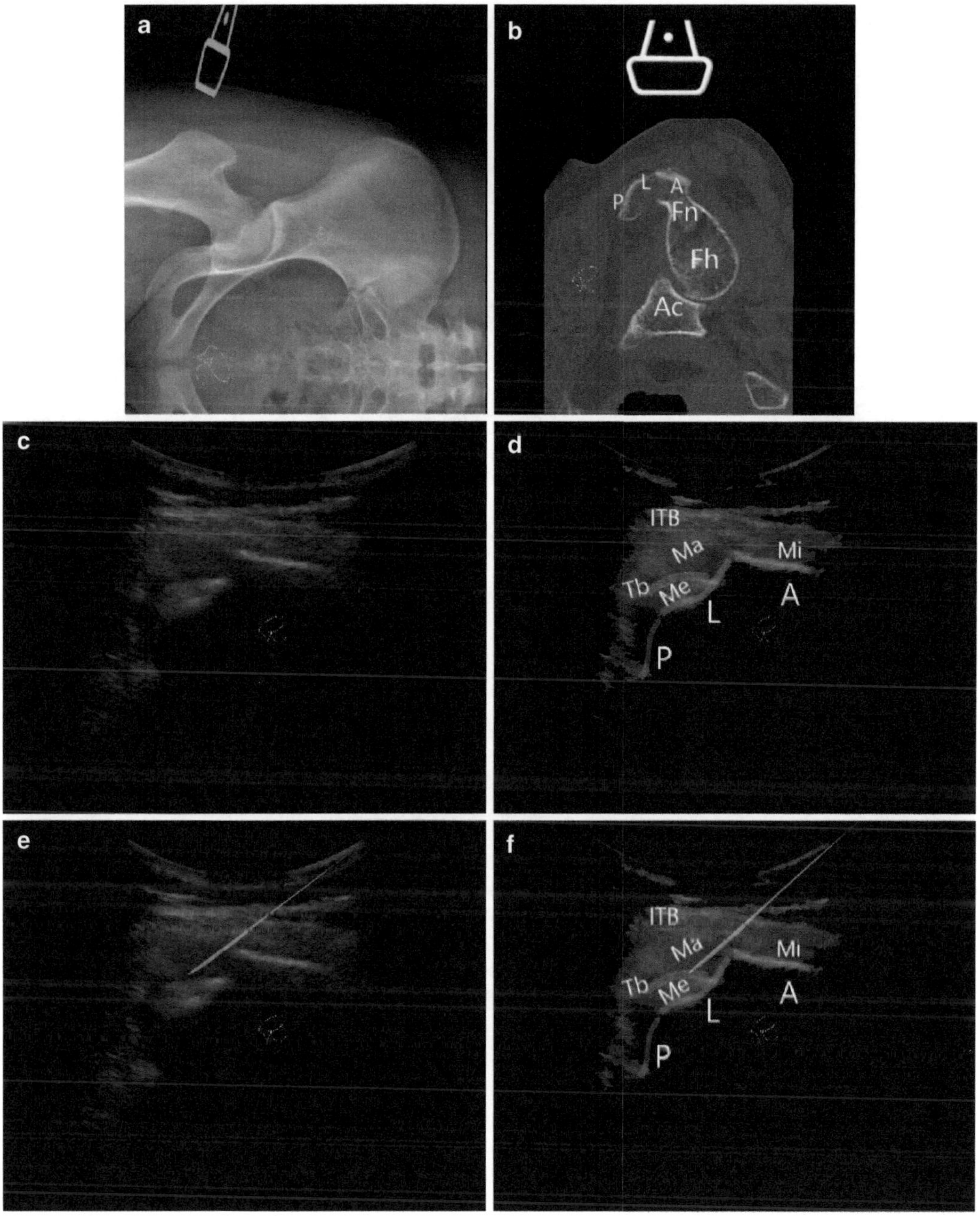

Fig. 5.7 Short axis at the level of the greater trochanter. The composite image is constructed from six distinct panels, each providing an in-depth medical imaging perspective of the hip region, focusing on the greater trochanter and surrounding anatomical structures. Panel (**a**) features an X-ray of the hip, presenting the greater trochanter with a probe positioned in a short-axis view. Panel (**b**) is a CT scan of the hip, also depicted in the short-axis view, offering enhanced visualization of the bony anatomy. This image includes labeled key anatomical landmarks: P (Posterior facet of the greater trochanter), L (Lateral facet of the greater trochanter), A (Anterior facet of the greater trochanter), Fn (Femoral Neck), Fh (Femoral Head), and Ac (Acetabulum). Panels (**c**) and (**d**) consist of short-axis ultrasound images of the greater trochanter. The ultrasound in panel (**d**) is both color-coded and annotated, emphasizing essential anatomical structures, such as ITB (Iliotibial Band), Tb (Trochanteric Bursa), Ma (Gluteus Maximus), Me (Gluteus Medius), Mi (Gluteus Minimus), A (Anterior facet of the greater trochanter), L (Lateral facet of the greater trochanter), and P (Posterior facet of the greater trochanter). These ultrasound images play a crucial role in assessing the integrity of soft tissues, identifying tendon pathologies, and diagnosing bursitis. Panels (**e**) and (**f**) replicate the ultrasound images found in panels (**c**) and (**d**), with the additional trajectory of the needle used in interventional procedures.

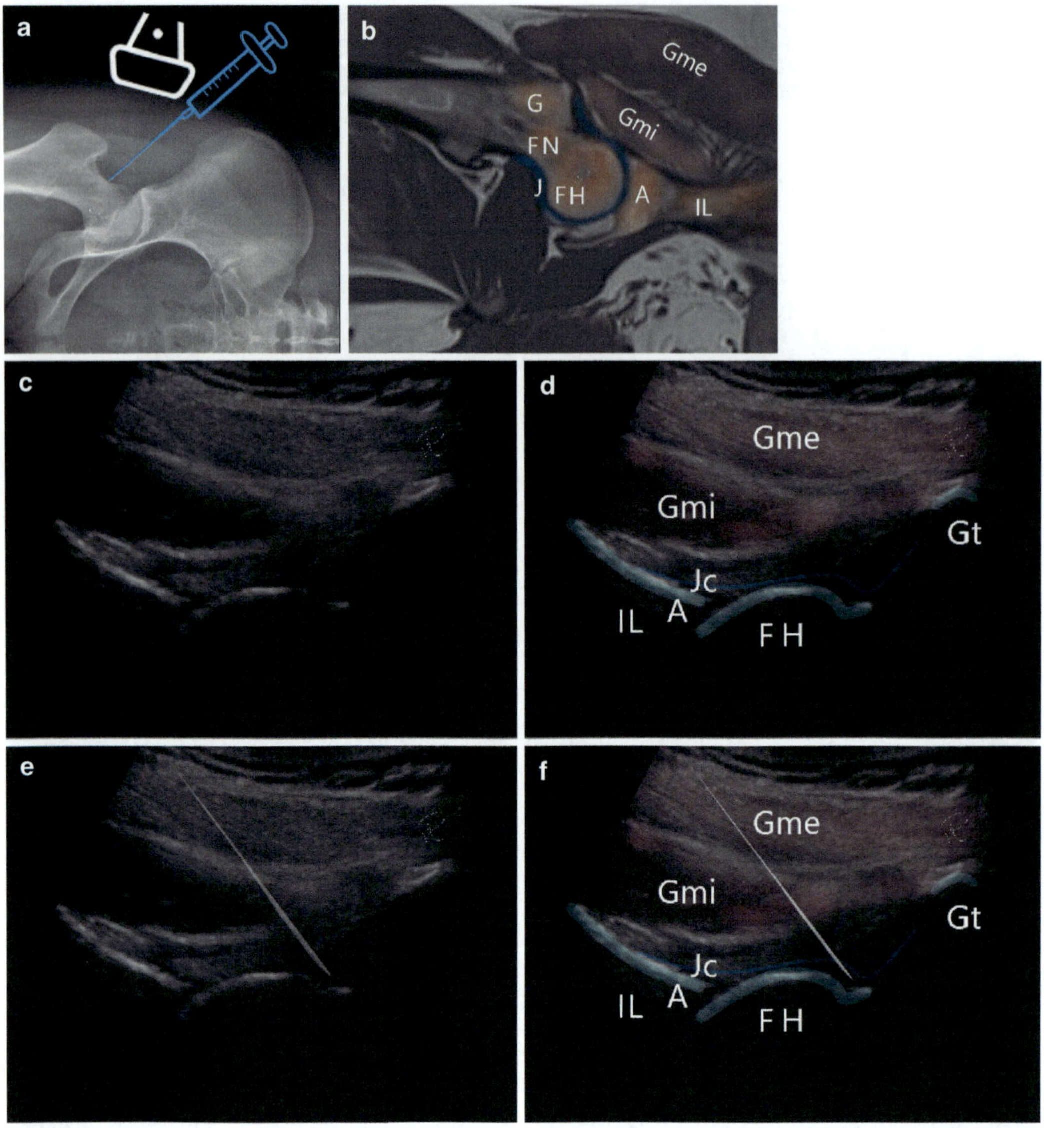

Fig. 5.8 The image is a composite of six panels illustrating hip joint anatomy and ultrasound imaging. Panel (**a**) shows a diagram of a hip joint with a syringe indicating an injection site. Panel (**b**) is a labeled anatomical diagram of the hip joint, highlighting structures such as the gluteus medius (Gme), gluteus minimus (Gmi), femoral neck (FN), and acetabulum (A). Panels (**c**) and (**e**) display ultrasound images of the hip joint without labels. Panels (**d**) and (**f**) are the same ultrasound images with anatomical labels, showing the gluteus medius (Gme), gluteus minimus (Gmi), greater trochanter (Gt), and femoral head (FH). The images demonstrate the correlation between anatomical structures and their ultrasound representations. (© Reza Roghani 2024. All Rights Reserved)

facets of the greater trochanter. Careful assessment of these sites is important for identifying potential signs of tendinopathy, tears, or other pathological alterations. (Fig. 5.8c, d). As the ultrasound probe is moved in a proximal direction, various anatomical structures become visible, including the femoral head and neck junction, the femoral head itself, acetabulum, labrum, and joint capsule. These structures are vital for evaluating joint integrity, detecting effusion, and diagnosing potential intra-articular pathologies. (Fig. 5.8e, f). For any interventional procedures, this proximal area serves as an ideal site for hip joint injections. The recommended approach is an in-plane injection from a proximal direction, allowing for precise needle placement and enhanced visualization of the target area. This technique is designed to improve accuracy while minimizing the risk of neurovascular injury.

5.4 Posterior Hip

5.4.1 Anatomy

(Fig. 5.9a) [9]. These anatomical features are particularly relevant in the context of conditions such as sacroiliac joint dysfunction and intervention in inflammatory or enthesopathy changes in patients presenting with chronic posterior hip or low back pain. Conversely, the axial oblique plane at the level of the sciatic nerve reveals essential muscular structures, including the gluteus maximus and piriformis muscles, alongside the sciatic nerve itself. The sciatic nerve, characterized by its hypoechoic appearance and fascicular pattern, is situated deep in the piriformis muscle, making it a common site for compression, often associated with piriformis syndrome. Utilizing ultrasound in these anatomical regions can significantly aid in diagnosing a range of conditions, such as gluteal tendinopathy, piriformis syndrome, sciatic nerve entrapment, and sacroiliac joint dysfunction. Furthermore, it serves as a guide for various therapeutic interventions, including injections, nerve blocks, and perineural hydro dissection. (Fig 5.9b) [10].

5.4.2 Scan

5.4.2.1 Short Axis at the Level of Sacroiliac Joint (Video 5.7)

Patient Position: Ensure the patient is comfortably positioned prone on the examination table. A small pillow can be placed under the abdomen to reduce lumbar lordosis and enhance visualization. (Fig. 5.10a).

Probe Position: When placing the ultrasound probe, position it longitudinally along the lumbosacral spine to locate the S1 spinous process. Once identified, rotate the probe 90° to obtain a transverse view for further assessment. [11].

Scanning: When scanning in the sagittal plane of the lumbosacral spine, multiple humps will be observed, corresponding to the lumbar spinous processes. The first upsloping hyperechoic structure without a significant hump is the S1 (Fig. 5.10c, d). Slide the probe distally to bring S1 spinous process in the middle of the ultrasound screen. Once it is properly aligned, rotate the probe 90 degrees while ensuring the structure remains centered in the image. Adjust the pressure and angle of the probe as necessary to maintain visibility of the spinous process throughout the rotation.. Then, slide to the side of interest until you see the S1 foramen, a broken line in the hyperechoic sacrum cortex relatively close to the spinous process (Fig. 5.10e, f). Then slide distally to observe the S2 foramen. Finally, continue scanning to the side to observe the second broken line between the sacrum and ilium, representing the sacroiliac joint (Fig. 5.10g, h). The optimal technique for injecting into the sacroiliac (SI) joint involves utilizing an in-plane, medial-to-lateral approach under ultrasound guidance. Initially, the practitioner should insert a 22- to 25-gauge, 3.5-inch needle from the medial aspect, maintaining clear visualization of the needle's trajectory throughout the process. It is essential to advance the needle carefully over the S2 foramen, utilizing bony landmarks for accurate placement while taking precautions to avoid neurovascular structures. Fine adjustments should be made as the needle approaches the SI joint to enhance its positioning. Upon confirming that the needle tip is within the joint space, the injection can be administered, ensuring the injectate is evenly distributed. The preferred composition of the injectate comprises one cc of steroid and one cc of lidocaine, which provide synergistic anti-inflammatory and anesthetic effects, thereby facilitating patient relief.

5.4.2.2 Axial Oblique at the Level of the Sciatic Nerve (Video 5.8)

Patient Position: Position the patient comfortably in a prone position on the examination table. A small pillow may be placed under the abdomen to reduce lumbar lordosis and improve visibility.

Probe Position: Place the ultrasound probe in the middle of the buttock, aligning it along an imaginary line between the greater trochanter and the sacrum while the patient is in a prone position. Ensure firm but gentle contact with the skin to optimize image quality. Adjust the probe angle slightly as needed to enhance visualization

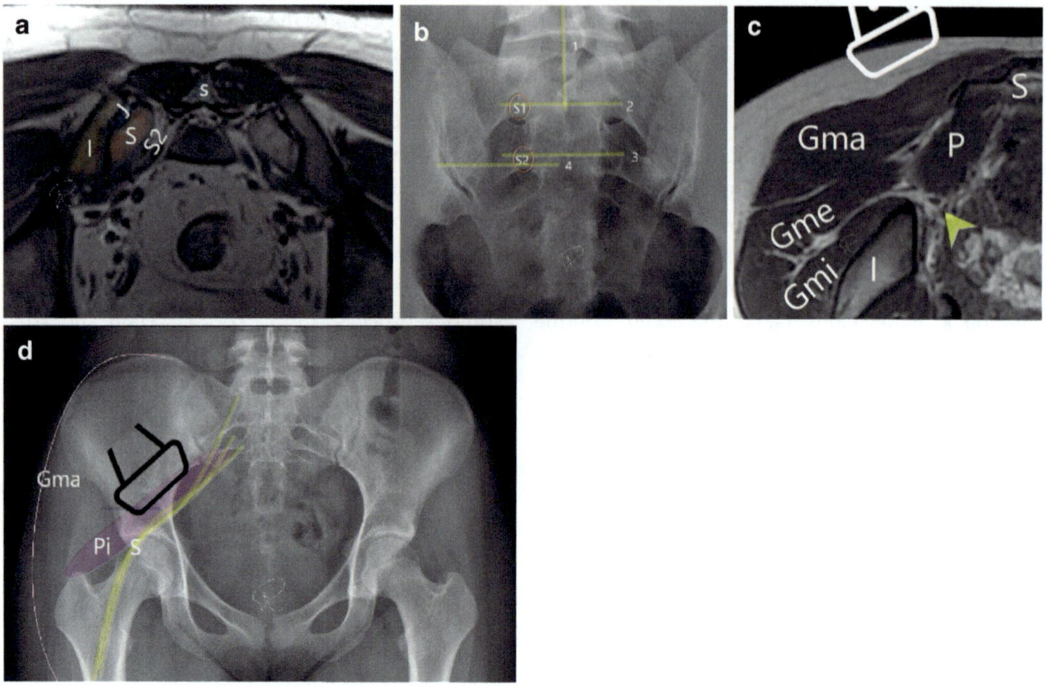

Fig. 5.9 Posterior hip anatomy: The visual representation comprises four distinct panels, each illustrating various anatomical perspectives of the pelvis and adjacent structures. These anatomies are pivotal for musculoskeletal evaluations and ultrasound-guided interventions. Panel (**a**) features an axial MRI scan that highlights crucial anatomical landmarks such as the sacral bone (S), sacral spinous process (s), S2 foramen (S2), sacroiliac joint (J), and iliac bone (I). In Panel (**b**), an X-ray of the pelvis is presented with marked horizontal lines indicating the S1 and S2 vertebral levels. The image includes four yellow lines denoting various probe position locations: (1) the spinous process of the lower lumbar and upper sacral, (2) the S1 vertebra, (3) the S1 foramen, and (4) the S2 foramen. These delineated probe positions are integral for ultrasound assessments and planning interventions such as sacral nerve blocks or sacroiliac joint injections. Panel (**c**) offers another axial MRI scan, this time concentrating on the soft tissue components, specifically the gluteus maximus (Gma), gluteus medius (Gme), gluteus minimus (Gmi), and piriformis (P) muscles and sacral bone (S). A yellow arrow indicates the position of the sciatic nerve, which is essential for diagnosing sciatic nerve entrapment and piriformis syndrome and for guiding perineural injections. Finally, Panel (**d**) presents an X-ray featuring overlaid illustrations that trace the anatomical pathways of the gluteus maximus (Gma), piriformis (Pi), and the sciatic nerve (S). This overlay provides a visual depiction of the sciatic nerve's positioning relative to the surrounding musculature, enhancing the understanding of posterior hip anatomy and interventional techniques to alleviate sciatic pain and address piriformis-related disorders. (© Reza Roghani 2024. All Rights Reserved)

Fig. 5.10 Short axis at the level of sacroiliac joint: L4 to S1: The image series features various medical scans and diagrams that illustrate the sacral region, highlighting probe placement and anatomical landmarks for ultrasound-guided procedures. Image (**a**) showcases an X-ray with labeled lines from 1 to 4, demonstrating a step-by-step approach to probe placement. The S1 and S2 foramina are identified, marking the posterior sacral foramina at the S1 and S2 levels. Image (**b**) presents a long-axis ultrasound scan of the spinous processes of the lower lumbar and upper sacral vertebrae, serving as an anatomical reference. Images (**c**) and (**d**) include short-axis ultrasound scans taken at the level of the S1 spinous process, with annotations that highlight S1 spinous process and the surrounding structures for clearer visualization. Images (**e**) and (**f**) offer short-axis ultrasound scans at the level of the S1 foramen, with image (**f**) being color-coded and labeled to enhance anatomical clarity. Image (**g**) features a CT scan of the sacroiliac (SI) joint at the level of S2, illustrating the probe position and needle insertion technique for interventional procedures. Image (**h**) presents a short-axis ultrasound scan of the SI joint, annotated to indicate the needle pathway through the SI joint for procedural guidance. Anatomical references included in the images span the spinous processes from L4 to S1, the sacroiliac joint (SI), the S1 foramen (S1f), and the sacral foramina at S1 and S2 levels. Other structures depicted are the sacrum (S), ilium (I), and the SI joint (J). The sequence of probe positioning adheres to four essential steps: first, positioning on the spinous process; second, aligning with the S1 vertebra; third, targeting the S1 foramen; and fourth, final placement at the S2 foramen. (© Reza Roghani 2024. All Rights Reserved)

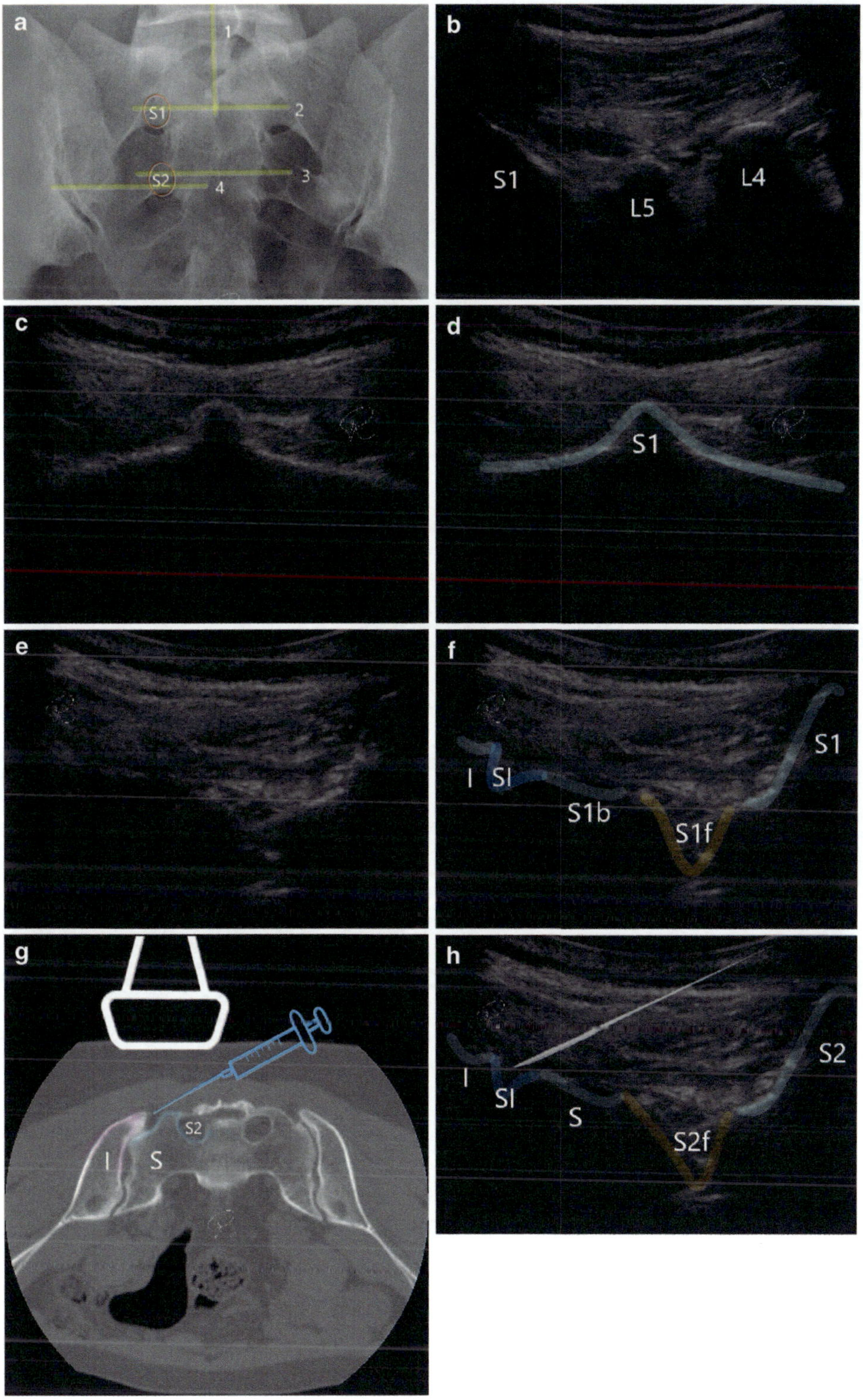
a
1
S1
2
S2
3
4
b
S1
L5
L4
c
d
S1
e
f
S1
I
SI
S1b
S1f
g
S2
I
S
h
S2
I
SI
S
S2f

of the sciatic nerve, which typically appears as a honeycomb, oval-shaped structure deep to the gluteus maximus and piriformis muscles and lateral to the iliac bone. (Fig. 5.11a).

Scanning: During neuromusculoskeletal ultrasound scanning of the posterior hip, the gluteus maximus is portrayed superficially as a prominent hypoechoic structure. Beneath it, the piriformis muscle is identifiable as another hypoechoic fascicular structure extending laterally from the sacrum to the greater trochanter. The sciatic nerve, characterized by its relatively large, honeycomb-like

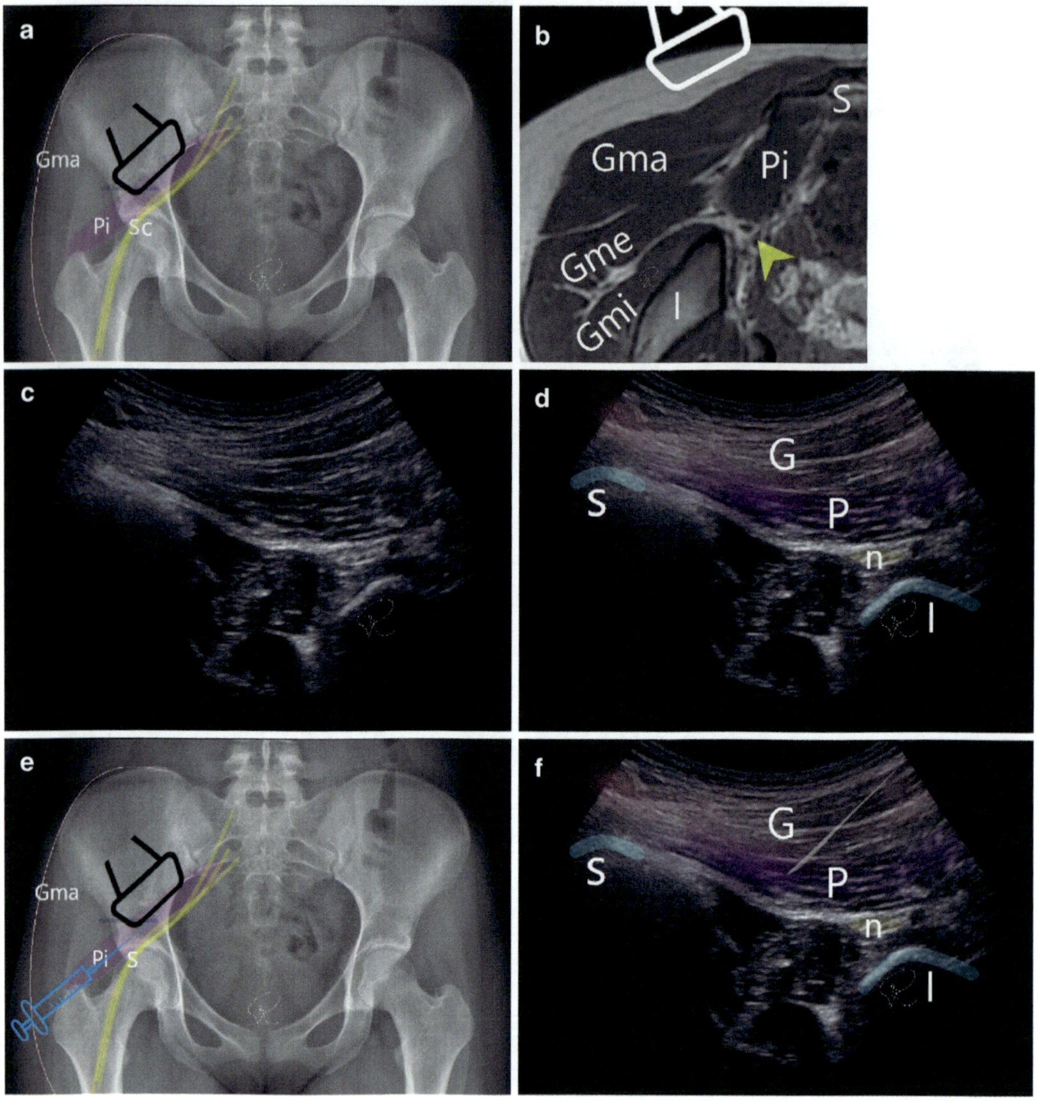

Fig. 5.11 Axial oblique at the level of the sciatic nerve. The image comprises six panels illustrating medical imaging of the sciatc nerve region. Panel (**a**) features an X-ray with annotations identifying the gluteus maximus (Gma), piriformis (Pi), and sciatic nerve (Sc). Panel (**b**) presents a cross-sectional MRI, labeling the gluteus medius (Gme), gluteus minimus (Gmi), piriformis (Pi), iliac crest (I), and sacrum (S), with a yellow solid arrowhead directing attention to the sciatic nerve. Panel (**c**) displays an ultrasound image of the sciatic nerve, devoid of annotations. Panel (**d**) presents the same ultrasound image with labels for the sacrum (S), gluteus maximus(G), piriformis (P), and sciatic nerve (n). Panel (**e**) repeats the X-ray, incorporating an illustration of a syringe to indicate needle insertion from the distal and lateral side in an in-plane approach. Finally, panel (**f**) showcases an ultrasound image featuring the needle, labeled similarly to panel (d), which illustrates the needle path for accurate targeting. (© Reza Roghani 2024. All Rights Reserved)

hyperechoic appearance, is located deep at the midpoint of the piriformis muscle (Fig. 5.11c, d). The recommended technique for administering piriformis muscle injections is an in-plane, distal-to-proximal approach. The needle should be inserted at the distal and lateral end of the probe, advancing under continuous ultrasound guidance to ensure accurate targeting and avoid neurovascular structures. Maintaining a safe distance from the sciatic nerve is essential to optimize both safety and efficacy during the delivery of the injectate [12].

References

1. Gupton M, Imonugo O, Black AC, Launico MV, Terreberry RR. Anatomy, bony pelvis and lower limb, knee. In: StatPearls. StatPearls Publishing; 2024. http://www.ncbi.nlm.nih.gov/books/NBK500017/.
2. Rodriguez JA, Kamara E, Cooper HJ. Applied anatomy of the direct anterior approach for femoral mobilization. JBJS Essent Surg Tech. 2017;7(2):e18. https://doi.org/10.2106/JBJS.ST.16.00099.
3. Zhu J, Zhao Y, Liu F, Huang Y, Shao J, Hu B. Ultrasound of the lateral femoral cutaneous nerve in asymptomatic adults. BMC Musculoskelet Disord. 2012;13(1):227. https://doi.org/10.1186/1471-2474-13-227.
4. Probyn L, Flores D, Rowbotham E, Cresswell M, Atinga A. High-resolution ultrasound in the evaluation of the adult hip. J Ultrason. 2023;23(95):e223–38. https://doi.org/10.15557/jou.2023.0031.
5. Weintraub MT, Barrack TN, Burnett RA, Serino J, Bhanot SS, Della Valle CJ. Ultrasound-guided iliopsoas bursal injections for management of iliopsoas bursitis after total hip arthroplasty. J Arthroplast. 2023;38(7 Suppl 2):S426–30. https://doi.org/10.1016/j.arth.2022.12.015.
6. Bardowski EA, Byrd JWT. Ultrasound-guided intra-articular injection of the hip: the Nashville sound. Arthrosc Tech. 2019;8(4):e383–8. https://doi.org/10.1016/j.eats.2018.11.016.
7. Lespasio MJ. Lateral hip pain: relation to greater trochanteric pain syndrome. Perm J. 2022;26(2):83–8. https://doi.org/10.7812/TPP/21.110.
8. Rowbotham EL, Grainger AJ. Ultrasound-guided intervention around the hip joint. AJR Am J Roentgenol. 2011;197(1):W122–7. https://doi.org/10.2214/AJR.10.6344.
9. Wong M, Sinkler MA, Kiel J. Anatomy, abdomen and pelvis, sacroiliac joint. In: StatPearls. StatPearls Publishing; 2024. http://www.ncbi.nlm.nih.gov/books/NBK507801/.
10. Chang C, Jeno SH, Varacallo M. Anatomy, bony pelvis and lower limb: piriformis muscle. In: StatPearls. StatPearls Publishing; 2024. http://www.ncbi.nlm.nih.gov/books/NBK519497/.
11. Chang W-H, Lew HL, Chen CPC. Ultrasound-guided sacroiliac joint injection technique. Am J Phys Med Rehabil. 2013;92(3):278. https://doi.org/10.1097/PHM.0b013e318278d108.
12. Aquino-Jose VM, Blinder V, Johnson J, Havryliuk T. Ultrasound-guided trigger point injection for piriformis syndrome in the emergency department. J Am Coll Emerg Physicians Open. 2020;1(5):876–9. https://doi.org/10.1002/emp2.12153.

Knee

6

Geet Paul, Reza Salman Roghani, Joseph Mouhanna, Jose Juan Diaz, Jasmine Sidhu, and Hein Linn Thant

6.1 Introduction

Ultrasound imaging plays a pivotal role in the assessment of knee pathologies, providing high-resolution, real-time visualization of musculoskeletal structures. For a thorough evaluation, the knee is divided into anterior, posterior, medial, and lateral compartments, with each region examined using proximal, mid, and distal scanning echniques. This chapter presents a comprehensive overview of knee sonoanatomy and the most commonly encountered pathologies, with a particular focus on the quadriceps tendon, suprapatellar recess, patellar tendon, and Hoffa's fat pad in the anterior compartment. The medial compartment is explored in detail, emphasizing the medial meniscus, medial collateral ligament (MCL), medial genicular nerves, and the pes anserine tendons and bursa—all vital for joint stability and sensory function. In the lateral compartment, the evaluation includes the lateral joint line, lateral collateral ligament (LCL), lateral meniscus, iliotibial band (ITB), and popliteus tendon, all of which are frequently associated with overuse syndromes, particularly among active individuals. The posterior region highlights important neurovascular and musculoskeletal structures, such as the popliteus tendon, tibial nerve, and common peroneal nerve. By presenting a structured, region-specific scanning protocol, this chapter aims to enhance diagnostic accuracy and improve the clinical application of musculoskeletal ultrasound in the evaluation and management of knee disorders

Supplementary Information The online version contains supplementary material available at https://doi.org/10.1007/978-3-031-81037-4_6.

G. Paul
Division of Pain Medicine, Department of Anesthesiology and Critical Care Medicine, George Washington University, Washington, DC, USA
e-mail: gpaul@mfa.gwu.edu

R. S. Roghani (✉) · J. Sidhu · H. L. Thant
Department of Physical Medicine and Rehabilitation, Larkin Community Hospital, Nova Southeastern University, Miami, FL, USA

J. Mouhanna
Division of Pain Medicine, Department of Anesthesiology, Larkin Community Hospital, Nova Southeastern University, South Miami, FL, USA
e-mail: drm@miamipain.com

J. J. Diaz
Department of Physical Medicine and Rehabilitation, Larkin Community Hospital, Nova Southeastern University, Miami, FL, USA

Integrative Spine and Sports, Fort Lauderdale, FL, USA

R. S. Roghani, J. J. Diaz (eds.), *Video Atlas of Neuromusculoskeletal Ultrasound*,
https://doi.org/10.1007/978-3-031-81037-4_6

6.1.1 Knee Ultrasound Protocol

Anterior Compartment

- **Suprapatellar Region**
  - Midsagittal View: Quadriceps Tendon and suprapatellar recess
  - Transverse View: Quadriceps tendon and suprapatellar recess
- **Infrapatellar Region**
  - Midsagittal View: Patellar tendon, Hoffa's fat pad, and prepatellar bursa
  - Transverse View: Patellar tendon, Hoffa's fat pad, and anterior knee joint space

Medial Compartment

- Coronal View (Central Knee): Medial joint line, medial meniscus, medial collateral ligament (MCL), medial genicular nerves, and pes anserine tendons
- Axial View (Superior Knee): Saphenous nerve
- Coronal View (Inferior Knee): Inferior medial genicular nerve

Lateral Compartment

- Coronal View: Lateral joint line, lateral meniscus, lateral collateral ligament (LCL), iliotibial band (ITB), and popliteus tendon.

Posterior Compartment

- **Posterolateral Region**
  - Sagittal View: Lateral joint line, lateral meniscus, and lateral head of the gastrocnemius
  - Transverse View: Tibial nerve and common peroneal nerve
- **Posteromedial Region**
  - Sagittal View: Semimembranosus tendon, medial belly of the gastrocnemius, and Baker's cyst

6.2 Anterior Knee

6.2.1 Anatomy

The anterior compartment of the knee contains vital neuromusculoskeletal structures, particularly the quadriceps muscles and their associated tendinous attachments, which are essential for knee extension and stability. The quadriceps—the rectus femoris, vastus medialis, vastus lateralis, and vastus intermedius—converge at the patella to form the quadriceps tendon (Fig. 6.1a) [1]. This tendon is the primary link between the quadriceps muscles and the patella, facilitating effective force transmission during movement. Above the patella lies the suprapatellar recess, an extension of the knee joint capsule that enables fluid dynamics within the joint. This recess is surrounded by a fat pad that provides cushioning and structural support [2]. The prepatellar bursa, located anteriorly over the lower portion of the patella and patellar tendon, functions as a friction-reducing structure, minimizing stress during repetitive knee flexion and extension. The patellar tendon, a robust ligamentous structure, extends from the inferior pole of the patella to the tibial tuberosity, anchoring the patella and playing a crucial role in knee mechanics. Hoffa's fat pad is deep to the patellar tendon (Fig. 6.1b), a highly vascularized and innervated fatty structure that absorbs shock and facilitates smooth patella movement. This area is critical in clinical evaluations, as inflammation or impingement of Hoffa's fat pad can lead to anterior knee pain. Musculoskeletal ultrasound provides a dynamic and high-resolution assessment of these structures, enhancing the diagnosis and management of anterior knee pathologies, including tendinopathies, bursitis, and fat pad impingement (Fig. 6.1b) [1–3].

6.2.2 Scan: Suprapatellar

6.2.2.1 Midsagittal: Quadriceps Tendon and Suprapatellar Recess (Video 6.1)

Patient Position: Lying down on the bed in the supine position. Have the patient bend the knee with a pillow under the knee.

Probe Position: When the knee is partially flexed, position the probe above the kneecap in the sagittal plane (Fig. 6.1a, b).

To obtain a clear ultrasound image of the anterior knee in the mid-sagittal plane, begin by placing the probe longitudinally along the anterior thigh, aligning it with the quadriceps tendon and patella. Gradually slide the probe proximally

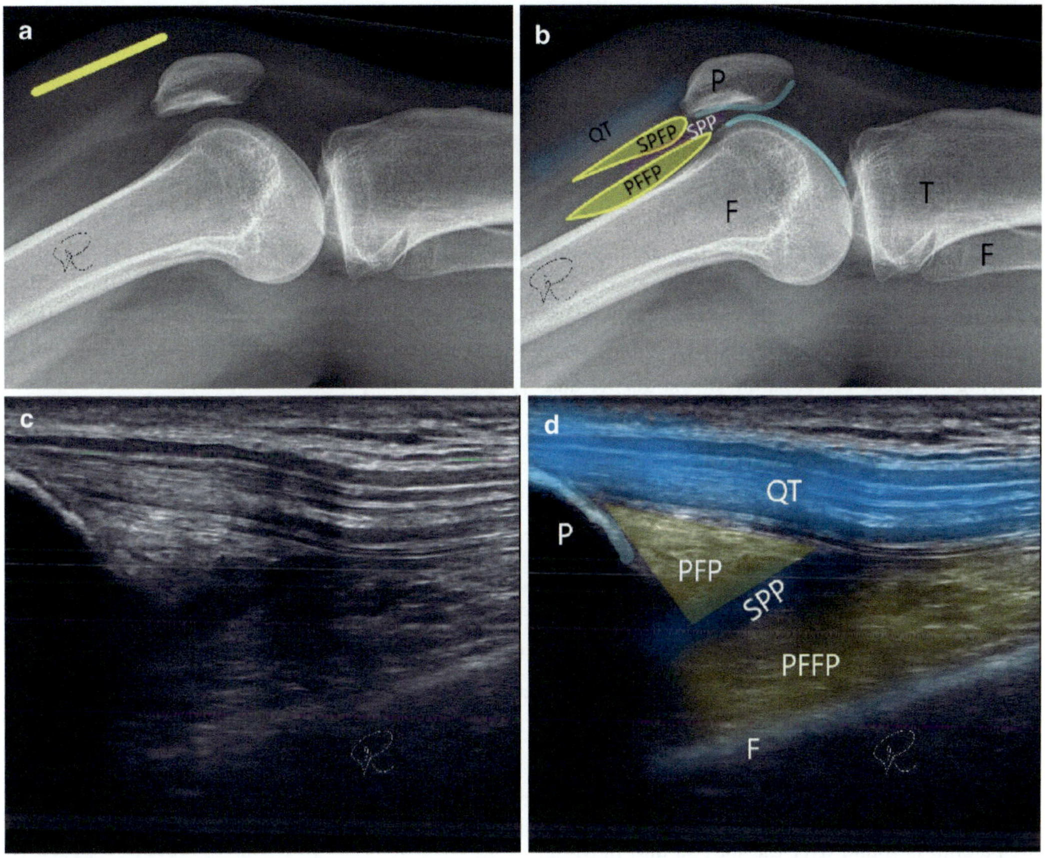

Fig. 6.1 Anterior superior midsagittal knee ultrasound scan. This figure comprises four images that illustrate the anatomical relationships and ultrasound visualization of the anterior knee structures. Image (**a**) features an X-ray representing patient position and highlights the quadriceps tendon (QT), with a yellow line indicating the optimal position of the ultrasound probe for imaging clarity. Image (**b**) provides a labeled schematic drawing over the same x-ray of the anterior knee, pinpointing key structures: the quadriceps tendon (QT), suprapatellar pouch (SPP), prefemoral fat pad (PFFP), suprapatellar fat pad (SPFP), tibia (T), and femur (F). Image (**c**) presents an unlabeled mid-sagittal ultrasound view of the superior anterior knee, offering a clear depiction of the anatomical structures without annotations. Image (**d**) reiterates the view from (**c**) but includes labels to identify the quadriceps tendon (QT), suprapatellar pouch (SPP), preprefemoral fat pad (PFFP), suprapatellar fat pad (SFP), and femur (F). Together, these images comprehensively illustrate the anatomical relationships, positioning, and sonographic appearance of the anterior knee structures, facilitating accurate identification and clinical assessment.

until the patella appears at the edge of the image, ensuring an optimal field of view for assessing key anatomical structures. Upon imaging, the quadriceps tendon is observed as a fibrillar, hyperechoic structure attaching to the superior pole of the patella. Directly beneath the tendon, the suprapatellar fat pad appears as a hyperechoic region, cushioning the tendon and contributing to smooth patellar movement. Deeper to the fat pad lies the suprapatellar recess, a hypoechoic structure representing an extension of the knee joint capsule. This area is clinically significant as it serves as a reservoir for joint effusion and synovial hypertrophy, commonly evaluated in inflammatory and degenerative conditions. Further in-depth, the prefemoral fat pad is visible, providing an additional layer of soft tissue between the suprapatellar recess and the femur. The deepest and brightest structure in the image is the femoral cortex, appearing as a continuous, hyperechoic line, signifying the bone's reflective surface. Maintaining probe orientation and optimizing depth settings allow for a comprehensive evaluation of these structures, aiding in the detection of pathology such as tendinopathy, bursitis, and joint effusion (Fig. 6.1d) [4, 5].

6.2.2.2 Transverse: Quadriceps Tendon and Suprapatellar Recess (Video 6.2)

Patient Position: Lying down on the bed in the supine position. Have the patient bend the knee with a pillow under the knee.

Probe Position: Place the probe in a transverse position on the patella and slide proximally until the patellar cortex has disappeared (Fig. 6.2a, b).

Scanning: Gradually advance the probe proximally until the patellar cortex is no longer visible, allowing for clear visualization of the deeper anatomical structures. The femoral cortex, visible as the deepest and brightest hyperechoic line, serves as the primary bony landmark. Just above this, the prefemoral fat pad appears as a relatively hypoechoic structure. Superficial to the fat pad, the hypoechoic linear area represents the suprapatellar recess, which is crucial for assessing joint effusion, synovial thickening, and intra-articular pathology. Above the suprapatellar recess lies the suprapatellar fat pad, which is relatively hypoechoic and functions as a cushioning structure. The quadriceps tendon, identifiable as a well-organized fibrillar structure extending from the quadriceps muscle to the patella, is found over the fat pad and plays an essential role in knee extension (Fig. 6.2c, d). The suprapatellar recess is often the preferred site for intra-articular knee injections, including steroid injections, viscosupplementation, and platelet-rich plasma (PRP) therapy. For optimal accuracy and safety, a medial in-plane approach is recommended. This technique allows for real-time needle visualization, ensuring precise placement of the injectate within the joint space. Proper probe positioning and anatomical identification significantly enhance diagnostic accuracy and procedural efficacy, making this technique vital for clinicians conducting musculoskeletal ultrasound evaluations and intervention (Fig. 6.2e, f).

6.2.3 Scan: Infrapatellar

6.2.3.1 Midsagittal: Patellar Tendon, Hoffa's Fat Pad and Pre Patellar Bursa (Video 6.3)

Patient Position: Lying down on the bed in the supine position. Have the patient bend the knee with a pillow under the knee.

Probe Position: When the knee is partially flexed, position the probe on top of the patella in the sagittal plane (Fig. 6.3a, b).

Scanning: To achieve a comprehensive longitudinal assessment of the patellar tendon and its surrounding structures, the ultrasound probe should be positioned on the patella. The probe is then gradually moved distally until the patella is positioned on one side of the image and the tibial tuberosity on the opposite side. This maneuver allows for the visualization of the entire length of the patellar tendon, alongside adjacent soft tissue structures. The patellar tendon, characterized as a dense, hyperechoic fibrous structure, extends from the inferior pole of the patella to the tibial tuberosity. It functions as an extension of the quadriceps tendon, facilitating the transmission of forces from the quadriceps muscles to enable knee extension. In a healthy tendon, the fibers should appear continuous and uniform; any observed disruptions, thickening, or hypoechoic regions may suggest conditions such as tendinopathy, partial tears, or post-traumatic changes. Superficially, the prepatellar bursa, located just beneath the skin over the lower half of the patella, represents a potential space that is typically non-visible in healthy individuals. However, in instances of bursitis, this bursa may become distended and hypoechoic. In cases of inflammation, the bursae often exhibit anechoic or complex fluid collections, with possible internal septations and synovial thickening. Chronic conditions may lead to calcifications or thickening of bursal walls, resulting from repetitive irritation or trauma. On a deeper level, Hoffa's fat pad, also referred to as the infrapatellar fat pad, appears as a relatively hypoechoic and homogenous structure situated between the patellar tendon and the anterior knee joint capsule. This fat pad plays an essential role in shock absorption and the reduction of friction within the knee joint. Pathological changes arising from issues such as fat pad impingement, or Hoffa's syndrome, can present as localized swelling, increased vascularity observable through Doppler imaging, and pain experienced during knee extension. For a thorough evaluation, it is advisable to scan both in longitudinal and transverse planes, ensuring a comprehensive assessment of tendon

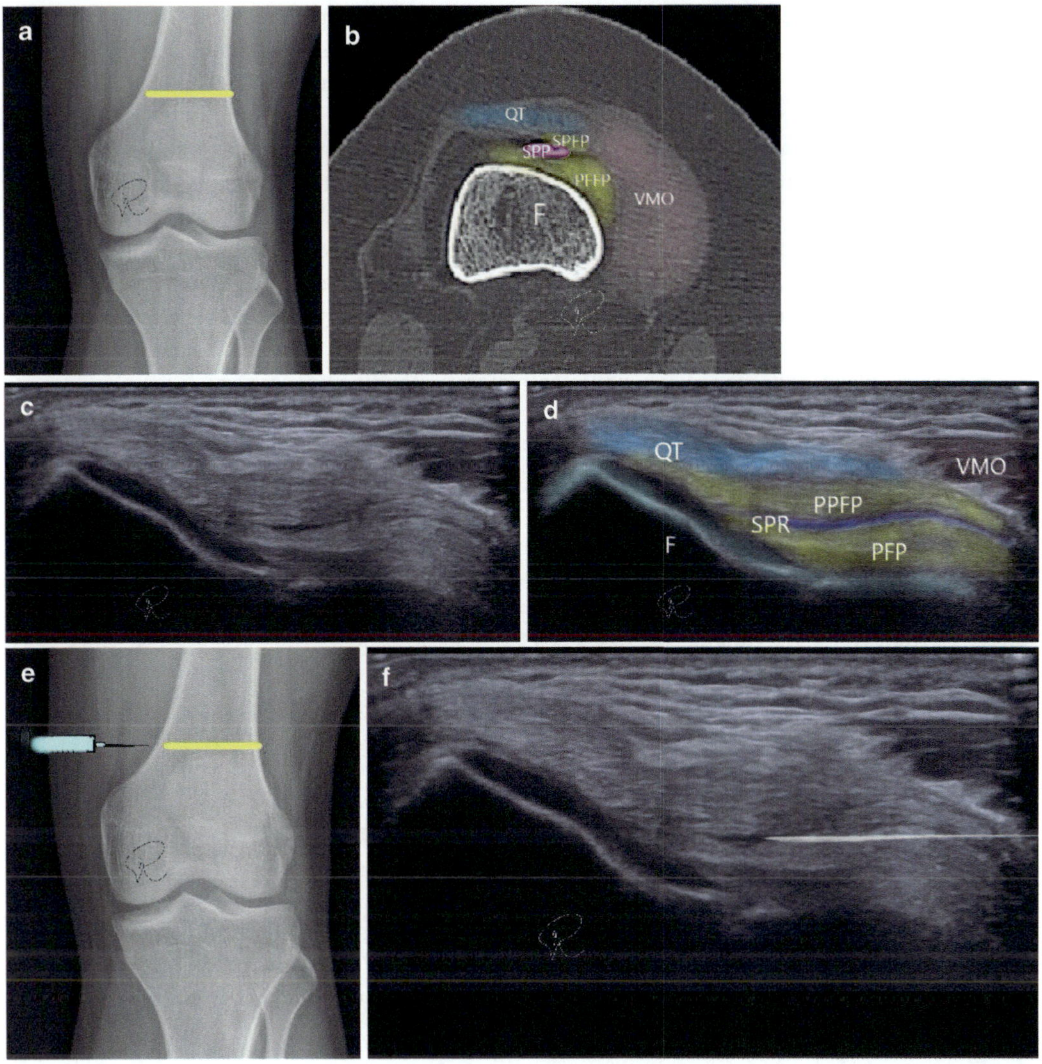

Fig. 6.2 Anterior superior knee transverse ultrasound scan. This composite image consists of six panels illustrating various imaging modalities and anatomical landmarks of the knee. Panel (**a**) features an X-ray of the knee, with a yellow line indicating the position of the ultrasound probe in the short-axis orientation. Panel (**b**) presents a cross-sectional MRI, annotated to highlight key anatomical structures for enhanced visualization and correlation with other imaging techniques. Panels (**c**) and (**d**) display ultrasound images of the knee, with panel (**d**) labeled to identify important sonoanatomical structures, including the suprapatellar fat pad (SPFP), pre-femoral fat pad (PFFP), suprapatellar recess (SPR), femur (F), and vastus medialis obliquus (VMO). Panel (**e**) shows another X-ray image, which includes an illustrated syringe to demonstrate the in-plane injection approach and indicate the recommended needle insertion point for intra-articular procedures. Finally, panel (**f**) provides an ultrasound-guided image of the knee, using the same d image featuring a visible needle to highlight the precision of ultrasound guidance for interventional procedures. These six panels offer a comprehensive overview of knee imaging, facilitating anatomical understanding, pathology assessment, and procedural guidance for ultrasound-guided interventions.

integrity, fat pad morphology, and any potential bursal inflammation. Power Doppler imaging may provide further insights into increased vascularity, which could indicate active inflammation, Hoffa's fat pad syndrome, or early-stage tendinopathy. Furthermore, ultrasound-guided procedures, including aspiration of prepatellar bursitis, corticosteroid injections aimed at treating Hoffa's fat pad inflammation, and needling techniques for addressing tendinopathy, can be executed with real-time imaging guidance to ensure accurate needle placement (Fig 6.3c) [4, 6].

6.2.3.2 Transverse: Patellar Tendon and Hoffa's Fat Pad, Knee Joint (Video 6.4)

Patient position: Lying down on the bed in the supine position. Have the patient bend the knee with a pillow under the knee.

Probe position: Place the probe on the patella's transverse plane and scan down until the patellar cortex disappears.

Scanning: To obtain a comprehensive transverse view of the patellar tendon and Hoffa's fat pad, it is imperative to position the ultrasound probe perpendicular to the long axis of the tendon. This should be done at the midpoint between the inferior pole of the patella and the tibial tuberosity, which allows for a clear cross-sectional assessment of the patellar tendon, the surrounding soft tissues, and the underlying knee joint structures. In the transverse plane, the patellar tendon is an oval, hyperechoic fibrillar structure that exhibits uniform thickness and echotexture. Notable changes, such as the presence of focal hypoechoic areas, may signify tendinosis or partial tears, while an increase in thickness may indicate chronic patellar tendinopathy. Additionally, calcifications can arise in degenerative conditions or enthesopathy, and any loss of the normal fibril-

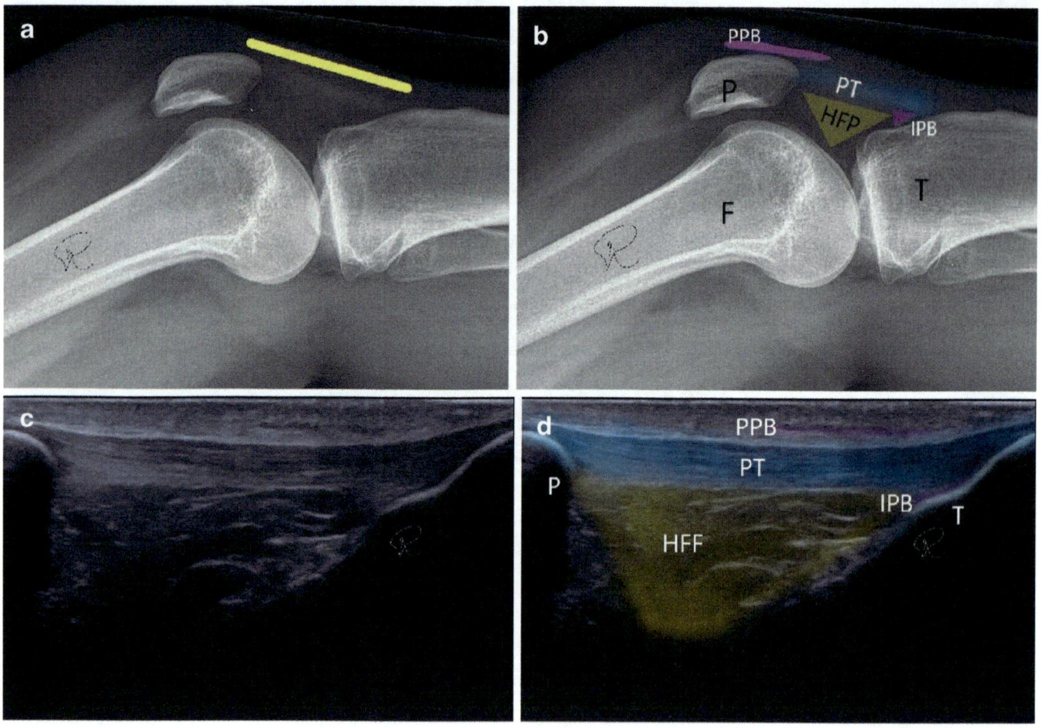

Fig. 6.3 Anterior inferior midsagittal knee ultrasound scan. The image features four panels that illustrate various imaging modalities of the knee joint, including X-ray, illustration, and ultrasound. Panel (**a**) displays an X-ray of the knee, with the patella highlighted and a yellow line indicating the probe's position for ultrasound imaging. Panel (**b**) presents an annotated X-ray, labeling key structures such as the patella (P), femur (F), tibia (T), prepatellar bursa (PPB), patellar tendon (PT), and Hoffa's fat pad (HFP). These anatomical structures are enhanced with colored overlays to improve visualization. Panel (**c**) showcases an ultrasound image of the knee joint, capturing important soft tissue and bony landmarks. Panel (**d**) features an annotated version of the ultrasound image, marking the same structures as in panel (**b**), along with additional colored overlays. This panel also includes the infrapatellar bursa (IPB) and Hoffa's fat pad (HFP), providing a more comprehensive view of the anatomical relationships within the knee. (© Reza Roghani 2024. All Rights Reserved)

lar pattern could hint at tendon injury or degeneration. Implementing dynamic scanning while having the patient contract their quadriceps muscles can further assist in assessing tendon mobility and revealing subtle abnormalities that may not be visible in static imaging. Hoffa's fat pad, situated deeper than the patellar tendon, typically appears hypoechoic and homogeneous, effectively filling the anterior compartment of the knee between the patellar tendon and the joint capsule. This fat pad maintains a uniform echotexture in a healthy knee without compressible areas. However, when viewed under Doppler imaging, inflammatory conditions, such as Hoffa's syndrome, may present with increased thickness, hypoechoic regions, or hypervascularity. Applying direct transducer compression to this area may reproduce pain, particularly in the inferomedial or inferolateral regions of the knee. The transverse view is particularly beneficial for guiding ultrasound procedures, such as administering corticosteroid or platelet-rich plasma injections for Hoffa's fat pad impingement (Fig. 6.4b).

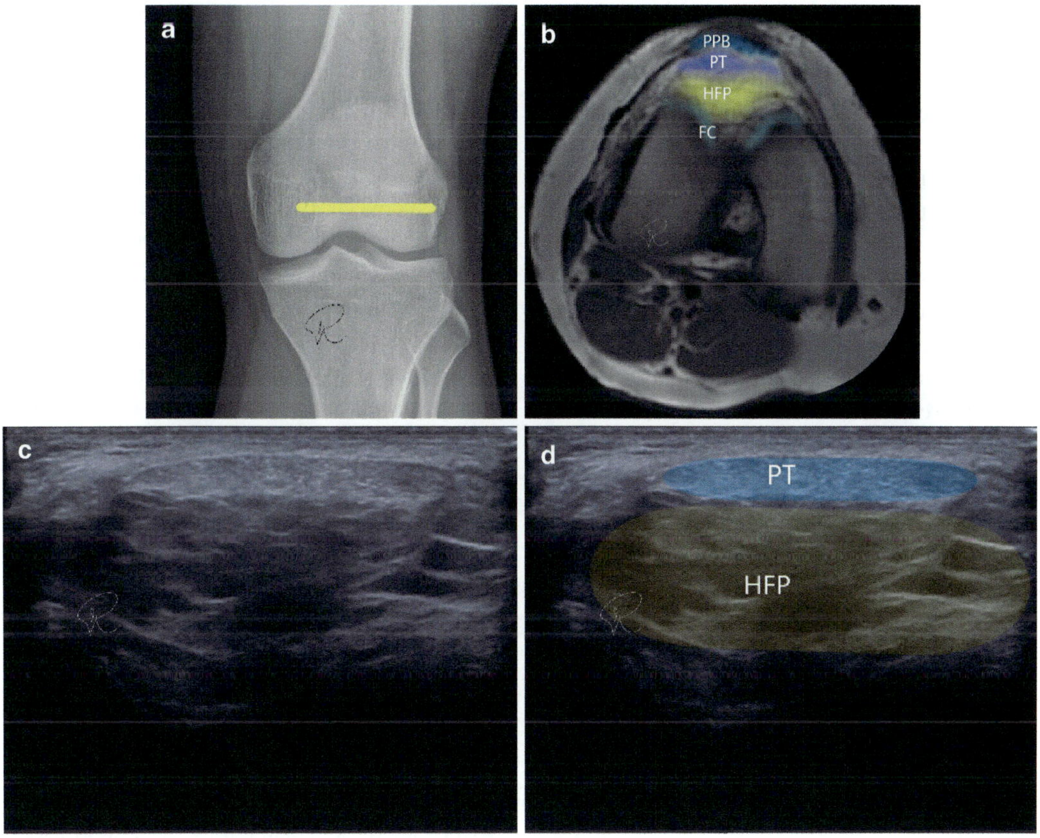

Fig. 6.4 Anterior inferior axial knee ultrasound scan. A composite image showcases four medical scans alongside an illustration of the anterior inferior knee compartment, each emphasizing different imaging modalities and anatomical structures. Image (**a**) features an X-ray marked with a yellow line that indicates the optimal probe positioning for ultrasound assessment. Image (**b**) is an MRI scan with distinct anatomical structures labeled and color-coded, such as the prepatellar bursa (PPB), patellar tendon (PT), Hoffa's fat pad (HFP), and femoral condyle (FC). Image (**c**) presents an unlabeled ultrasound scan of the knee, providing a grayscale representation of the relevant anatomical components. Image (**d**) is a corresponding ultrasound image that includes color-coded labels, identifying the patellar tendon (PT) in blue and Hoffa's fat pad (HFP) in yellow. These images illustrate the relationships between key structures in the anterior inferior knee in the short axis and their appearances across different imaging modalities, offering a comprehensive visual guide for clinical assessment and ultrasound-guided interventions. (© Reza Roghani 2024. All Rights Reserved)

6.3 Medial Knee

6.3.1 Anatomy

When examining the medial side of the knee, several vital anatomical structures must be considered for diagnostic and interventional considerations. The medial collateral ligament (MCL) spans from the medial condyle of the femur to the medial condyle of the tibia, serving a significant role in maintaining the stability of the knee joint by resisting valgus forces. Ultrasound imaging provides valuable insights into the fibrillar structure of the MCL and is crucial for identifying potential injuries such as sprains or tears [6]. Another important structure in the medial knee is the medial joint space, which houses the medial meniscus. While ultrasound predominantly visualizes the outer contour of the meniscus, it is instrumental in detecting joint effusions, synovial hypertrophy, and meniscal extrusion. Adjacent to this joint space is the pes anserinus complex, formed by the tendinous insertions of the sartorius, gracilis, and semitendinosus muscles. This composite tendon crosses over the MCL before its insertion on the anteromedial aspect of the tibia. Beneath it lies the pes anserine bursa, which can become inflamed, often resulting in pes anserine bursitis—a common etiology of medial knee pain (Fig. 6.5b) [7, 8]. The saphenous nerve, the terminal sensory branch of the femoral nerve, traces the path of the femoral artery within the sub sartorial (adductor) canal before emerging approximately four inches above the knee joint. It subsequently gives rise to the infrapatellar branch, providing sensory innervation to the anteromedial knee before extending down the leg. Understanding the saphenous nerve's trajectory is essential for minimizing the risk of iatrogenic injury during medial knee injections or nerve blocks [9, 10]. Moreover, the medial genicular nerves, which consist of superior and inferior branches, typically originate from the tibial nerve. In certain anatomical variations, these nerves may also receive contributions from the saphenous nerve. Their role in the innervation of the knee joint is significant, as they are frequently targeted in radiofrequency ablation procedures to manage chronic knee pain [11].

6.3.2 Scan

6.3.2.1 Medial-Central Knee Scan in the Coronal Plane: Joint Line, Medial Meniscus and Medial Collateral Ligament, Medial Genicular Nerves, Pes Anserine Tendons (Video 6.5)

Patient position: Lying down on the bed in the supine position. Have the patient bend the knee.

Probe position: Place the probe on the medial side of the knee in the coronal plane (Fig. 6.5a, b).

Scanning: Position the probe to visualize a V-shaped interruption in the deeper structures, located between two bright hyperechoic lines corresponding to the medial condyle of the femur and the medial condyle of the tibia, centrally displayed on the screen (Fig. 6.5c, d). This V-shaped structure represents the knee joint space. A wedge-shaped hypoechoic structure within this space can be seen, corresponding to the medial meniscus. To thoroughly assess the medial meniscus, scan both the anterior and posterior regions, looking for irregularities, tears, or signs of degenerative changes. The joint capsule and medial collateral ligament (MCL) are visible, overlaying the medial meniscus. The MCL, a crucial stabilizer of the medial knee, appears as a superficial hyperechoic fibrillar structure extending between the medial femoral and medial tibial condyle. Proper visualization of these structures is vital for assessing ligamentous integrity and identifying potential injuries, such as MCL sprains, meniscal degeneration, or joint effusion.

6.3.2.2 Medial-Superior Parasagittal Plane; Superior Medial Genicular Nerve (Video 6.6)

Patient position: Lying on the bed in the supine position, ask the patient to bend their knee.

Probe position: Place the probe on the medial side of the knee in the parasagittal plane (Fig. 6.6a, b).

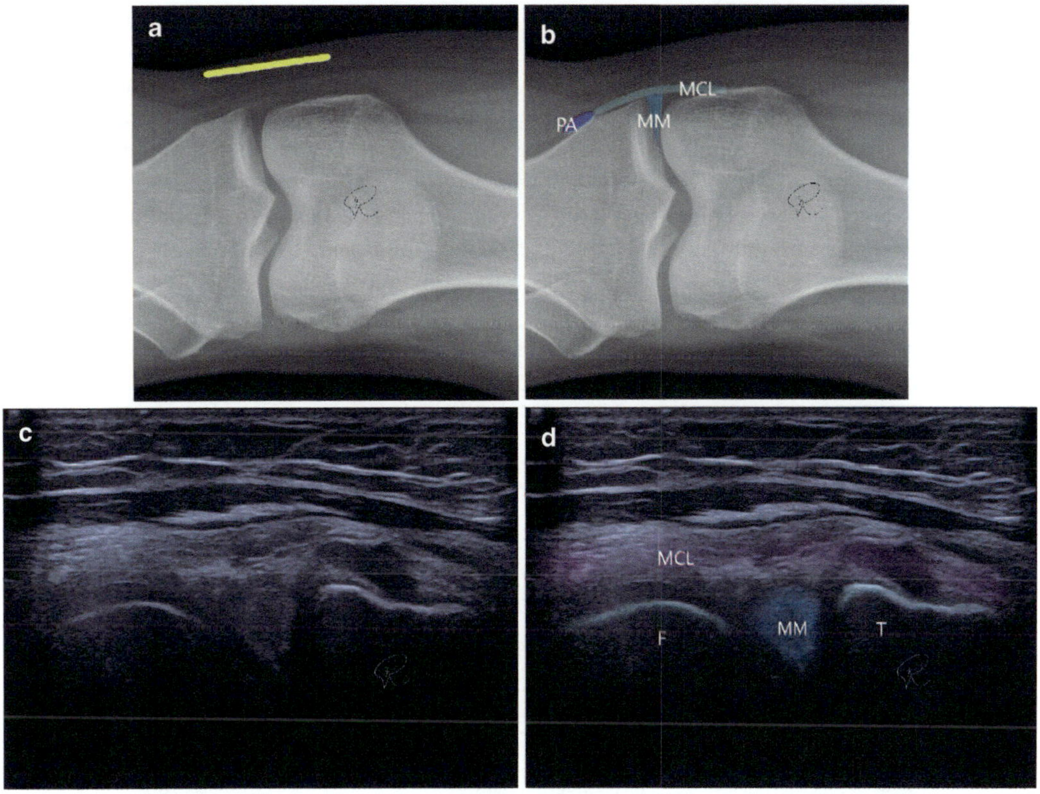

Fig. 6.5 Medial-central knee scan in the coronal plane. The composite image meticulously illustrates a comparative analysis of X-ray and ultrasound imaging techniques utilized for the evaluation of the medial knee joint. Panel (**a**) presents an X-ray image with a distinct yellow line that marks the precise location of the ultrasound probe during scanning. In panel (**b**), another X-ray is displayed, annotated with critical anatomical landmarks including the patella (PA), medial collateral ligament (MCL), and medial meniscus (MM), facilitating an understanding of the region's anatomy. Panel (**c**) showcases an unannotated ultrasound scan of the medial knee, allowing for an assessment of the imaging technique itself. Finally, panel (**d**) complements the previous ultrasound image with color overlays and labeled structures, emphasizing the medial collateral ligament (MCL), medial meniscus (MM), femur (F), and tibia (T). (© Reza Roghani 2024. All Rights Reserved)

Scanning: The medial superior genicular nerve and artery can be located at the junction of the femoral shaft and the medial femoral condyle. To visualize these structures, position the ultrasound probe in a parasagittal orientation along the medial aspect of the knee. The medial superior genicular artery typically appears as a pulsatile, hypoechoic circular, or tubular structure, depending on probe orientation. In contrast, the medial superior genicular nerve, a branch of the tibial nerve, is identified as a small, hyperechoic fascicular structure adjacent to the artery. Careful adjustment of the probe's angle and depth is essential to optimize visualization, as these structures are often closely associated with surrounding connective tissue and the vastus medialis muscle (Fig. 6.6c, d).

6.3.2.3 Medial-Superior Knee Scan in the Axial Plane; Saphenous Nerve (Video 6.7)

Patient position: Lying on the bed in the supine position, the patient is asked to bend their knee.

Probe position: Place the probe in the axial plane about 3–4 in. above the medial side of the knee (Fig. 6.7a, b).

Scanning: When conducting an ultrasound scan of the medial superior knee, identify the sartorius muscle. This hypoechoic, semi-oval structure is located in the superficial layer and serves as a crucial landmark for locating deeper neurovascular structures. A small, hyperechoic, honeycomb-like structure—the saphenous nerve—is positioned anterolaterally at the distal tip of the sartorius muscle. This nerve is the largest cutaneous branch of the femoral nerve, providing sensory innervation to the medial side of the knee and the lower leg. Beneath the saphenous nerve, you will observe a well-defined, round, hypoechoic structure exhibiting pulsatile movement. This structure represents the femoral artery, which is vital for providing vascular supply to the lower limb and can be easily recognized by its rhythmic pulsations during Doppler imaging. Next to the femoral artery, the femoral vein appears slightly larger and more oval-shaped. Unlike the artery, the vein is non-pulsatile and displays compressibility when gentle pressure is applied with the ultrasound probe. The proximity of these structures is particularly significant when performing ultrasound-guided interventions, such as nerve blocks or vascular access procedures (Fig. 6.7c, d).

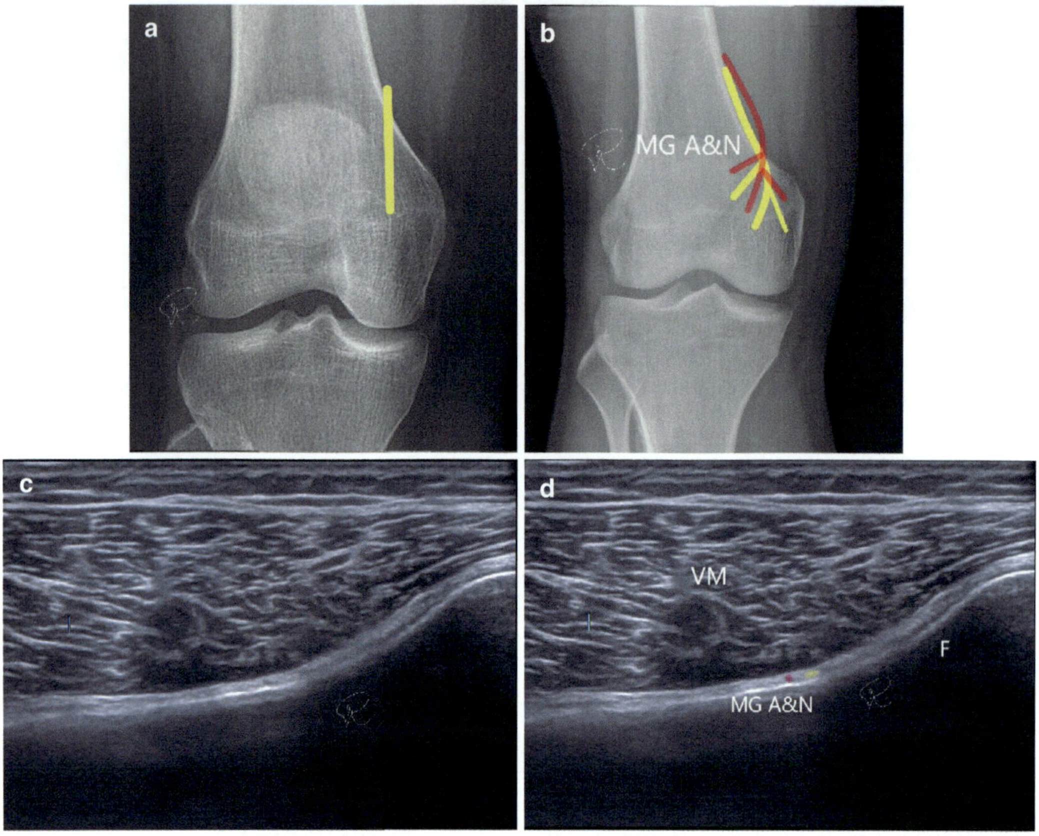

Fig. 6.6 Medial-superior knee scan in the coronal plane. The four-panel composite medical image presents knee scans utilizing various imaging modalities and orientations. Panel (**a**) features an X-ray of the knee, marked with a vertical yellow line that indicates the placement of the probe in a parasagittal long-axis orientation, thereby outlining the scanning plane. Panel (**b**) showcases another X-ray, emphasizing the medial genicular artery and nerve (MG A&N), marked with red and yellow lines to illustrate their anatomical trajectory. Panel (**c**) offers an ultrasound image of the knee, providing an unobstructed view of soft tissue structures without labels. Panel (**d**) presents a labeled and color-enhanced ultrasound image, identifying key anatomical features such as the vastus medialis (VM), the femur (F), and the medial genicular artery and nerve (MG A&N), which are identified as tiny red and yellow circles. (© Reza Roghani 2024. All Rights Reserved)

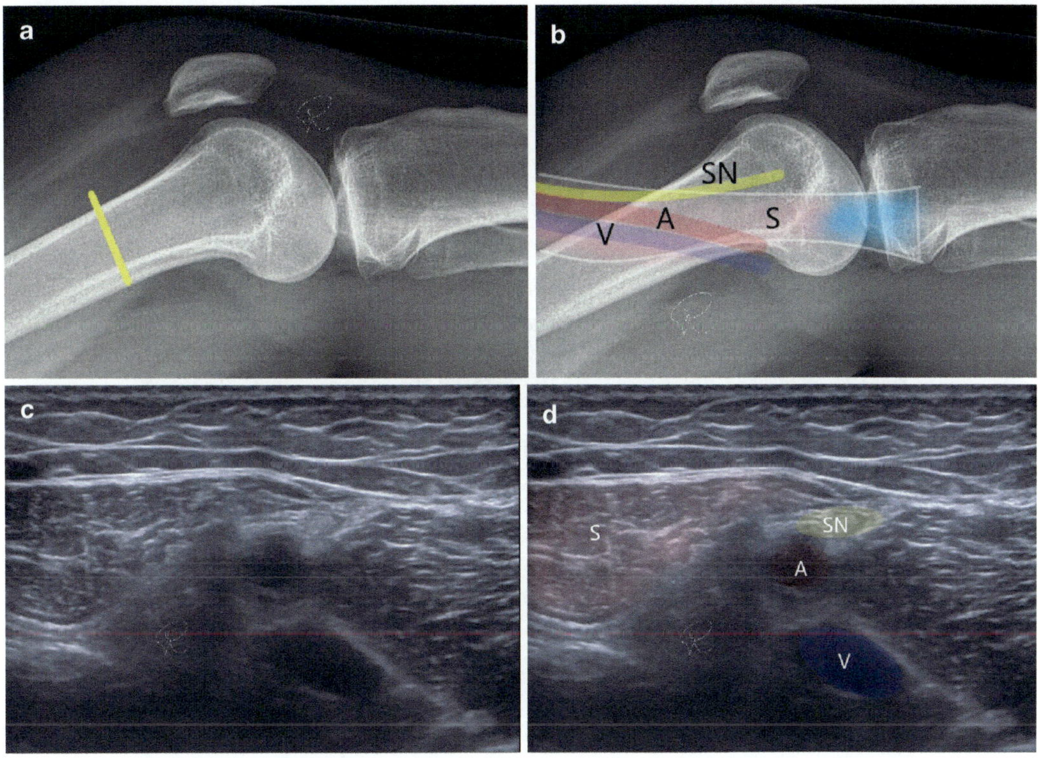

Fig. 6.7 Medial-superior knee axial scan. The image comprises four panels that offer a comparative view of the medial superior knee using various imaging modalities. Panel (**a**) displays a lateral X-ray of the knee, with a yellow line marking the probe placement for ultrasound scanning. Panel (**b**) features the same X-ray, enhanced with colored overlays that highlight essential anatomical structures, including the saphenous nerve (SN), artery (A), vein (V), and sartorius muscle (S), which aids in anatomical orientation. Panels (**c**) and (**d**) present ultrasound images of the medial superior knee in the short axis. In panel (**d**), color-coded overlays correspond to those in panel (**b**), effectively labeling the SN, A, V, and S for improved visualization of the neural, vascular, and muscular structures.

6.3.2.4 Medial-Inferior Knee Scan in the Coronal Plane; Medial Inferior Genicular Nerve (Video 6.8)

Patient position: Lying on the bed in the supine position, ask the patient to bend their knee.

Probe position: Put the probe in the mid-coronal plane, below the knee joint (Fig. 6.8a, b).

Scanning: To identify the medial inferior genicular artery and nerve, begin your examination at the junction of the tibial shaft and the medial condyle. The medial inferior genicular artery, a branch of the popliteal artery, travels along the posterior aspect of the tibial condyle before curving anteriorly to supply the medial structures of the knee. Accompanying the artery is the medial inferior genicular nerve, a branch of the tibial nerve, which follows a similar path and plays a crucial role in providing sensory innervation to the knee joint. On ultrasound, both structures appear as small, closely associated tubular or circular formations, depending on the orientation of the probe; the artery is hypoechoic while the nerve appears hyperechoic. [12, 13]. Continuing in the same scanning plane and moving distally, you will observe the pes anserinus, formed by the confluence of three tendons: the sartorius, gracilis, and semitendinosus. These tendons insert onto the anteromedial aspect of the proximal tibia, creating a distinct triangular shape on ultrasound. They are represented as hyperechoic fibrillar structures, best visualized in the longitudinal plane. Between the pes anserine tendons and the underlying medial tibia lies the pes anserine bursa, a potential space that reduces friction between the tendons and the bone. Under normal conditions, the bursa may not be easily visible; however, in cases of bursitis, it can be identified as a hypoechoic or anechoic fluid-filled area, often with thickening of the bursal walls (Fig. 6.8c, d).

6.4 Lateral Knee

6.4.1 Anatomy

When assessing the lateral aspect of the knee, it is crucial to identify several key anatomical structures for a comprehensive evaluation. The lateral collateral ligament (LCL) extends from

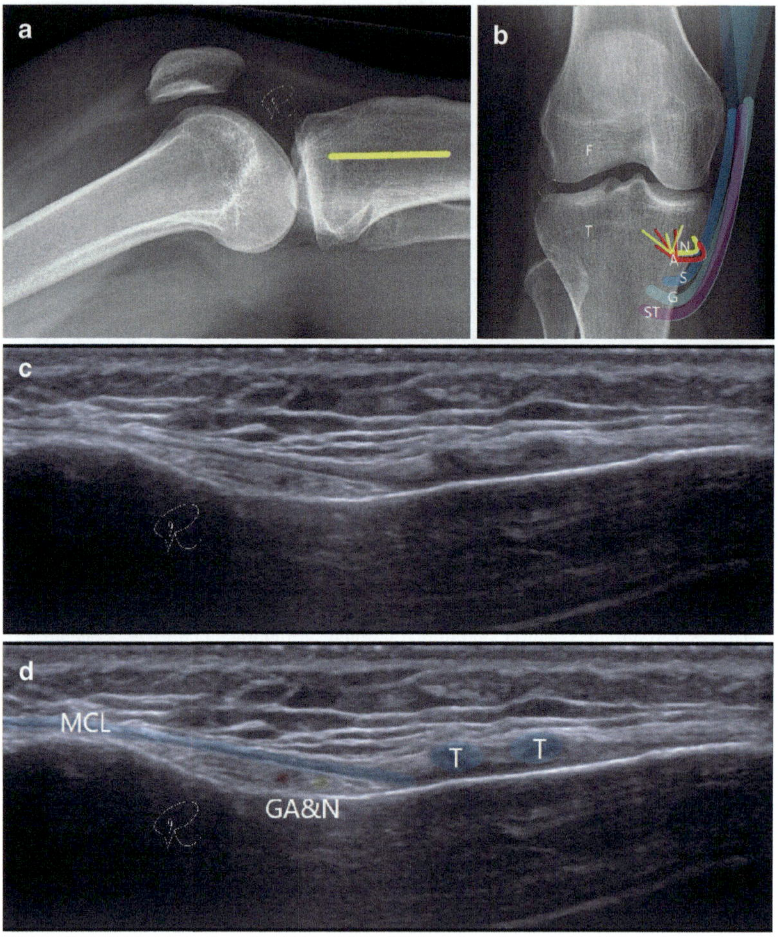

Fig. 6.8 Medial inferior knee ultrasound scan in the coronal plane. The image is composed of four panels, and it provides a detailed view of the medial inferior knee region through X-ray and ultrasound imaging. Panel (**a**) features a lateral X-ray of the knee joint, with a yellow line indicating the probe position to denote the scanning plane. This effectively highlights the joint space and the key bony landmarks of the femur and tibia. Panel (**b**) showcases an anteroposterior X-ray of the knee, enhanced with colored overlays that outline critical anatomical structures, including the femur (F), tibia (T), genicular nerve (N), and genicular artery (A). Additionally, the tendons of the sartorius (S), gracilis (G), and semitendinosus (ST) muscles converge at the pes anserinus insertion, illustrating their anatomical relationships within the medial knee. Panel (**c**) presents an ultrasound image of the medial inferior knee, capturing the medial inferior genicular artery and nerve (MIG A&N) alongside the pes anserinus area. The vascular and neural elements are displayed in relation to the surrounding soft tissue structures. Panel (**d**) offers the same ultrasound image, now labeled with key anatomical structures. The medial collateral ligament (MCL), medial inferior genicular artery and nerve (MIG A&N), and the pes anserinus tendons (T) are identified.

the lateral femoral condyle to the head of the fibula, providing essential lateral stability to the knee joint. In contrast to the medial collateral ligament, the LCL does not have a direct attachment to the meniscus, allowing for greater lateral mobility. Within the lateral joint space lies the lateral meniscus, a shock absorber between the femoral and tibial surfaces. While ultrasound can visualize the outer margin of the meniscus, its deeper portions may be less distinguishable without advanced imaging techniques such as MRI. The iliotibial band (ITB) is another important structure that runs over the lateral femoral condyle and attaches to Gerdy's tubercle on the anterolateral aspect of the tibia. As the most superficial structure in this region, the ITB plays a significant role in lateral knee stabilization and movement, especially during activities involving repetitive knee flexion and extension, such as running and cycling. The biceps femoris tendon, part of the hamstring muscle group, inserts onto the head of the fibula and aids in knee flexion and external rotation. Due to its anatomical location, it is particularly vulnerable to injury, especially in athletes participating in high-impact sports. Beneath the LCL lies the popliteus muscle, which originates from the lateral femoral condyle and runs obliquely toward the posteromedial aspect of the tibial shaft. This muscle is vital for knee stability as it unlocks the knee joint from full extension and helps control rotational movements. Some of its fibers attach to the lateral meniscus, facilitating its dynamic movement during knee motion. Understanding the intricate relationships between these structures is essential for diagnosing lateral knee pain, evaluating the integrity of ligaments and tendons, and informing interventional procedures when needed [14, 15].

6.4.2 Scan

6.4.2.1 Lateral Knee in Coronal Plane: Lateral Joint Line, Lateral Collateral Ligament (LCL), Lateral Meniscus, Iliotibial Band (ITB), Popliteus Tendon (Video 6.9)

Patient position: Lying down on the bed in the supine position. Have the patient bend the knee with a pillow under the knees.

Probe position: Place the probe on the lateral side of the knee in the coronal plane (Fig. 6.9a, b).

Scanning: Position the ultrasound probe to visualize a V-shaped interruption in the deep, bright lines, representing the lateral condyle of the femur and the lateral condyle of the tibia, located at the center of the screen. Within this V-shaped space is a triangular hypoechoic structure—the lateral meniscus—a crucial shock absorber between the femoral and tibial surfaces. Superficial to the lateral meniscus is a thin, fibrillar hyperechoic band that extends proximally from the lateral thigh and inserts into Gerdy's tubercle on the tibia; this structure is known as the iliotibial band (ITB). As the most superficial lateral structure of the knee, the ITB plays an essential role in lateral knee stabilization and movement. Just proximal to the joint line, within a distinct groove on the femoral bone, lies an oval-shaped hypoechoic structure—the popliteus tendon. The popliteus muscle serves as a key dynamic stabilizer of the knee, particularly in controlling rotation and assisting in unlocking the knee from full extension (Fig 6.9c,d) [16, 17].

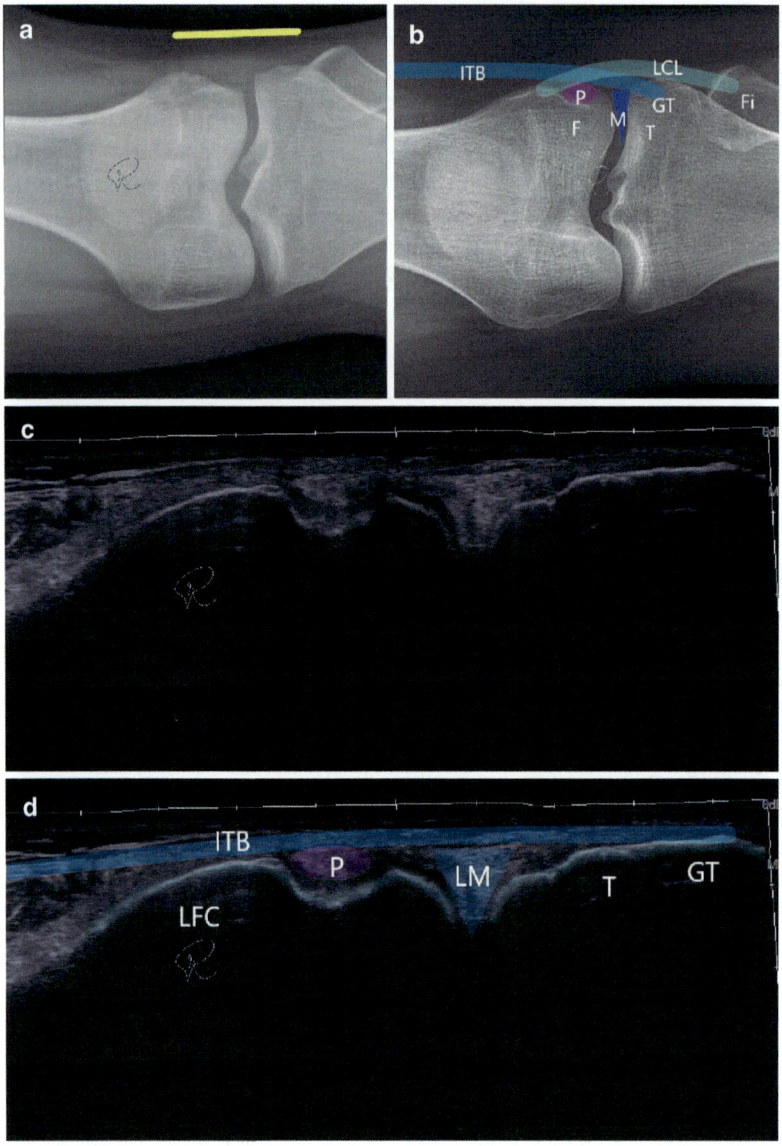

Fig. 6.9 Lateral knee ultrasound scan in the coronal plane. The image features four panels that provide a comprehensive view of the lateral knee joint using different imaging modalities. Panel (**a**) displays a lateral knee X-ray with a yellow line indicating the probe's position for ultrasound scanning. This serves as a reference to understand the scanning plane utilized in the subsequent ultrasound images. Panel (**b**) includes another X-ray that identifies key anatomical landmarks: the Tibial bone (T), Femur (F), Lateral Collateral Ligament (LCL), Gerdy's Tubercle (GT), Fibula (Fi), Popliteus (P), and Lateral Meniscus (LM). These annotations help recognize the significant bony and soft tissue structures important for the lateral knee's stability and function. Panel (**c**) presents a panaromic ultrasound image of the lateral knee, showcasing soft tissue structures and their relation to bony landmarks. This image offers a detailed perspective on structures not visible in x-rays, such as tendons, ligaments, and menisci. Panel (**d**) features a labeled same (c) ultrasound image that highlights essential anatomical components, including the Iliotibial Band (ITB), Lateral Femoral Condyle (LFC), Popliteus Tendon (P), Lateral Meniscus (LM), Tibia (T), and Gerdy's Tubercle (GT). (© Reza Roghani 2024. All Rights Reserved)

6.5 Posterior Knee

6.5.1 Anatomy

The posterior aspect of the knee is home to several crucial anatomical structures, including muscles, tendons, bursae, blood vessels, and nerves, all of which play significant roles in the function, stability, and circulation of the knee joint. Among these structures, the semimembranosus-gastrocnemius bursa, often referred to as baker's cyst, is of particular clinical importance. This fluid-filled sac is located in the medial popliteal fossa, nestled between the medial head of the gastrocnemius muscle and the semimembranosus tendon. Its primary function is to minimize friction between these anatomical components. However, it can become pathologically enlarged, resulting in posterior knee pain and limited mobility. The vascular network in this area is primarily composed of the popliteal artery and vein, which traverse the popliteal fossa. The popliteal artery is a continuation of the femoral artery and is vital for supplying blood to the lower leg. Surrounding this artery are various muscular branches that either connect to or originate from deeper vascular structures. These branches supply essential blood to the hamstrings, gastrocnemius, and popliteus muscles, making them critical for proper circulation. Conditions such as popliteal artery entrapment syndrome and deep vein thrombosis warrant careful evaluation of these vessels. The sciatic nerve follows a posterior course along the thigh before reaching the popliteal fossa, where it bifurcates approximately five centimeters above the knee crease into two major branches. The tibial nerve continues down the posterior leg, innervating the calf muscles and the plantar surface of the foot. Conversely, the common fibular (peroneal) nerve moves around the head of the fibula, supplying the anterior and lateral compartments of the lower leg. These nerves are essential for both motor and sensory functions of the lower limb, and their compression or injury may lead to neuropathies, muscle weakness, or foot drop. Additionally, the hamstring tendons offer structural support to the posterior knee. The biceps femoris tendon, representing the lateral hamstring, inserts into the fibular head and is integral for knee flexion and external rotation. On the medial side, the semitendinosus and semimembranosus tendons insert into the tibia, assisting in knee flexion and internal rotation. The popliteus muscle, situated deep within the fossa, acts as a dynamic stabilizer of the knee, originating from the posterior tibia and inserting onto the lateral femoral condyle, playing a crucial role in unlocking the knee from full extension by internally rotating the tibia. A comprehensive understanding of posterior knee anatomy is essential for diagnosing various clinical conditions, including Baker's cysts, popliteal artery aneurysms, deep vein thrombosis, hamstring tendon injuries, and nerve entrapments [18–20] (Fig. 6.11).

6.5.2 Scan: Posterolateral

6.5.2.1 Posterolateral Knee in Sagittal Plane: Joint Line and Lateral Meniscus, Lateral Head of the Gastrocnemius (Video 6.10)

Patient position: Have the patient lie prone and extend the knee.

Probe position: Position the probe on the lateral side of the popliteal fossa in the sagittal plane (Fig. 6.10a, b).

Scanning: Ultrasound examination of the posterolateral knee reveals two prominent convex structures representing the femoral and tibial condyles, with the joint line distinctly visible between them. At the center of the image, you can identify the lateral meniscus, which appears as a well-defined triangular cartilage structure that is essential for joint stability and shock absorption. Positioned directly above the meniscus is the lateral head of the gastrocnemius muscle, recognizable as a relatively hypoechoic structure due to its muscular composition [21, 22] (Fig. 6.10c, d).

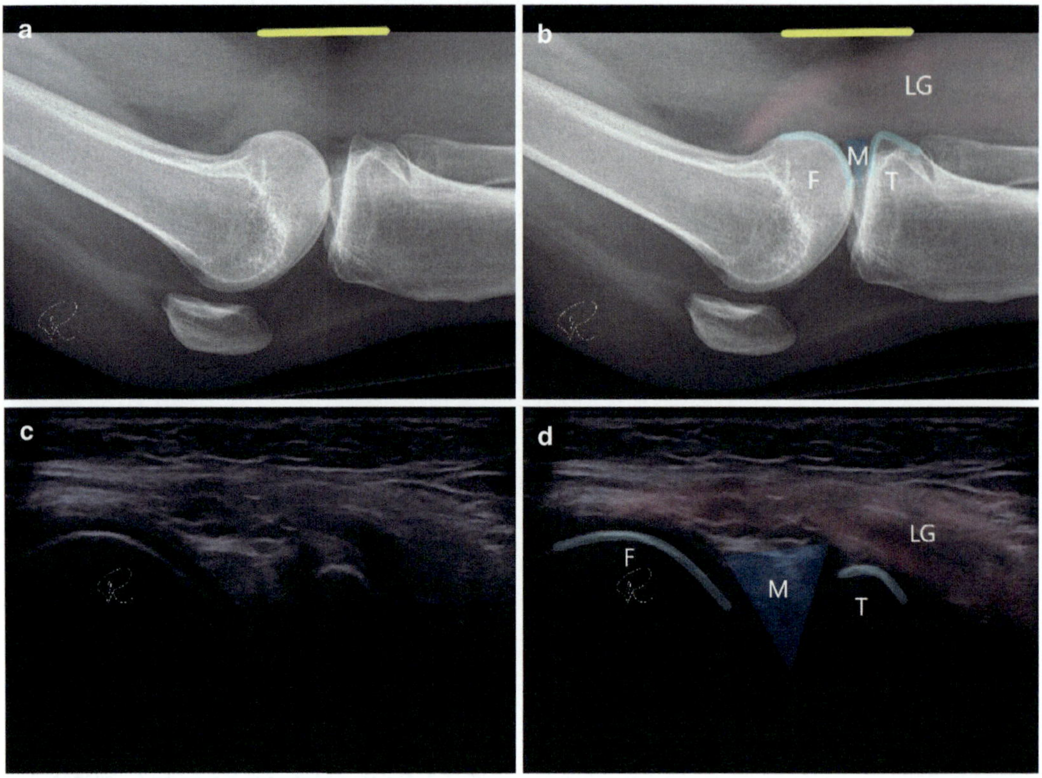

Fig. 6.10 Posterior lateral knee ultrasound scan in the sagittal plane. The image consists of four panels that offer a detailed view of the posterior knee joint through X-ray, illustration, and ultrasound imaging. Panel (**a**) features a standard knee X-ray showing the femur and tibia, with a yellow line indicating the probe's position for ultrasound scanning. Panel (**b**) presents an annotated X-ray that highlights key anatomical structures, including the femur (F), tibia (T), meniscus (M), and lateral gastrocnemius (LG), which helps to illustrate the relationship between the bony and soft tissue components. Panel (**c**) displays an ultrasound image of the posterior knee, revealing soft tissue structures such as the popliteal vessels, hamstring tendons, and gastrocnemius muscle. Finally, panel (**d**) provides the corresponding annotated ultrasound image, labeling the femur (F), tibia (T), meniscus (M), and lateral gastrocnemius (LG), which offers a thorough depiction of the anatomical landmarks and their spatial relationships. (© Reza Roghani 2024. All Rights Reserved)

6.5.2.2 Posterolateral Knee in Transverse Plane: Tibial Nerve, Common Peroneal Nerve (Video 6.11)

Patient position: Have the patient lie prone and extend the knee.

Probe position: Place the probe on the popliteal fossa lateral side in the sagittal plane as above, then rotate it 90°.

Scanning: Deep in the image, you will see a pulsatile vascular structure, the popliteal artery; on top of that, a compressible non-pulsatile hypo density, the popliteal vein; and above it, two honeycomb structures [23, 24]. The lateral one is the common peroneal nerve, and the medial one is the tibial nerve (Fig. 6.11).

6.5.3 Scan: Posteromedial Knee

6.5.3.1 Posteromedial Knee in Sagittal Plane; Semimembranosus Tendon, Gastrocnemius Medial Belly, Backer Cyst (Video 6.12)

Patient position: Have the patient lie prone and extend the knee.

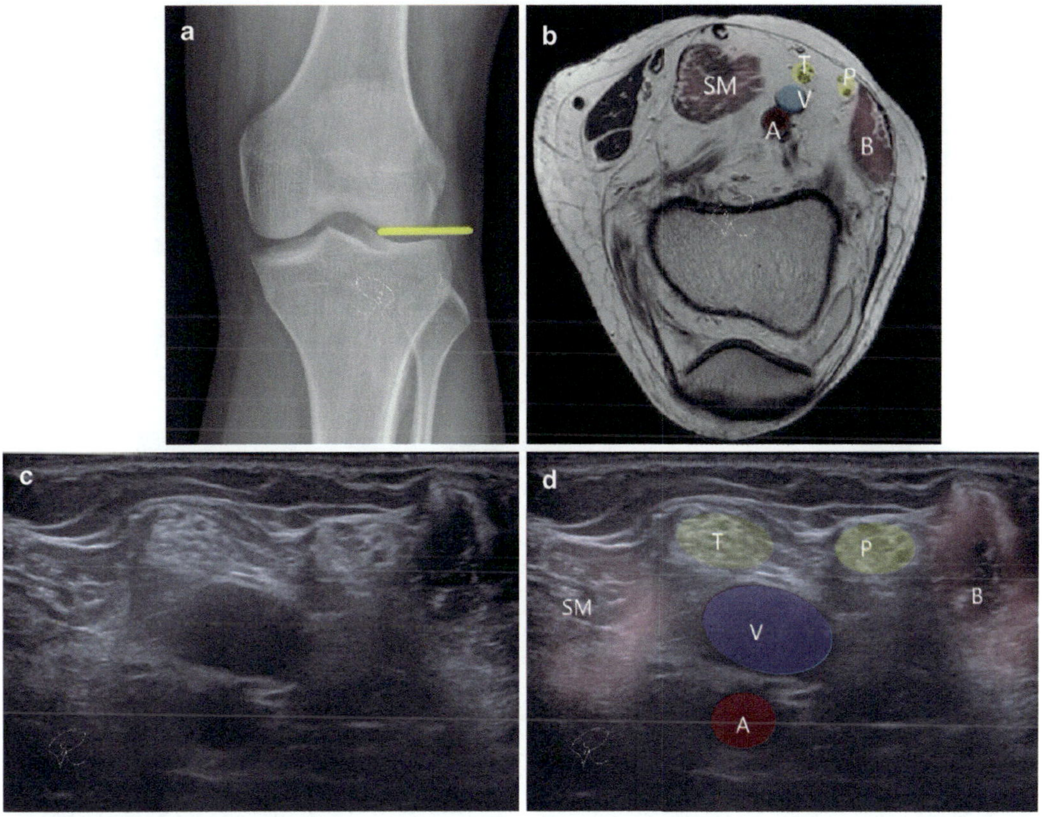

Fig. 6.11 Posterior lateral knee ultrasound scan in the axial plane. The image set offers a cross-sectional axial anatomical assessment of the knee joint utilizing various imaging modalities. Panel (**a**) displays an X-ray in the anteroposterior (AP) view, illustrating the knee joint with a yellow line indicating the probe positions for ultrasound scanning. Panel (**b**) features an MRI cross-section that provides a high-resolution visualization of both soft tissue and neurovascular structures. Key anatomical components are labeled, including the semimembranosus muscle (SM), popliteal artery (A), popliteal vein (V), peroneal nerve (P), tibial nerve (T), and biceps femoris (B). Panel (**c**) presents an unlabeled ultrasound scan, showing real-time soft tissue structures without annotations. In contrast, Panel (**d**) is a labeled ultrasound image that highlights crucial elements such as the semimembranosus (SM), tibial nerve (T), peroneal nerve (P), popliteal vein (V), popliteal artery (A), and biceps femoris (B). (© Reza Roghani 2024. All Rights Reserved)

Probe position: Place the probe in the sagittal plane on the popliteal fossa medial side.

Scanning: You will see two convex structures and the joint line in between. The medial meniscus is a triangular cartilage located at the center of this image. The medial head of the gastrocnemius and semimembranosus are found on top of the tibial condyle. Then, rotate the probe 90°. This image shows the musculotendinous junction of the medial belly of the gastrocnemius on the lateral side and the semimembranosus tendon on the medial side. In between is the potential site of baker's cyst (Fig. 6.12) [18, 25, 26].

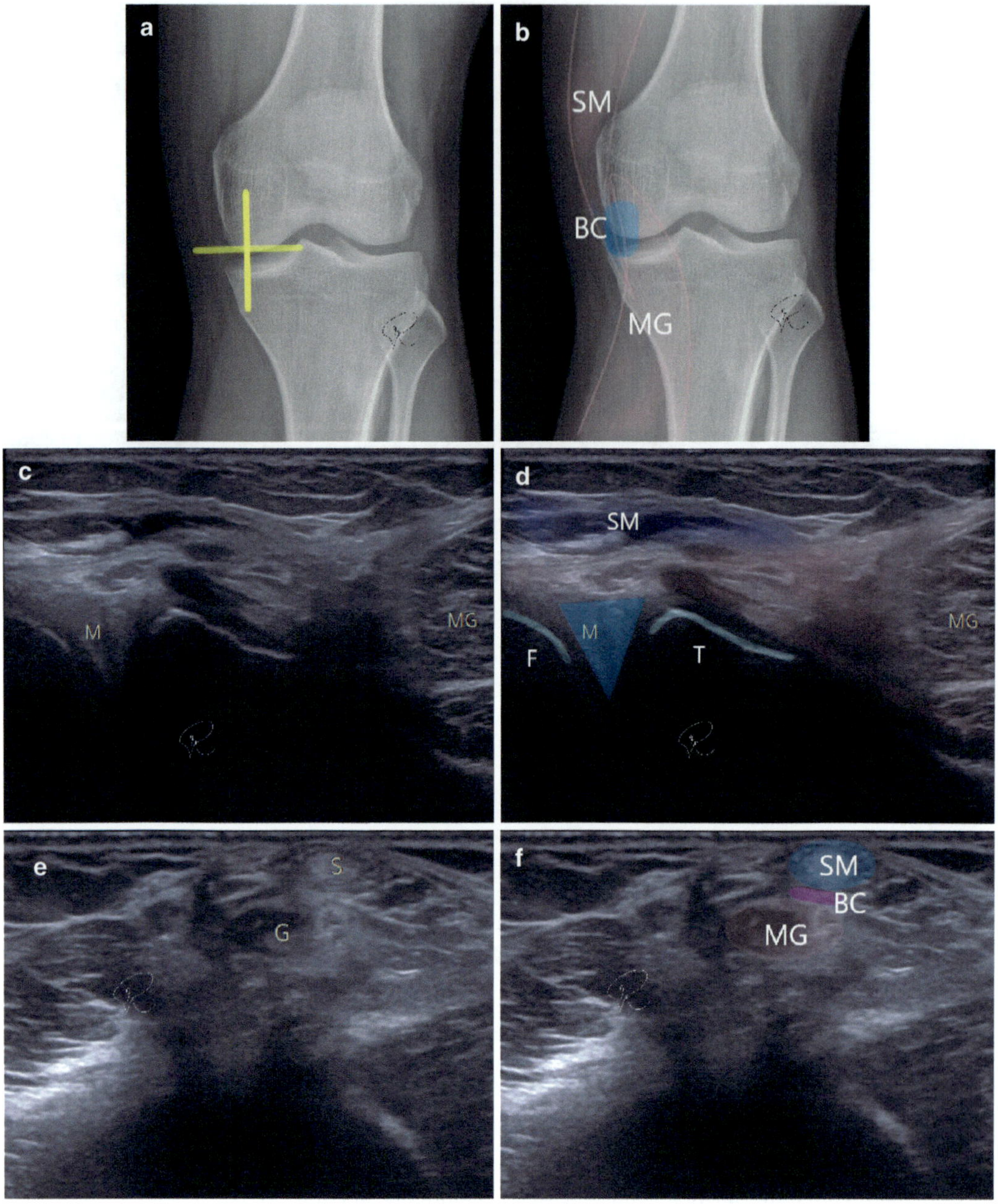

Fig. 6.12 Posteromedial knee scan. The image set consists of six panels that provide a detailed examination of the knee joint through X-ray and ultrasound imaging. Panels (**a**) and (**b**) feature X-ray images, with panel (**a**) emphasizing the knee joint and probe positioning via yellow lines. Panel (**b**) annotates key anatomical structures, which include the semimembranosus muscle (SM), baker's cyst (BC), and medial gastrocnemius (MG). Panels (**c**) and (**d**) offer long-axis ultrasound views, while panels (**e**) and (**f**) present short-axis ultrasound perspectives. Panel (**c**) identifies the meniscus (M) along with the medial gastrocnemius (MG). Panel (**d**) enhances visualization with color overlays, labeling the semimembranosus (SM), meniscus (M), femur (F), tibia (T), and medial gastrocnemius (MG). Panel (**e**) focuses on the semimembranosus (SM) and gastrocnemius (G). Finally, panel (**f**) further highlights semimembranosus (SM), the potential site of baker's cyst (BC), and medial gastrocnemius (MG), incorporating additional color overlays to illustrate their anatomical relationships clearly. (© Reza Roghani 2024. All Rights Reserved)

References

1. Gupton M, Imonugo O, Black AC, Launico MV, Terreberry RR. Anatomy, bony pelvis, and lower limb, knee. In: StatPearls. StatPearls Publishing; 2024. http://www.ncbi.nlm.nih.gov/books/NBK500017/.
2. Vaienti E, Scita G, Ceccarelli F, Pogliacomi F. Understanding the human knee and its relationship to total knee replacement. Acta Biomed. 2017;88(Suppl 2):6–16. https://doi.org/10.23750/abm.v88i2-S.6507.
3. Pinskerova V, Vavrik P. Knee anatomy and biomechanics and its relevance to knee replacement. In: Rivière C, Vendittoli P-A, editors. Personalized hip and knee joint replacement. Cham: Springer; 2020. p. 159–68. https://doi.org/10.1007/978-3-030-24243-5_14.
4. Basha MAA, Eldib DB, Aly SA, Azmy TM, Mahmoud NEM, Ghandour TM, Aly T, Mostafa S, Elaidy AM, Algazzar HY. Diagnostic accuracy of ultrasonography in the assessment of anterior knee pain. Insights Imaging. 2020;11:107. https://doi.org/10.1186/s13244-020-00914-2.
5. Wu W-T, Chang K-V, Nanka O, Mezian K, Ricci V, Wang B, Özçakar L. Ultrasound imaging of the articularis genus muscle: implications for ultrasound-guided suprapatellar recess injection. Diagnostics. 2024;14(2):183. https://doi.org/10.3390/diagnostics14020183.
6. Draghi F, Ferrozzi G, Urciuoli L, Bortolotto C, Bianchi S. Hoffa's fat pad abnormalities, knee pain, and magnetic resonance imaging in daily practice. Insights Imaging. 2016;7(3):373–83. https://doi.org/10.1007/s13244-016-0483-8.
7. Amis AA, Robinson JR. The anatomy and biomechanics of the medial collateral ligament and posteromedial corner of the knee. In: Bonnin M, Amendola A, Bellemans J, MacDonald S, Ménétrey J, editors. The knee joint: surgical techniques and strategies. Paris: Springer; 2012. p. 23–30. https://doi.org/10.1007/978-2-287-99353-4_3.
8. Dasari SP, Kerzner B, Fortier LM, Gursoy S, Chahla J. Key surgically relevant anatomy of the medial and lateral aspects of the knee. Oper Tech Sports Med. 2022;30(2):150908. https://doi.org/10.1016/j.otsm.2022.150908.
9. Ghosh A, Chaudhury S. Morphology of saphenous nerve in cadavers: a guide to saphenous block and surgical interventions. Anat Cell Biol. 2019;52(3):262–8. https://doi.org/10.5115/acb.19.031.
10. Herman DC, Vincent KR. Saphenous neuropathy—a masquerading cause of anteromedial knee pain. Curr Sports Med Rep. 2018;17(6):177. https://doi.org/10.1249/JSR.0000000000000488.
11. Roberts SL, Stout A, Dreyfuss P. Review of knee joint innervation: implications for diagnostic blocks and radiofrequency ablation. Pain Med. 2020;21(5):922–38. https://doi.org/10.1093/pm/pnz189.
12. Tan YL, Neo EJR, Wee TC. Ultrasound-guided genicular nerve blockade with pharmacological agents for chronic knee osteoarthritis: a systematic review. Pain Physician. 2022;25(4):E489–502.
13. Wong J, Bremer N, Weyker PD, Webb CAJ. Ultrasound-guided genicular nerve thermal radiofrequency ablation for chronic knee pain. Case Rep Anesthesiol. 2016;2016:8292450. https://doi.org/10.1155/2016/8292450.
14. James EW, LaPrade CM, LaPrade RF. Anatomy and biomechanics of the lateral side of the knee and surgical implications. Sports Med Arthrosc Rev. 2015;23(1):2–9. https://doi.org/10.1097/JSA.0000000000000040.
15. Park J-G, Han S-B, Rhim HC, Jeon OH, Jang K-M. Anatomy of the anterolateral ligament of the knee joint. World J Clin Cases. 2022;10(21):7215–23. https://doi.org/10.12998/wjcc.v10.i21.7215.
16. Falkowski AL, Jacobson JA, Gandikota G, Lucas DR, Magerkurth O, Zaottini F. Imaging characteristics of the proximal lateral collateral ligament of the knee: findings on ultrasound and MRI with histologic correlation. J Ultrasound Med. 2022;41(4):827–34. https://doi.org/10.1002/jum.15761.
17. Rocha de Faria JL, Crespo B, Guesser MW, da Silva Araújo JH, Feitosa Bezerra PÊ, Menegassi ZJB, de Souza SAL, Pereira HM, Mozella AP, LaPrade RF, Guimarães JAM. Ultrasound with stress for assessing injuries to the medial and lateral collateral ligaments of the knee. Arthrosc Tech. 2024;13:103009. https://doi.org/10.1016/j.eats.2024.103009.
18. Leib AD, Roshan A, Foris LA, Varacallo M. Baker's cyst. In: StatPearls. StatPearls Publishing; 2024. http://www.ncbi.nlm.nih.gov/books/NBK430774/.
19. Greenwood K, van Zyl R, Keough N, Hohmann E. Defining the popliteal fossa by bony landmarks and mapping the courses of the neurovascular structures for application in popliteal fossa surgery. Anat Cell Biol. 2021;54(1):10–7. https://doi.org/10.5115/acb.20.179.
20. Nichols JS, Ashford RU. Surgical anatomy & pathology of the popliteal fossa. Orthop Trauma. 2013;27(2):113–7. https://doi.org/10.1016/j.mporth.2013.02.011.
21. Sekiya JK, Swaringen JC, Wojtys EM, Jacobson JA. Diagnostic ultrasound evaluation of posterolateral corner knee injuries. Arthroscopy. 2010;26(4):494–9. https://doi.org/10.1016/j.arthro.2009.08.023.
22. Wu W-T, Onishi K, Mezian K, Nanka O, Wang B, Su DC-J, Ricci V, Chang K-V, Özçakar L. Ultrasound imaging of the posterior lateral corner of the knee: a pictorial review of anatomy and pathologies. Insights Imaging. 2024;15(1):39. https://doi.org/10.1186/s13244-024-01606-x.
23. Singh AP, Chandak S, Agarwal A, Malhotra A, Jain A, Khan AA. Utility of high-resolution sonography for evaluation of knee joint pathologies as a screening tool. J Diagn Med Sonogr. 2021;37(6):556–67. https://doi.org/10.1177/87564793211035773.

24. Stoianov AG, Patrascu JM, Hogea BG, Andor B, Florescu S, Misca LC, Laza R, Fericean RM, Mavrea A, Terzi A, Patrascu JM. Point-of-care ultrasound for the evaluation and management of posterior cruciate ligament injuries: a systematic review. Diagnostics. 2023;13(14):2352. https://doi.org/10.3390/diagnostics13142352.
25. Frush TJ, Noyes FR. Baker's cyst. Sports Health. 2015;7(4):359–65. https://doi.org/10.1177/1941738113520130.
26. Li TY. The sonographic spectrum of baker cysts. J Diagn Med Sonogr. 2018;34(1):38–48. https://doi.org/10.1177/8756479317733750.

Ankle and Foot

7

Yashar Eshraghi, Reza Salman Roghani,
Mihir Nakrani, Ceci Guerrero, Nicole Schneider,
and Shravan Gupta

7.1 Introduction

The ankle represents a complex and dynamic region of the musculoskeletal system, encompassing multiple interconnected joints—including the ankle joint and subtalar joint—alongside a sophisticated network of tendons, ligaments, muscles, and nerves. It is essential to have a thorough understanding of anatomy to conduct precise ultrasound evaluations. To optimize scanning and maintain a systematic approach, the ankle is typically divided into four primary anatomical zones: anterior, medial, posterior, and lateral. Often, it is essential to extend the examination into the foot to enhance diagnostic accuracy and support comprehensive pain management strategies.

Key ligamentous structures, such as the anterior talofibular ligament and the deltoid ligament, can be visualized using high-resolution ultrasound, thereby improving the precision of structural assessments. The real-time assessment of the Achilles tendon and plantar fascia aids in identifying tendinopathies and fasciopathies in clinical practice. Additionally, focused scanning of the tibial nerve provides valuable insights into entrapment syndromes and neuropathic conditions affecting the ankle and foot.

This chapter also addresses ultrasound-guided interventions, including joint injections for the ankle and subtalar joints, tendinitis injections targeting structures like the Achilles tendon, and nerve blocks for the tibial nerve and its branches. Step-by-step scanning protocols and detailed interventional techniques aim to facilitate targeted treatments and improve patient outcomes in the diagnosis and management of ankle-related disorders.

Supplementary Information The online version contains supplementary material available at https://doi.org/10.1007/978-3-031-81037-4_7.

Y. Eshraghi
Division of Pain Medicine, Department of Anesthesiology and Critical Care Medicine, Ochsner Health System, University of Queensland Ochsner Medical School, New Orleans, LA, USA

R. S. Roghani (✉) · M. Nakrani · C. Guerrero
Department of Physical Medicine and Rehabilitation, Larkin Community Hospital, Nova Southeastern University, Miami, FL, USA

N. Schneider
Dr. Kiran C. Patel College of Osteopathic Medicine, Nova Southeastern University, Fort Lauderdale, FL, USA

S. Gupta
Coastal Interventional Pain & Spine Center, Seminole, FL, USA

7.1.1 Ankle Cross-Sectional Anatomy

The right ankle joint's top-down cross-section view reveals several important anatomical structures. The extensor hallucis longus is located at the top (noon position), the anterior tibialis ten-

R. S. Roghani, J. J. Diaz (eds.), *Video Atlas of Neuromusculoskeletal Ultrasound*,
https://doi.org/10.1007/978-3-031-81037-4_7

don is on its medial side, and the tendon complex of the extensor digitorum longus is on its lateral side. Below the extensor hallucis longus and above the talus lies a neurovascular complex that houses the anterior tibial artery and the deep peroneal nerve (Fig. 7.1) [1].

Starting from the 3 o'clock position and moving clockwise, we encounter the lateral malleolus. Positioned behind it, from 4 to 6 o'clock, are the tendons of the peroneus brevis and longus as well as a neurovascular complex comprising the sural nerve, lateral peroneal artery, and vein. The Achilles tendon is located at 6 o'clock, with the flexor hallucis longus tendon deep within it. Moving toward the medial and anterior, a neurovascular bundle containing the tibial nerve, posterior tibial artery, and vein can be found. Situated at the 8 and 9 o'clock positions are the flexor digitorum longus and posterior tibialis tendons, and anterior to that, we see the medial malleolus. Finally, to complete the circle, we can pinpoint the saphenous nerve and superficial vein at the 10–11 o'clock position (Fig. 7.1) [2–4].

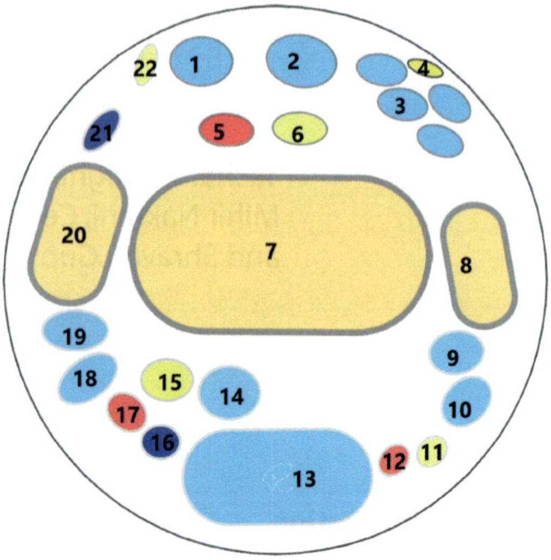

Fig. 7.1 Ankle schematic cross-sectional anatomy. A circular diagram featuring various colored and numbered sections illustrates a cross-section of the ankle at the level of the talus dome. The central sections, labeled 7, 8, and 20, are highlighted in yellow-orange to represent the bony structures of the ankle. Surrounding these central sections are smaller segments, color-coded to differentiate the anatomical components: blue for tendons, yellow for nerves, red for arteries, and purple for veins. Each structure is numbered sequentially as follows: (1) Anterior tibialis tendon, (2) Extensor hallucis longus, (3) Extensor digitorum longus, (4) Superficial peroneal nerve, (5) Dorsalis pedis artery, (6) Deep peroneal nerve, (7) Talus, (8) Lateral malleolus, (9) Peroneus brevis, (10) Peroneus longus, (11) Sural nerve, (12) Lateral ankle artery, (13) Achilles tendon, (14) Flexor hallucis longus, (15) Tibial nerve, (16) Tibial vein, (17) Tibial artery, (18) Flexor digitorum longus, (19) Posterior tibialis, (20) Medial malleolus, (21) Saphenous vein, (22) Saphenous nerve. This labeled cross-section serves as a detailed anatomical reference, clearly illustrating the spatial relationships between bones, tendons, nerves, arteries, and veins within the ankle joint. (© Reza Roghani 2024. All Rights Reserved)

7.1.2 Ankle Ultrasound Protocol

Anterior Compartment

- **Sagittal View:** Evaluate the ankle joint space, anterior tibia, and talar dome.
- **Transverse View:** Visualize the dorsalis pedis artery and nerve, extensor tendons (extensor hallucis longus and extensor digitorum longus), and the anterior joint capsule.

Medial Compartment

- **Short-Axis View:** Assess the tibialis posterior tendon, flexor digitorum longus tendon, flexor hallucis longus tendon, tibial nerve, posterior tibial artery, and deltoid ligament complex.

Posterior Compartment

- **Sagittal View:** Visualize the Achilles tendon, subtalar joint, posterior ankle joint, and tibial nerve.
- **Transverse View:** Evaluate the Achilles tendon, retrocalcaneal bursa, and tibial nerve.

Lateral Compartment

- **Short-Axis View at the Level of the Lateral Malleolus:** Identify the peroneus longus and peroneus brevis tendons, sural nerve, and subtalar joint.

- **Short-Axis View Anterior and Distal to the Lateral Malleolus:** Assess the sinus tarsi and surrounding ligamentous structures.

7.1.3 Foot Ultrasound Protocol

Plantar Aspect
- **Long-Axis View:** Examine the plantar fascia, particularly for thickening or tears.
- **Short-Axis View:** Focus on the plantar fascia insertion at the calcaneus for enthesopathy or fasciitis.

Dorsal Aspect
- **Sagittal View**: Evaluate the metatarsophalangeal (MTP) and proximal interphalangeal (PIP) joints.
- **Transverse View:** Assess the interdigital nerves for neuroma or entrapment.

7.2 Anterior Ankle

7.2.1 Anatomy

The anterior ankle region is composed of bones, muscles, tendons, ligaments, nerves, and blood vessels that work together to support movement and stability. The primary bony structures include the distal tibia and fibula, which form the superior and lateral aspects of the ankle mortise, and the talus, which articulates with them at the talocrural joint. The inferior tibiofibular joint, a syndesmotic joint between the tibia and fibula, is stabilized by the anterior inferior tibiofibular ligament.The anterior compartment of the leg houses several muscles that contribute to dorsiflexion and toe movement. The tibialis anterior originates from the lateral tibia and interosseous membrane and inserts on the medial cuneiform and first metatarsal, playing a key role in dorsiflexion and inversion. The extensor hallucis longus, originating from the anterior fibula and interosseous membrane, extends the great toe and assists in dorsiflexion. The extensor digitorum longus, which arises from the lateral tibial condyle, fibula, and interosseous membrane, extends the lateral four toes and contributes to dorsiflexion. The fibularis tertius, if present, originates from the distal fibula and inserts on the base of the fifth metatarsal, aiding in dorsiflexion and eversion.Ligaments in this region include the anterior inferior tibiofibular ligament, which supports the syndesmosis, and the anterior talofibular ligament, which is the most commonly injured ligament in ankle sprains.The deep peroneal nerve runs through this region, providing motor innervation to the anterior compartment muscles and sensory innervation to the first web space of the foot. The anterior tibial artery, which courses alongside the deep peroneal nerve, supplies blood to this area before continuing as the dorsalis pedis artery.In a cross-sectional view at the level of the anterior ankle, the tibialis anterior is positioned medially, while the extensor hallucis longus and extensor digitorum longus lie centrally and laterally, respectively. The deep peroneal nerve and anterior tibial artery are located between the extensor hallucis longus and tibialis anterior. Laterally, the fibula and the anterior talofibular ligament provide structural support, while the tibia and the anterior inferior tibiofibular ligament are found medially. Understanding this anatomical layout is essential for diagnosing and managing conditions such as anterior ankle impingement, tendonitis, andfractures [4].

7.2.2 Scan (Videos 7.1 and 7.2)

Patient position: The patient should lie on their back with their knees bent at a 90° angle and the soles of their feet resting on the bed.

Probe position: Position the ultrasound probe on the skin's surface at the midpoint of the ankle in a sagittal plane (Fig. 7.2a) to visualize the dome of the talus. Then, place the talus neck at the center and rotate the probe 90° to a transverse plane (Fig. 7.2b).

Scanning: This positioning will allow visualization of the tibialis anterior tendon far medially, followed by the extensor hallucis longus tendon lateral to it. More laterally, the extensor digitorum longus tendon will be displayed. Below the extensor hallucis longus, the pulsatile hypoechoic

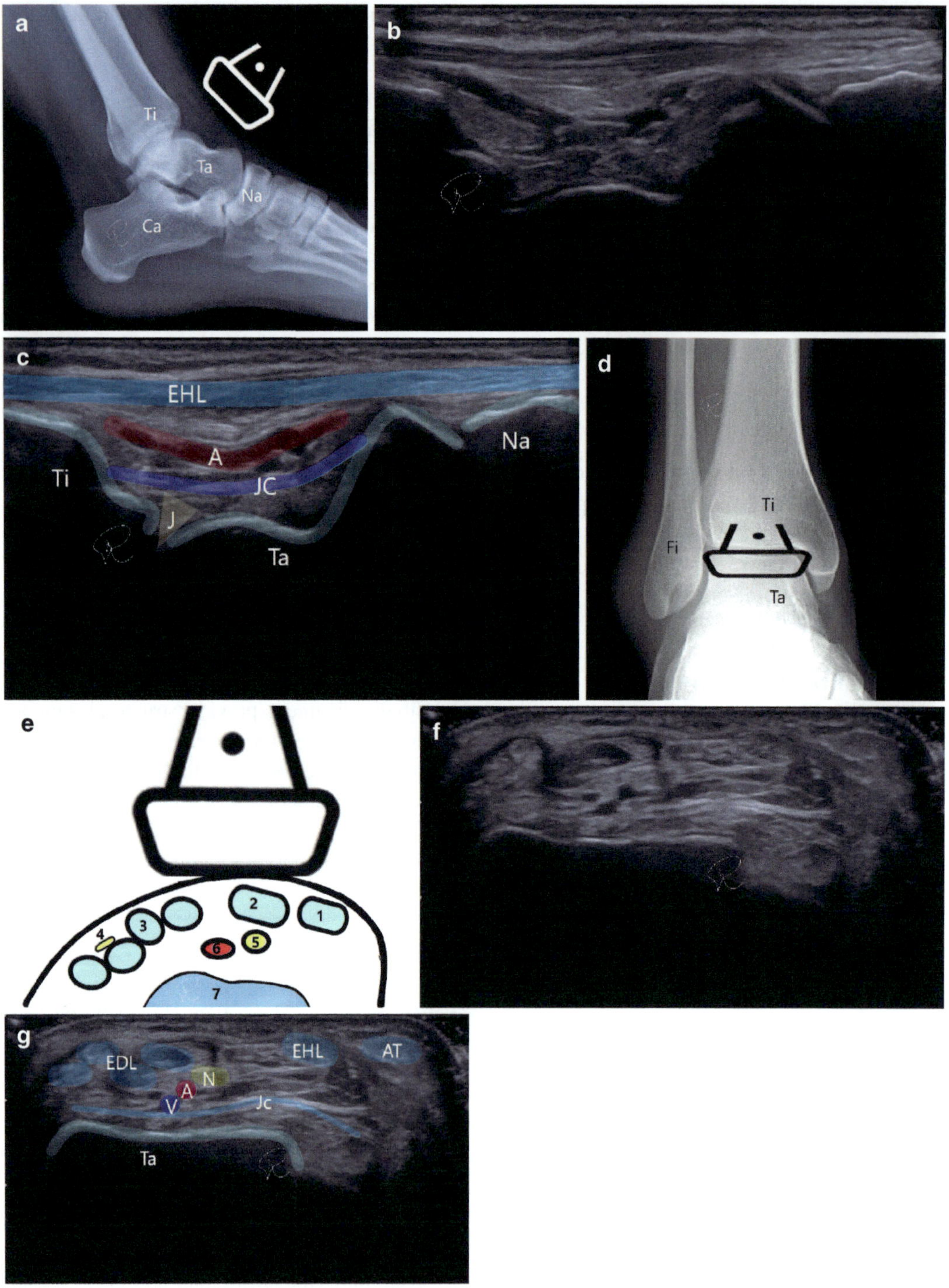

Fig. 7.2 Anterior ankle scanning, sagittal and axial scan. The image presents a detailed overview of the ankle region through a composite of seven panels incorporating various imaging techniques and schematic representations. Panel (**a**) features a lateral X-ray of the ankle, clearly marked with the tibia (Ti), talus (Ta), navicular (Na), and calcaneus (Ca). The ultrasound probe's position at the center illustrates the long-axis view probe placement. In Panel (**b**), an ultrasound image of the ankle is showcased, emphasizing real-time visualization of the

structure of the anterior tibial artery and the deep peroneal nerve honeycomb structure will be visible (Fig. 7.2g, h). Above the previously mentioned tendons lie the extensor retinaculum, which appears as a relative hyperechoic band stretching from the anterior border of the tibial bone to the fibula (Fig. 7.2h).

7.2.3 Procedure

7.2.3.1 Anterior Tarsal Tunnel (Video 7.3)

Anterior Tarsal Tunnel Syndrome (ATTS) is a condition characterized by the irritation or compression of the deep peroneal nerve as it traverses the tarsal tunnel located at the front of the ankle. Although it is less common than other entrapment neuropathies, such as posterior tarsal tunnel syndrome, ATTS can lead to significant discomfort and functional impairment if not accurately diagnosed and treated. The anterior tarsal tunnel serves as a narrow passage for tendons, nerves, and blood vessels. The deep peroneal nerve runs through this tunnel and can become compressed in the anterior region of the ankle. Various factors can contribute to the onset of anterior tarsal tunnel syndrome, including anatomical variations, trauma or injury, overuse, tumors or cysts, and inflammation. Patients typically experience sharp or burning pain on the top of the foot or ankle, which may radiate toward the toes. Activities such as walking or running often exacerbate this pain. Diagnosing anterior tarsal tunnel syndrome generally involves a comprehensive medical history and physical examination. A crucial diagnostic test is Tinel's sign, where percussion over the deep peroneal nerve can elicit a tingling or shock-like sensation along the nerve's pathway. Imaging modalities like ultrasound or MRI may be utilized to identify anatomical abnormalities, tumors, or cysts that are compressing the nerve. Treatment approaches vary based on the severity of symptoms and the underlying cause. Initially, conservative measures—such as rest, ice application, nonsteroidal anti-inflammatory drugs (NSAIDs), and physical therapy—are often effective. Modifications to footwear or the use of orthotics can also help reduce pressure on the nerve. In certain cases, corticosteroid injections into the tarsal tunnel may be employed to diminish inflammation and alleviate symptoms [5].

The procedure involves using a fine-gauge needle and a small syringe to inject a local anesthetic, such as lidocaine or bupivacaine, and a corticosteroid if needed. The injection is typically guided by ultrasound in the transverse plane to accurately target the suspected site of DPN nerve entrapment (see Fig. 7.3). The needle is carefully inserted beneath the tibialis anterior tendon and guided in-plane using real-time ultrasound imaging to approach the deep peroneal nerve. The ultrasound offers continuous feedback, ensuring precise needle placement while avoiding adjacent structures. Once the needle reaches the targeted area near the nerve, the injectate is administered slowly and accurately to the site of nerve entrapment or inflammation. Following the injection, the needle is removed, and a sterile dressing is applied to the injection site to reduce the risk of infection and maintain

Fig. 7.2 (continued) anatomical structures within the region. Panel (**c**) takes the ultrasound image from Panel (**b**). It applies color-coding to highlight better key anatomical elements, including the extensor hallucis longus (EHL), anterior tibial artery (A), joint capsule (JC), tibia (Ti), talus (Ta), navicular (Na), and the ankle joint (J), improving clarity for the viewer. Panel (**d**) provides an anteroposterior X-ray view of the ankle, with noted structures such as the tibia (Ti), fibula (Fi), and talu (Ta). The ultrasound probe's position at the center illustrates the short-axis view probe placement. Panel (**e**) provides a schematic representation of ankle anatomy, featuring numbered labels (1–7) that indicate the various components of the tendon and neurovascular bundle located at the anterior aspect of the ankle. This comprehensive breakdown is further clarified with numbered labels corresponding to specific structures: (1) Anterior tibialis tendon, (2) Extensor hallucis longus, (3) Extensor digitorum longus, (4) Superficial peroneal nerve, (5) Deep peroneal nerve, (6) Dorsalis pedis artery, and (7) Talus bone. Panel (**f**) contains another ultrasound image of the anterior ankle in the short axis. The image represented in Panel (**g**) is an enhanced version of image (**f**), utilizing a color-coded scheme to label key anatomical structures effectively. Among these are the extensor digitorum longus (EDL), extensor hallucis longus (EHL), anterior tibialis tendon (AT), artery (A), vein (V), nerve (N), talus (Ta), and joint capsule (Jc).

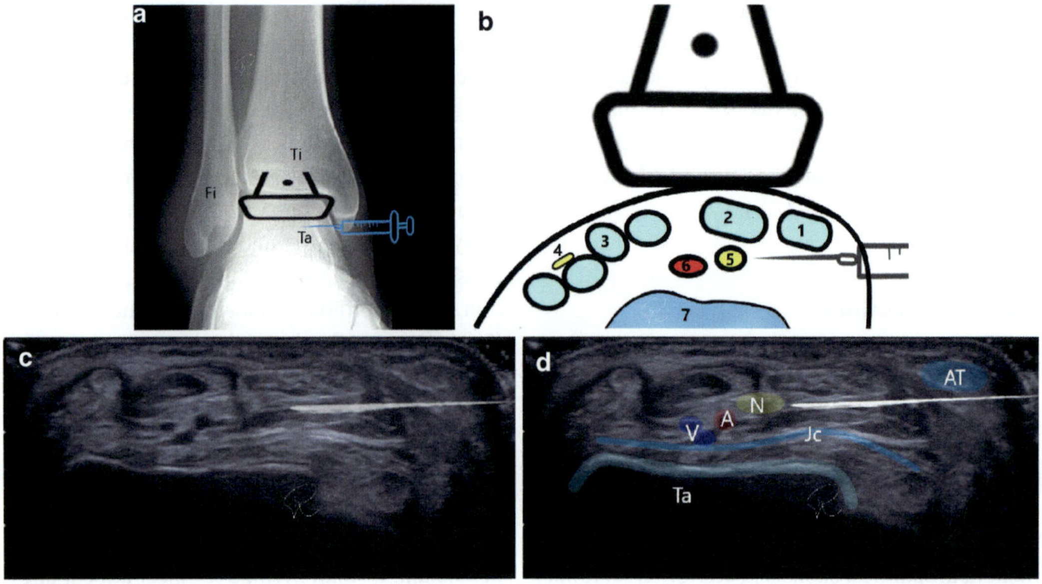

Fig. 7.3 Anterior tarsal tunnel ultrasound-guided needle approach. The image comprises four panels that illustrate the anterior tarsal tunnel injection procedure. Panel (**a**) features an X-ray of the ankle, clearly labeling the bones—the tibia (Ti), fibula (Fi), and talus (Ta)—and displaying the probe's position to demonstrate the ideal alignment for the procedure. The syringe in the image indicates the needle insertion point and highlights the in-plane approach necessary for accurate delivery of the injectate. Panel (**b**) presents a cross-sectional ankle diagram with numbered and color-coded structures outlining the injection path. Panels (**c**) and (**d**) consist of ultrasound images capturing real-time guidance during the procedure. Specifically, panel (**c**) shows the trajectory of the needle. In contrast, panel (**d**) emphasizes relevant anatomical structures, including the vein (V), artery (A), nerve (N), joint capsule (Jc), and anterior tibialis tendon (AT). The structures are numbered as follows: (1) Anterior tibialis tendon, (2) Extensor hallucis longus, (3) Extensor digitorum longus, (4) Superficial peroneal nerve, (5) Dorsalis pedis artery, (6) Deep peroneal nerve, and (7) Talus bone. Overall, these panels provide a thorough visual guide for executing the anterior tarsal tunnel injection procedure, offering anatomical context and proper technique.

cleanliness. The patient is typically monitored for any immediate adverse reactions before being discharged.

7.2.3.2 Ankle Joint (Videos 7.4 and 7.5)

Ankle joint pain can originate from a multitude of conditions, ranging from acute injuries to chronic disorders. Among the most prevalent causes of ankle pain are sprains and strains, which occur when the ligaments or muscles surrounding the ankle are overstretched or ripped, frequently due to abrupt twisting motions or high-impact activities. A sprained ankle is the most common injury, predominantly affecting the lateral ligaments. Arthritis, encompassing osteoarthritis and rheumatoid arthritis, is another significant source of ankle pain. Osteoarthritis results from cumulative wear and tear, while rheumatoid arthritis is an autoimmune condition. Both types of arthritis contribute to joint pain, stiffness, and swelling. Ankle impingement is characterized by the pinching or compression of soft tissues around the ankle during movement, resulting in pain, swelling, and restricted mobility. Management of ankle pain may include the RICE protocol—rest, ice, compression, elevation—alongside anti-inflammatory medications, physical therapy, injections, or surgical intervention in severe cases. Moreover, injecting therapeutic agents into the anterior ankle joint is a commonly executed procedure to alleviate pain and inflammation associated with arthritis and synovitis. This procedure typically involves the administration of corticosteroids, local anesthetics, or other medications directly into the joint, facilitating a reduction in swelling, enhancement of mobility, and relief from chronic pain. Often performed under ultrasound guidance, this approach ensures precise needle placement, minimizing risk and optimizing therapeutic outcomes [6].

To minimize patient discomfort, a small-gauge needle, usually 22–25 gauge, and a syringe ranging from 3 to 5 mL are utilized for this injection. The injection contains a blend of local anesthetic and corticosteroid. The recommended entry point, when viewed from a transverse plane, is the medial side of the anterior tibialis tendon, which is sufficiently distant from the anterior neurovascular bundle. It is crucial to conduct a transverse plane scan of the anterior ankle to accurately locate the joint, neurovascular complex, and anterior tibialis tendon (refer to Fig. 7.4). While constantly monitoring with ultrasound, the needle should be inserted below and medial to the tibialis anterior tendon, approaching the joint in-plane under real-time ultrasound guidance.

The sagittal plane provides an alternative approach, as illustrated in the image below. Begin by scanning the joint in the axial plane to identify the anterior tibialis and extensor hallucis longus tendons, as detailed in Sect. 7.2.2. Center the space between these two tendons on the screen. Next, rotate the probe 90 degrees to shift to the sagittal plane. It is crucial to ensure that neither the tendon nor the neurovascular bundles are within your field of view. Insert the needle from the proximal aspect, guiding it towards the joint, as demonstrated in Sect. 7.5 (Fig. 7.5).

7.3 Medial Ankle

7.3.1 Anatomy

The medial ankle, particularly the tarsal tunnel, represents a significant anatomical region posterior to the medial malleolus, through which vital neurovascular and tendinous structures traverse a fibro-osseous tunnel. This tunnel's configuration

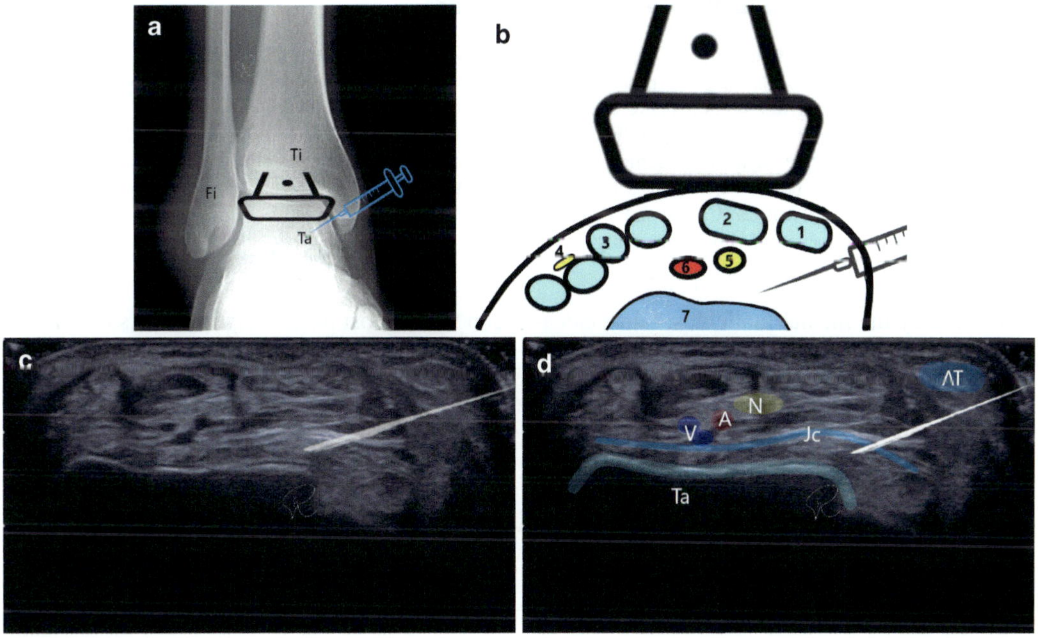

Fig. 7.4 Ankle joint injection. The image features four panels illustrating the ankle joint injection procedure. Panel (**a**) displays an X-ray of the ankle, with labeled anatomical structures: "Ti" for the tibia, "Fi" for the fibula, and "Ta" for the talus. Additionally, it includes a probe and syringe, indicating the site of needle insertion and demonstrating an in-plane approach. Panel (**b**) presents a schematic cross-sectional view of the ankle, showcasing numbered anatomical structures alongside a syringe representing the injection pathway into the ankle joint. Panels (**c**) and (**d**) consist of ultrasound images of the ankle. Panel (**c**) illustrates the trajectory of the needle as it approaches the joint. In contrast, panel (**d**) emphasizes the key anatomical structures with labels: "V" for vein, "A" for artery, "N" for nerve, "Jc" for joint capsule, and "AT" for the anterior tibialis tendon. (© Reza Roghani 2024. All Rights Reserved)

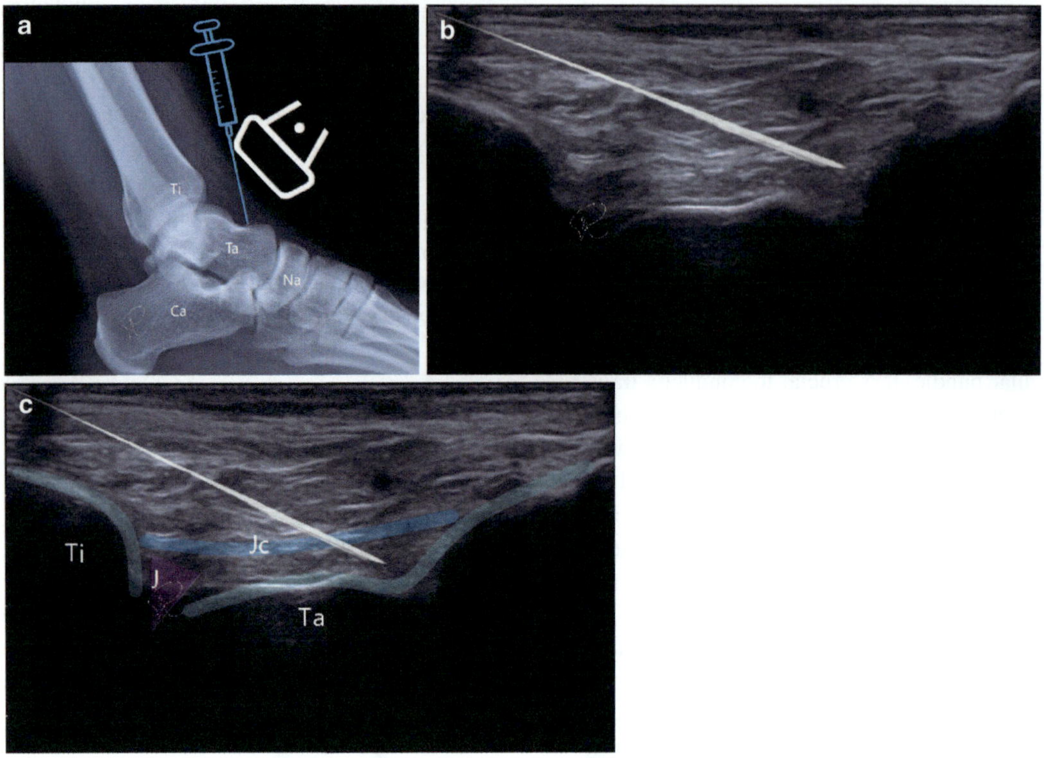

Fig. 7.5 Ankle joint approach in sagittal view. The image comprises three panels that illustrate the process of an ankle joint injection using the sagittal plane approach. Panel (**a**) features an X-ray of the ankle, highlighting the probe and syringe to indicate the needle insertion site and the in-plane approach. The bones are labeled as Ti (Tibia), Ta (Talus), Na (Navicular), and Ca (Calcaneus). Panel (**b**) presents an ultrasound image showing the trajectory of the needle as it enters the joint space. Panel (**c**) displays the same ultrasound image as panel (**b**) but with anatomical structures labeled, including Ti (Tibia), Ta (Talus), Jc (Joint Capsule), and J (Joint Space). These images effectively demonstrate the technique of performing a guided injection into the ankle joint. (© Reza Roghani 2024. All Rights Reserved)

is dictated by the medial malleolus, talus, calcaneus, and flexor retinaculum, which provides a structural roof over these critical components. Moreover, a robust ligamentous complex, the deltoid ligament, enhances stability at the medial ankle by connecting the tibia to the talus, calcaneus, and navicular bones. A labeled cross-sectional depiction of the tarsal tunnel illustrates the tibialis posterior tendon as the most anterior structure adjacent to the medial malleolus. Following this, the flexor digitorum longus tendon lies posterior to it. In contrast, the posterior tibial artery occupies a position between the flexor digitorum longus and flexor hallucis longus tendons, supplying blood to the plantar aspect of the foot. The tibial nerve parallels the posterior tibial artery, delivering sensory and motor innervation to the sole. The flexor hallucis longus tendon found most posteriorly in the tarsal tunnel, is near the calcaneus. The deltoid ligament, characterized by its deep and superficial fibers, also spans the medial ankle to confer essential stability. The superficial fibers extend from the medial malleolus to the navicular, calcaneus, and talus, while the deeper fibers connect the medial malleolus directly to the talus. This ligament is instrumental in resisting excessive eversion of the foot. It serves as a protective mechanism against valgus stress, which is crucial in maintaining ankle stability and functionality (Fig. 7.6a) [7]. Cross-sectional ultrasound imaging of the tarsal tunnel is invaluable for evaluating conditions such as tarsal tunnel syndrome, tenosynovitis, ligamentous injuries, or vascular pathologies. Furthermore, the deltoid ligament's integrity can be assessed for sprains, tears, or

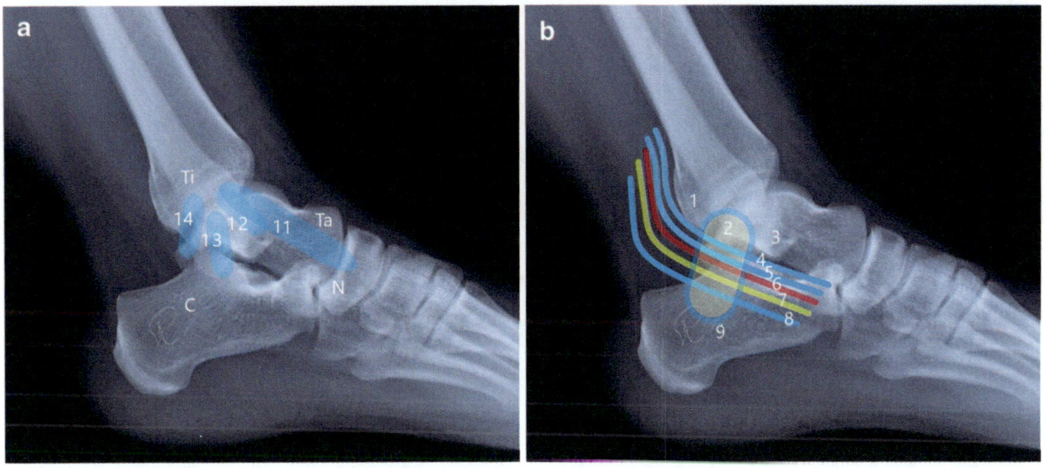

Fig. 7.6 Medial ankle ligaments and joints. The image consists of two lateral X-ray views of the ankle. Image (**a**) highlights key bony structures, including the tibia (Ti), talus (Ta), navicular (N), and calcaneus (C), with numbered markers (11 to 14) identifying components of the deltoid ligament. Image (**b**) presents an overlay of colored lines and numbered labels (1 to 9), illustrating the anatomical structures of the tarsal tunnel in relation to the bony framework. The structures depicted include the medial malleolus (1), flexor retinaculum (2), talus (3), posterior tibialis (4), flexor digitorum longus (5), tibial artery (6), tibial nerve (7), flexor hallucis longus (8), and calcaneus (9). The deltoid ligament components are labeled as the tibionavicular ligament (11), anterior tibiotalar ligament (12), tibiocalcancal ligament (13), and posterior tibiotalar ligament (14). (© Reza Roghani 2024. All Rights Reserved)

degenerative changes, which may contribute to medial ankle instability or discomfort.

7.3.2 Scan

7.3.2.1 Medial Ankle (Tarsal Tunnel) Scan (Video 7.6)

Patient positioning: To initiate the examination, the patient should lie supine on the table with a bent knee and keep the ankle relaxed in a neutral position.

Probe positioning: To capture the tarsal tunnel area, position the ultrasound probe in a short-axis, with one end placed on the medial malleolus and the other on the calcaneus.

Scanning: The ultrasound image offers a cross-sectional view of the medial ankle, showcasing key anatomical structures within the tarsal tunnel. Three distinct hyperechoic shadows are visible, representing the medial malleolus, calcaneus, and the cortexes of the talus, which serve as critical bony landmarks. Above these bony structures, the arrangement of soft tissue components follows a characteristic anterior-to-posterior sequence. The tibialis posterior tendon is located first, followed by the flexor digitorum longus tendon. Centrally positioned within the tarsal tunnel, the tibial nerve runs alongside the posterior tibial artery, forming a neurovascular bundle. The flexor hallucis longus tendon is identified posterior to these structures, completing the tendinous and neurovascular elements arrangement. This ultrasound view is invaluable for evaluating tarsal tunnel pathology, including nerve entrapment, tendon abnormalities, and vascular changes. The hyperechoic perineurium surrounding the tibial nerve and the anechoic lumen of the posterior tibial artery are clear sonographic landmarks for guided interventions, such as diagnostic nerve blocks or therapeutic injections (Fig. 7.7).

7.3.2.2 Deltoid Ligament (Videos 7.7 and 7.8)

The deltoid ligament, also known as the medial collateral ligament, is a strong, triangular structure located on the inner side of the ankle. It is essential for stability, as it helps prevent excessive eversion of the foot. This ligament is composed of four distinct components. The talonavicular ligament extends from the medial malleolus to the navicular bone, helping to support the medial lon-

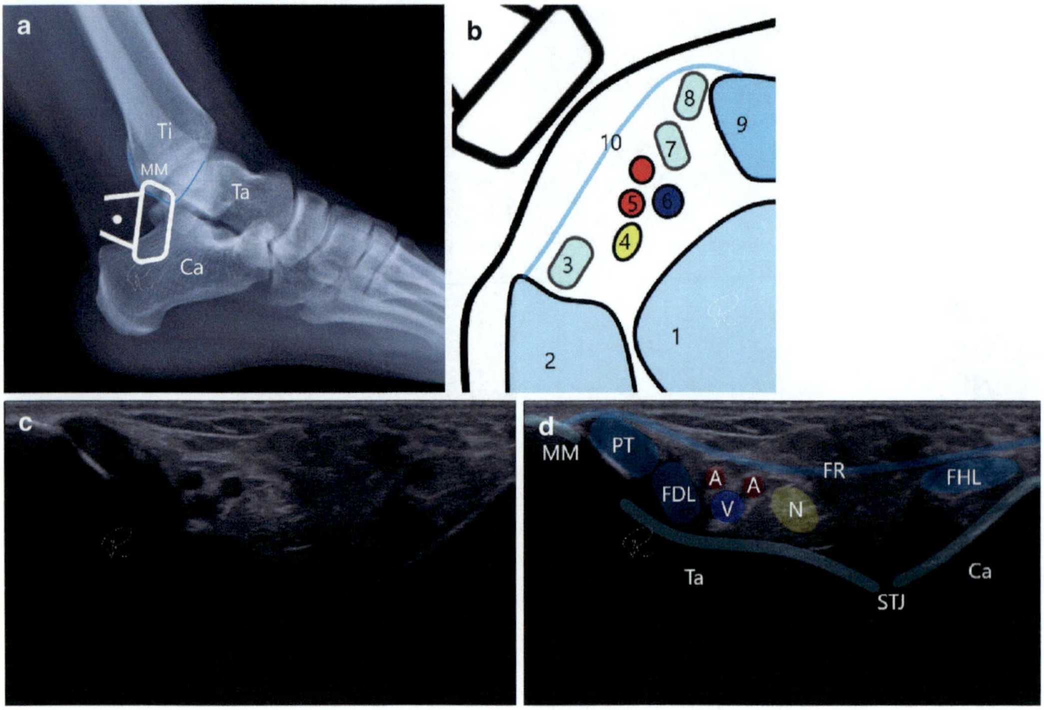

Fig. 7.7 Medial ankle (Tarsal tunnel) scanning. The illustration comprises four panels that detail the positioning, anatomy, and ultrasound imaging of the medial ankle. Panel (**a**) features a lateral X-ray of the ankle, emphasizing key bony landmarks, including the talus (Tal), calcaneus (Ca), medial malleolus (MM), and tibia (Ti), along with labeled probe position. Panel (**b**) presents a diagrammatic representation of the ankle joint, with numbered and color-coded regions that correspond to significant anatomical structures: (1) Talus bone, (2) Calcaneus, (3) Flexor hallucis longus, (4) Tibial nerve, (5) Tibial artery, (6) Tibial vein, (7) Flexor digitorum longus, (8) Posterior tibialis, (9) Medial malleolus, and (10) Flexor retinaculum. Panel (**c**) showcases an ultrasound scan of the medial ankle, capturing the soft tissue structures in their anatomical orientation. Panel (**d**) is an annotated version of the ultrasound image, labeling key structures with letters and employing color differentiation for clarity: A (Tibial artery), V (Tibial vein), N (Tibial nerve), FHL (Flexor hallucis longus), FDL (Flexor digitorum longus), PT (Posterior tibialis), FR (Flexor retinaculum), Ca (Calcaneus), Ta (Talus), MM (Medial malleolus), and STJ (Subtalar joint). Together, these panels provide a comprehensive view of the medial ankle, integrating radiographic, diagrammatic, and ultrasound perspectives to enhance anatomical understanding and facilitate clinical assessment. (© Reza Roghani 2024. All Rights Reserved)

gitudinal arch and stabilize the talonavicular joint. The anterior tibiotalar ligament runs from the medial malleolus to the anterior part of the talus, preventing excessive plantarflexion and eversion. The tibiocalcaneal ligament connects the medial malleolus to the sustentaculum tali of the calcaneus, providing vertical support to the medial aspect of the ankle. Finally, the posterior tibiotalar ligament extends from the medial malleolus to the posterior aspect of the talus, helping to prevent excessive dorsiflexion and eversion. These components collectively stabilize the ankle joint by limiting excessive movement and providing essential medial support.

Patient positioning: To initiate the examination, the patient should lie supine on the table with a bent knee and keep the ankle relaxed in a neutral position.

Probe positioning: To locate the anterior tibiotalar ligament, position the ultrasound probe obliquely between the medial malleolus and the talus bone in the medial ankle until the bright band connecting the two structures is visible [8].

To identify the posterior tibiotalar ligament, place the probe behind the medial malleolus in an oblique position between the medial malleolus and talus bone until the ligament appears as a bright band connecting those two points.

To identify the tibiocaneal ligament (Fig. 7.8c, d), position the ultrasound probe obliquely between the medial malleolus and the sustentaculum Tali of calcaneus until the bright band, deep in the image, connecting the tibia and calcaneus, is visible.

Finally, to identify the tibionavicular ligament (Fig. 7.8e, f), adjust the probe to a transverse plane and position it on the medial malleolus, moving it anteriorly until the bright ligament connecting the tibia and navicular bone is visualized.

7.3.3 Procedures (Video 7.9)

Tarsal tunnel syndrome is a neuropathic condition characterized by the compression of the tibial nerve as it traverses the tarsal tunnel, a confined anatomical space on the medial aspect of the ankle beneath the flexor retinaculum. This entrapment can lead to pain, tingling, burning sensations, and numbness localized to the foot's medial ankle, heel, and plantar surface. The medial malleolus, talus, and calcaneus define the tarsal tunnel's boundaries, with the flexor retinaculum functioning as the superior structure. Within this narrow passage, vital neurovascular and tendinous components are housed, including the tibial nerve, tibial artery, and tibial vein, along with the tendons associated with the posterior tibialis, flexor digitorum longus, and flexor hallucis longus muscles. Conditions that reduce the spatial dimensions of the tunnel—such as inflammation, varicosities, ganglion cysts, or traumatic injury—can precipitate tibial nerve compression. Patients typically present with clinically significant symptoms, including burning pain, tingling, and numbness along the medial ankle and the plantar aspect of the foot. These symptoms tend to be aggravated by prolonged standing, ambulation, or dorsiflexion of the foot. A positive Tinel's sign may be obtained by tapping over the tarsal tunnel, eliciting tingling along the course of the tibial nerve. In more severe instances, weakness in the intrinsic musculature of the foot may manifest. Management strategies are customized based on the severity and underlying cause of the condition. If the conservative treatment proves ineffective, interventional options such as ultrasound-guided tibial nerve hydro dissection may assist in alleviating adhesions. Additionally, regenerative therapies like platelet-rich plasma (PRP) injections are currently being investigated for their potential to promote nerve recovery [9].

During the procedure to treat Tarsal Tunnel Syndrome, a small-gauge needle is connected to a suitably sized syringe. The injectate typically comprises a local anesthetic and a corticosteroid to reduce inflammation and offer long-lasting relief. The injection is administered with the patient lying on their side, with a bent knee and foot resting on a table. An ultrasound probe is used, aligned longitudinally with the tarsal tunnel as described in Sect. 7.3.2.1. The needle is inserted using an in-plane technique, passing above the flexor hallucis longus and approaching the nerve under live ultrasound guidance (Fig. 7.9c, d).

7.4 Lateral Ankle

7.4.1 Anatomy

The lateral ankle comprises several essential anatomical structures, including bones, ligaments, tendons, and neurovascular components. The primary bony landmarks include the lateral malleolus (the distal fibula), talus, calcaneus, and the fifth metatarsal base. The lateral collateral ligaments play a crucial role in stabilizing the ankle joint and consist of the anterior talofibular ligament (ATFL), calcaneofibular ligament (CFL), and posterior talofibular ligament (PTFL). The structures are arranged in distinct layers in a cross-sectional view of the lateral ankle. The most superficial layers consist of skin and subcutaneous tissue, followed by the peroneal tendons (peroneus longus and brevis), which run posterior to the lateral malleolus. Beneath the peroneal tendons lie the lateral collateral ligaments, with the ATFL connecting the fibula to the talus, the CFL extending from the fibula to the calcaneus, and the PTFL providing reinforcement to the posterior aspect of the joint. The sural nerve and small saphenous vein are also found in this

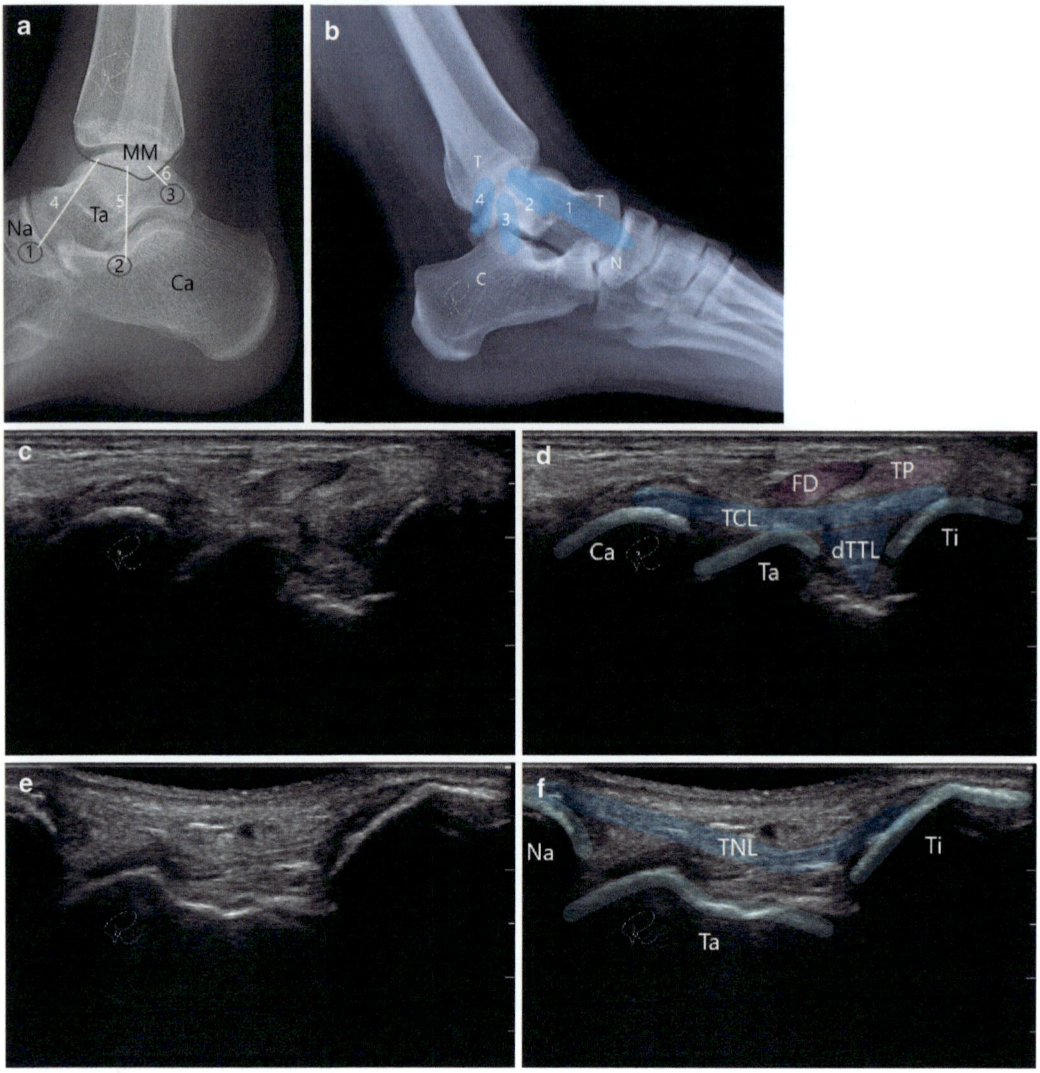

Fig. 7.8 Ligaments and joints of medial ankle. The composite Image provides a comprehensive overview of the anatomical structures of the ankle, which are revealed through X-ray and ultrasound imaging. Images (**a**) and (**b**) contain clearly labeled X-ray views that identify key bony landmarks, including the medial malleolus (MM), navicular (Na), talus (Ta), calcaneus (Ca), and tibia (T). Furthermore, Image (**a**) incorporates three distinctly marked white lines labeled 4 to 6, denoting the probe positions utilized to examine the tibionavicular, tibiocalcaneal, and tibiotalar ligaments. In reviewing the anatomical features in the provided Image, particularly Image (**b**), it is essential to note the presence of four blue tick lines, which signify the deltoid ligament. Images (**c**) and (**d**) concentrate on the tibiocalcaneal ligament, with Image (**d**) offering specific labeling of this structure. Similarly, images (**e**) and (**f**) showcase the tibionavicular ligament, with Image (**f**) providing detailed annotations for additional structures, including the tibionavicular ligament (TNL), flexor digitorum (FD), tibialis posterior (TP), deep tibiotalar ligament (dTTL), navicular (Na), tibia (Ti)and talus (Ta). Overall, the scans illustrate critical anatomical features of the ankle, such as the tibiotalar ligament, tibiocalcaneal ligament, and calcaneonavicular ligament, as well as the various joints in the region, including the ankle joint, subtalar joint, and talonavicular joint. Additional structures recognized comprise the talus bone (Ta), talocalcaneal ligament (TCL), calcaneus (Ca), and calcaneonavicular ligament (CNL). This integrated imaging further enhances understanding of the ankle's complex anatomy and ligamentous relationships.

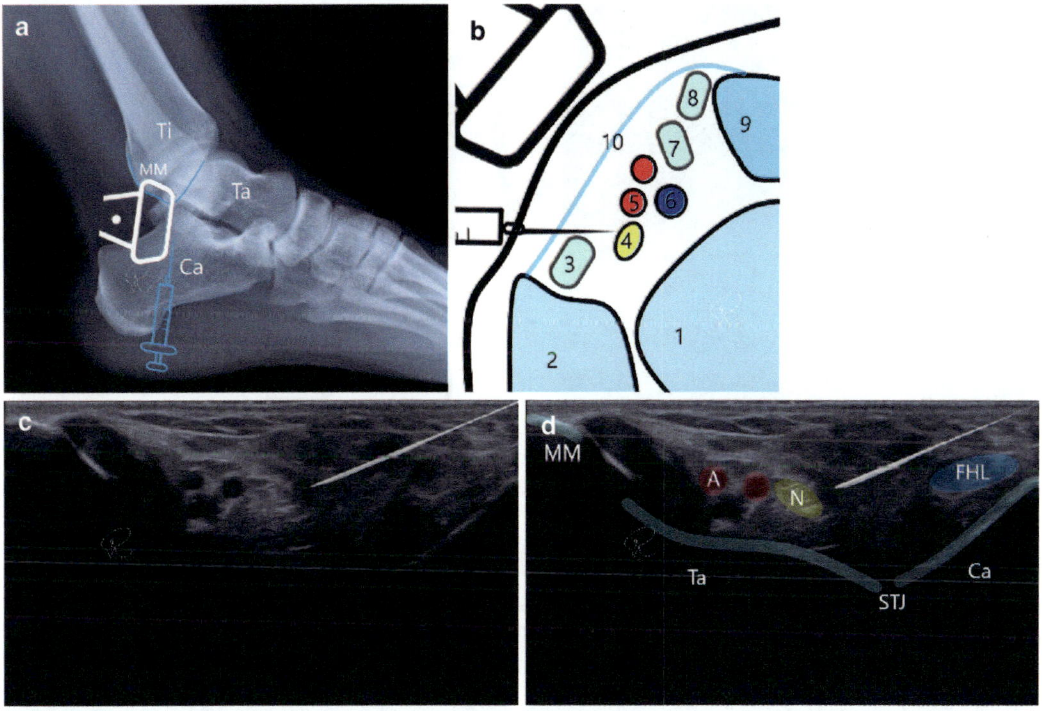

Fig. 7.9 Tarsal tunnel syndrome steroid injection. The illustration comprises four panels, each providing a different perspective on the anatomy, diagnostic evaluations, and procedural approaches related to the medial ankle. Panel (**a**) exhibits an X-ray of the ankle, clearly labeling the bony structures, including the tibia (Ti), talus (Ta), calcaneus (Ca), and medial malleolus (MM). A probe and syringe are strategically positioned to illustrate the probe placement, needle insertion site, and in-plane approach. Panel (**b**) presents a diagrammatic representation of the ankle joint, emphasizing key anatomical structures with numbered and color-coded sections for clarity: (1) Talus bone, (2) Calcaneus, (3) Flexor hallucis longus, (4) Tibial nerve, (5) Tibial artery, (6) Tibial vein, (7) Flexor digitorum longus, (8) Posterior tibialis, (9) Medial malleolus, and (10) Flexor retinaculum. Panel (**c**) displays an ultrasound image of the medial ankle, illustrating soft tissue structures and the trajectory of the needle as it approaches the tibial nerve. Panel (**d**) provides an annotated version of the panel (**c**), labeling the medial malleolus (MM), talus (Ta), calcaneus (Ca), flexor hallucis longus (FHL), artery (A), nerve (N), and subtalar joint (STJ). (© Reza Roghani 2024. All Rights Reserved)

region. Deep within the ankle joint, the talus articulates with the tibia and fibula, forming the ankle mortise. The subtalar joint between the talus and calcaneus facilitates inversion and eversion movements (Fig. 7.10b) [10].

7.4.2 Scan (Video 7.10)

Patient Position: The examination should start with the patient lying supine, with the knee flexed and the ankle placed neutrally on the table. The examiner should be facing the lateral aspect of the ankle.

Probe Position: The ultrasound probe needs to be positioned in a short-axis orientation over the lateral aspect of the ankle joint. One probe end should be aligned with the lateral malleolus, and the other should align with the calcaneus bone (Fig. 7.10a, b).

Scanning: As you position the ultrasound probe over the lateral ankle, ensure it is perpendicular to the skin to optimize visualization of essential anatomical structures. Begin by identifying the peroneus brevis and peroneus longus tendons, which run parallel to each other posterior to the lateral malleolus. The peroneus brevis tendon is more anteriorly, lying directly adjacent

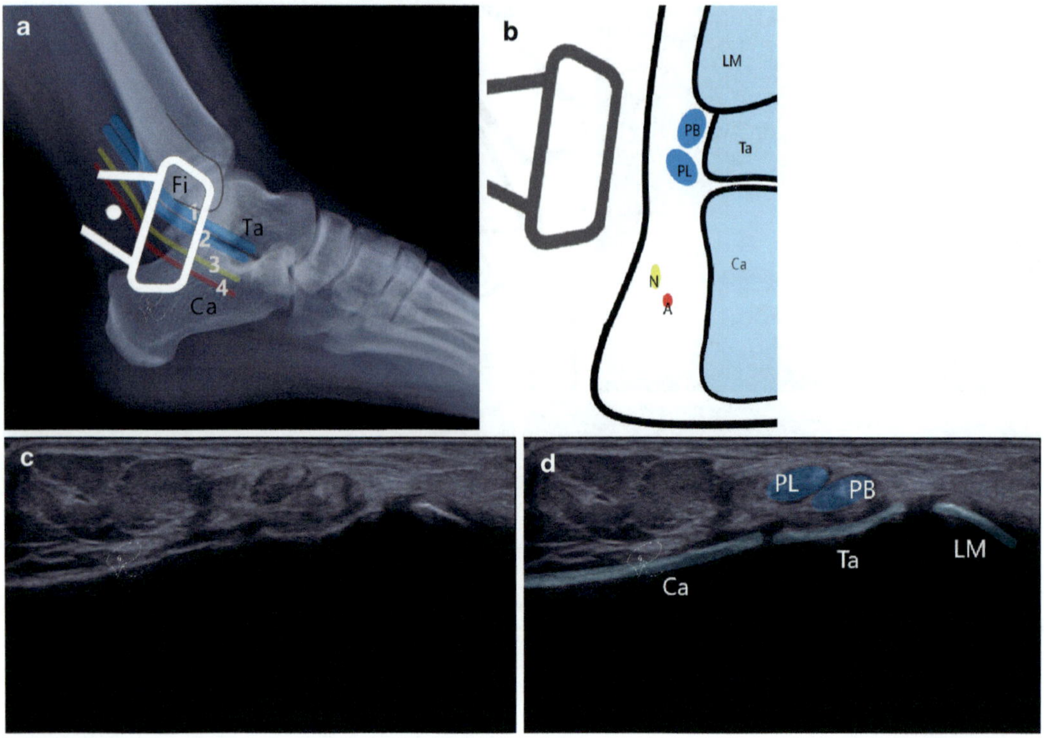

Fig. 7.10 Lateral ankle scanning. The image features four panels that illustrate the anatomical details and an ultrasound scan of the lateral ankle. Panel (**a**) displays a lateral X-ray of the ankle, showcasing the patient's positioning along with key bony landmarks, including the fibula (Fi), talus (Ta), and calcaneus (Ca). Colored lines numbered 1 to 4 demarcate different structures, and a probe is indicated to demonstrate the scanning position. The specific anatomical features identified include the peroneus brevis (1), peroneus longus (2), sural nerve (3), and sural artery (4). Panel (**b**) presents a schematic representation of the lateral ankle, labeling significant structures such as the lateral malleolus (LM), peroneus brevis (PB), peroneus longus (PL), talus (Ta), and calcaneus (Ca). This diagram also identifies the tibial nerve (N) and artery (A) essential for diagnostic and procedural considerations. Panels (**c**) and (**d**) illustrate ultrasound images of the lateral ankle. Panel (**c**) shows a general view of the ultrasound, while panel (**d**) emphasizes specific structures, including the peroneus longus (PL), peroneus brevis (PB), talus (Ta), lateral malleolus (LM), and calcaneus (Ca).

to the fibula, while the peroneus longus tendon is posterior to it. Proper angulation and a slight probe tilt can enhance the differentiation between these tendons and their surrounding soft tissue structures. Continuing the scan from anterior to posterior, you will observe the sural nerve and artery. The sural nerve, a sensory nerve, is positioned superficially and traverses along the posterior aspect of the lateral malleolus. It typically appears as a small hypoechoic oval structure with a hyperechoic border, indicative of its fascicular architecture. The sural artery, which runs parallel to the nerve, may be visualized as a pulsatile, anechoic structure, with color Doppler imaging confirming its vascular nature. Maintaining consistent probe pressure is crucial to prevent compression of the smaller structures, which could obscure their appearance. Additionally, performing a dynamic assessment by asking the patient to move their foot into eversion and inversion can facilitate the evaluation of tendon movement, confirm their integrity, and identify any signs of tendinopathy or subluxation (Fig. 7.10c, d).

7.4.3 Subtalar Joint Injection (Video 7.11)

To manage subtalar arthritis resulting from rheumatoid arthritis or osteoarthritis, a fine-gauge needle, accompanied by an appropriately sized syringe, delivers a combination of local anesthetic and corticosteroid. This mixture effectively reduces inflammation, alleviates pain, and enhances joint mobility. The patient is positioned in a lateral decubitus pose on the unaffected side to ensure that the affected ankle remains relaxed and easily accessible for the procedure.This proper positioning not only minimizes discomfort for the patient but also improves the accuracy of the injection. The procedure employs an in-plane ultrasound-guided technique to ensure precise needle placement while avoiding critical anatomical structures. Key landmarks such as the lateral malleolus and calcaneus bone are used to position the ultrasound probe accurately. By aligning the probe with the subtalar joint, real-time imaging facilitates the identification of the joint space, adjacent tendons, and neurovascular structures. The needle is introduced from the distal end of the probe, passing over the neurovascular bundle under live ultrasound monitoring and advancing toward the subtalar joint with careful attention to its trajectory. This approach ensures avoidance of the neurovascular bundle while optimizing the delivery of the injectate into the joint capsule. Continuous visualization during the needle's approach allows for real-time adjustments, thereby maintaining precision and preventing complications. Once optimally positioned, the local anesthetic and corticosteroid mixture is injected, providing targeted relief to the inflamed joint. Post-procedural care includes monitoring the patient for immediate pain relief and potential adverse reactions and offering recommendations for activity modification and follow-up care (Fig. 7.11).

7.4.4 Sinus Tarsi Injection (Video 7.12)

The sinus tarsi represents a morphologically significant tunnel-like structure between the talus and calcaneus within the foot. This anatomical compartment plays a vital conduit for several important ligamentous structures, including the interosseous talocalcaneal ligament. Furthermore, it houses vascular components essential for the overall functionality and stability of the foot. Inflammation or irritation of the sinus tarsi contents may manifest as localized pain and swelling, primarily along the lateral aspect of the ankle. This condition, commonly referred to as sinus tarsi syndrome, can arise from repetitive trauma, excessive stress, or inflammatory disorders such as arthritis. Patients often report that weight-bearing activities—such as running, walking, or pivoting—intensify the pain. A targeted injection into the sinus tarsi, employing corticosteroids or platelet-rich plasma (PRP), has emerged as an effective therapeutic intervention for alleviating the symptoms associated with this syndrome. The injection aims to mitigate inflammation within the tunnel, ameliorate pain, and facilitate healing. Corticosteroids deliver immediate anti-inflammatory effects, whereas PRP injections harness the patient's blood-derived growth factors to promote tissue repair and regeneration over a more extended period. Ultrasound guidance is typically employed to ensure precise needle placement when executing a sinus tarsi injection. This minimally invasive technique can yield substantial symptom relief, enhanced functional capacity, and a decreased dependence on oral medications or more invasive surgical options [11].

For an ultrasound-guided sinus tarsi injection, the precise positioning of the ultrasound probe and real-time imaging are crucial to achieving accurate needle placement while safeguarding critical anatomical structures. The patient should be positioned comfortably, supine, or in a lateral decubitus posture, with the affected foot slightly inverted. This positioning aids in optimizing the visualization of the sinus tarsi. The ultrasound probe is situated anterior to the lateral malleolus at an oblique angle, aligning with the natural trajectory of the sinus tarsi. To effectively center the sinus tarsi on the ultrasound imaging screen, key bony landmarks such as the talus and calcaneus must be identified. Additionally, the interosseous talocalcaneal ligament and the surrounding soft tissue structures within the sinus tarsi must be visualized to ensure precise targeting. After adequately identifying the anatomical structures, a fine-gauge needle is introduced using an in-plane technique, enhancing the visibility of the needle's trajectory. The needle is advanced from

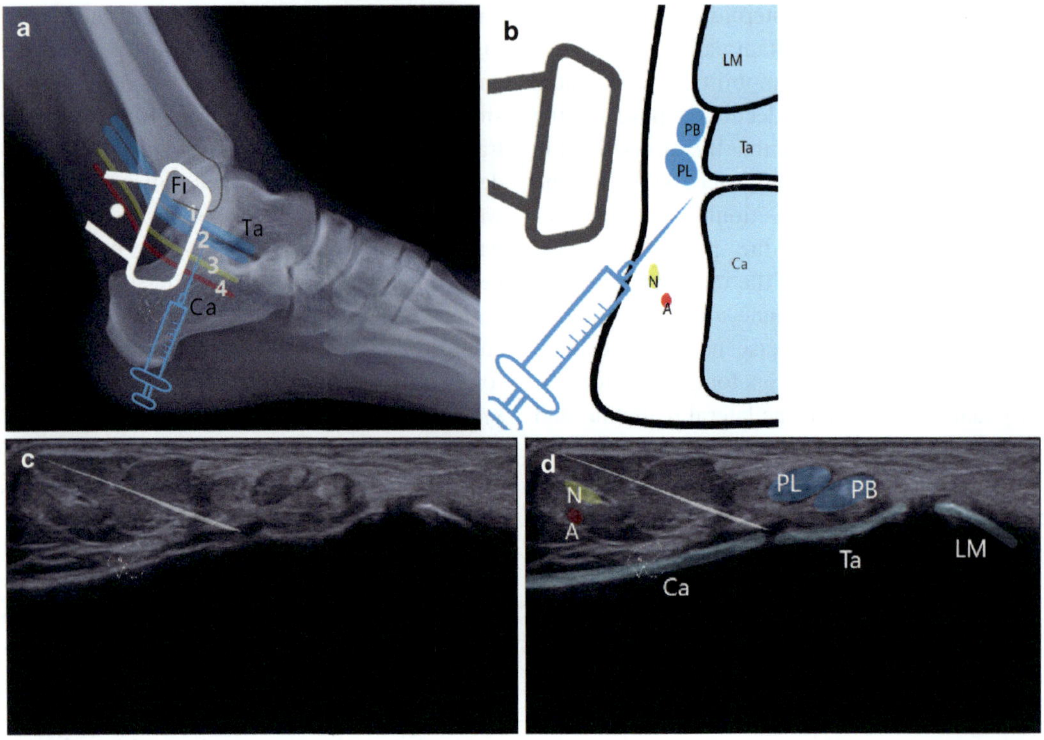

Fig. 7.11 Lateral ankle subtalar joint approach. The image features four panels that illustrate the anatomical details of the lateral ankle and subtalar joint injection ultrasound scan. Panel (**a**) displays a lateral X-ray of the ankle, showcasing the patient's positioning along with key bony landmarks, including the fibula (Fi), talus (Ta), and calcaneus (Ca). Colored lines numbered 1 to 4 demarcate different structures, a probe is indicated to demonstrate the scanning position, and a syringe demonstrates the needle insertion site and in-plane approach. The specific anatomical features identified include the peroneus brevis (1), peroneus longus (2), sural nerve (3), and sural artery (4). Panel (**b**) presents a schematic representation of the lateral ankle, labeling significant structures such as the lateral malleolus (LM), peroneus brevis (PB), peroneus longus (PL), talus (Ta), and calcaneus (Ca). This diagram also identifies the tibial nerve (N) and artery (A) essential for diagnostic and procedural considerations. Panels (**c**) and (**d**) illustrate ultrasound images of the lateral ankle. Panel (**c**) shows a general view of the ultrasound with the needle trajectory, while panel (**d**) emphasizes specific structures, including the peroneus longus (PL), peroneus brevis (PB), talus (Ta), lateral malleolus (LM), calcaneus (Ca), the tibial nerve (N) and artery (A). (© Reza Roghani 2024. All Rights Reserved)

the distal aspect, carefully traversing above the neurovascular bundle, and is directed proximally towards the sinus tarsi while continuously monitoring via live ultrasound imaging. This meticulous approach significantly reduces the risk of vascular or nerve injury while ensuring accurate deposition of the injectate into the targeted region. The composition of the injectate may vary based on the clinical indications; it could consist of a corticosteroid combined with a local anesthetic to alleviate inflammation and provide pain relief or platelet-rich plasma (PRP) to foster tissue healing. Once the needle tip's position within the sinus tarsi is confirmed through direct visualization, the injection is administered slowly. Post-injection, the patient requires monitoring to assess immediate responses to the treatment and provide post-procedural care instructions. These instructions may involve temporary modifications in activity, the application of ice, and a gradual resumption of weight-bearing activities. Furthermore, recommending appropriate rehabilitation exercises can aid in restoring ankle stability and functionality, thereby enhancing the long-term efficacy of the treatment (Fig. 7.12).

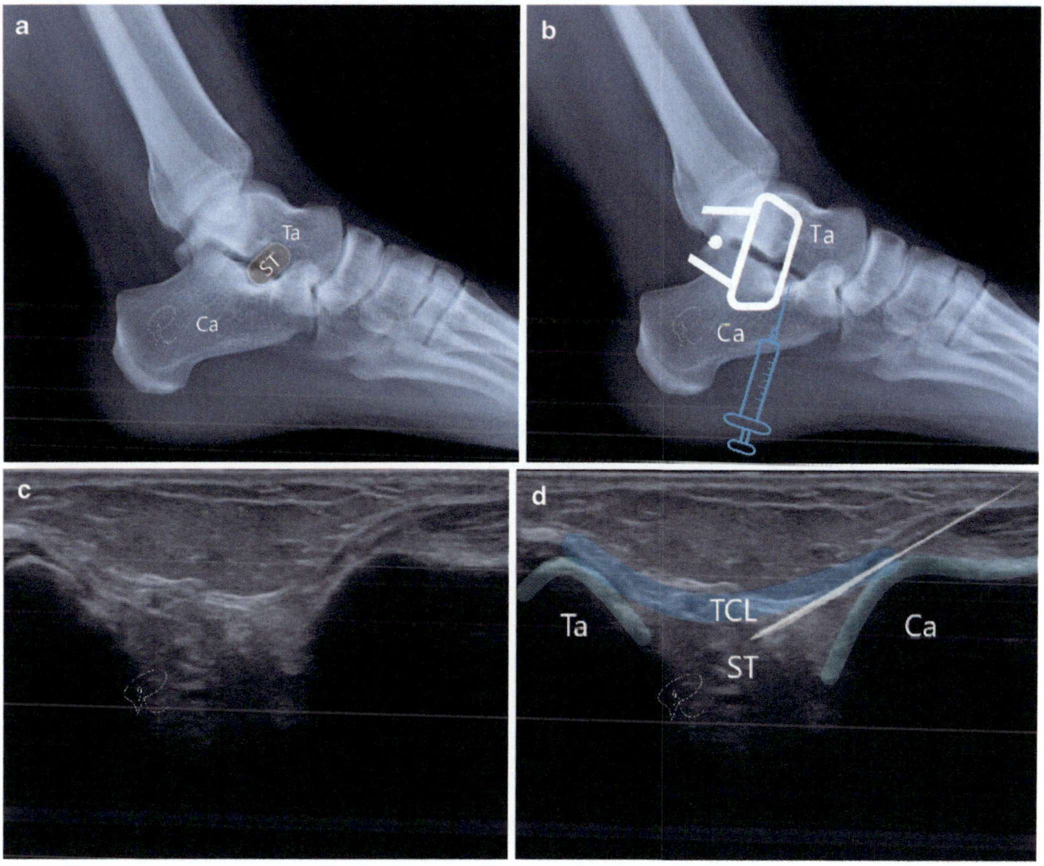

Fig. 7.12 Lateral ankle sinus tarsi approach. The image consists of four panels depicting the radiographic and ultrasound-guided visualization of the lateral ankle during a sinus tarsi injection. Panel (**a**) features an X-ray of the lateral ankle, distinctly highlighting key bony landmarks such as the talus (Ta), calcaneus (Ca), and the sinus tarsi (ST), which is the target area for the injection. Panel (**b**) presents an annotated version of the X-ray, incorporating a schematic overlay of the ultrasound probe and syringe. This illustration demonstrates the probe's positioning and the needle's trajectory as it approaches the sinus tarsi. Panel (**c**) showcases an ultrasound image of the sinus tarsi and the surrounding soft tissue structures. Panel (**d**) serves as an annotated version of the panel (**c**), labeling essential anatomical features, including the talus (Ta), calcaneus (Ca), sinus tarsi (ST), and talocalcaneal ligament (TCL). It also outlines the needle's trajectory, illustrating its path toward the sinus tarsi under live ultrasound guidance.

7.5 Posterior Ankle

7.5.1 Anatomy

The posterior ankle is a complex region that houses essential musculoskeletal and neurovascular structures integral to movement, stability, and overall function. At the forefront of these structures is the Achilles tendon, recognized as the thickest and strongest tendon in the human body. This tendon serves as the primary connection between the gastrocnemius and soleus muscles and the posterior surface of the calcaneus. The Achilles tendon plays a crucial role in locomotion by facilitating plantarflexion of the foot, which is vital for jumping, running, and walking. Given its significant load-bearing capacity, the Achilles tendon is susceptible to various overuse injuries, including tendinopathy and potential rupture, particularly among athletes and individuals with high physical activity levels. At the tendon's insertion point on the calcaneus, the retrocalcaneal bursa—a fluid-filled sac—diminishes friction and promotes smooth movement.

The superficial calcaneal bursa, located between the skin and the Achilles tendon, further cushions the area and alleviates stress during motion. Situated deeper and more toward the medial aspect of the Achilles tendon is the flexor hallucis longus (FHL) tendon. Originating from the posterior fibula, the FHL tendon traverses the posterior ankle. It passes beneath the sustentaculum tali of the calcaneus before inserting into the base of the distal phalanx of the great toe. During gait dynamics, this tendon is pivotal in toe flexion, balance, and the push-off phase. In addition to these muscular components, the tibial nerve occupies a critical position within the neurovascular bundle of the posterior ankle. Located deeper and more medially about the Achilles tendon, the tibial nerve travels through the tarsal tunnel, positioned posterior to the medial malleolus, and runs alongside the posterior tibial artery and vein. Its functions are multifaceted, as the tibial nerve innervates the foot's intrinsic muscles and contributes significantly to the sensory innervation of the sole, making it an essential structure for functional activities of the lower limb. Conversely, on the lateral side of the posterior ankle, the peroneal (fibular) tendons, which include the peroneus longus and peroneus brevis, are positioned toward the outer side of the Achilles tendon. These tendons traverse behind the lateral malleolus and follow the lateral aspect of the calcaneus before they insert into the foot. They are critical for foot eversion and contribute to stabilizing the ankle, particularly during dynamic movements such as cutting and pivoting (Fig. 7.13b) [12].

7.5.2 Scan (Video 7.13)

Patient position: The patient should be positioned prone on a table, allowing the foot to hang off the edge. A small cushion or towel can be placed under the shin for added comfort and stability.

Probe position: The examiner should carefully place the ultrasound probe on the back of the heel, aligned longitudinally with the Achilles tendon, to scan the posterior ankle in the long axis. This orientation provides a clear view of the tendon fibers, retrocalcaneal bursa, and their relationship to the calcaneus (Fig. 7.13a). The probe is then rotated 90 degrees perpendicular to the tendon to obtain a short-axis view (Fig. 7.13d).

Scanning: In the long-axis (longitudinal) view, the Achilles tendon presents as a robust fibrillar structure extending from the calcaneal bone to the musculotendinous junction. This view facilitates the assessment of the tendon's integrity, thickness, and any pathological changes, such as tendinosis or tears. The retrocalcaneal bursa, located between the Achilles tendon and calcaneus, can be examined for signs of inflammation or fluid accumulation. By sliding the probe proximally, one can inspect the musculotendinous junction, while a distal movement allows for a detailed evaluation of the calcaneal insertion (Fig. 7.13 b, c). In the short-axis (transverse) view, the Achilles tendon appears as a prominent hyperechoic oval structure situated superficially at the center of the screen. Deeper and slightly toward the medial side of the Achilles tendon lies the flexor hallucis longus tendon. Additionally, the tibial nerve, an important neural structure in the posterior ankle, is more profound and medially (Fig. 7.13e–f).

7.5.3 Procedures

7.5.3.1 Achilles Tendonitis (Video 7.14)

Ultrasound-guided injection is a commonly used procedure for treating Achilles tendinitis, characterized by inflammation and pain in the Achilles tendon [13]. During the procedure, a fine-gauge needle and a small syringe are utilized to administer a combination of local anesthetic and a corticosteroid. The injection is performed in the sagittal plane, with the patient typically lying in a prone position while the ultrasound probe is positioned over the posterior aspect of the ankle. The needle is inserted from the distal end, and with real-time ultrasound guidance, it is directed toward the tendon synovium. This method allows for the precise delivery of pain relief and the potential reduction of inflammation (Fig. 7.14). When encountering resistance during needle advancement or injection, it is essential to

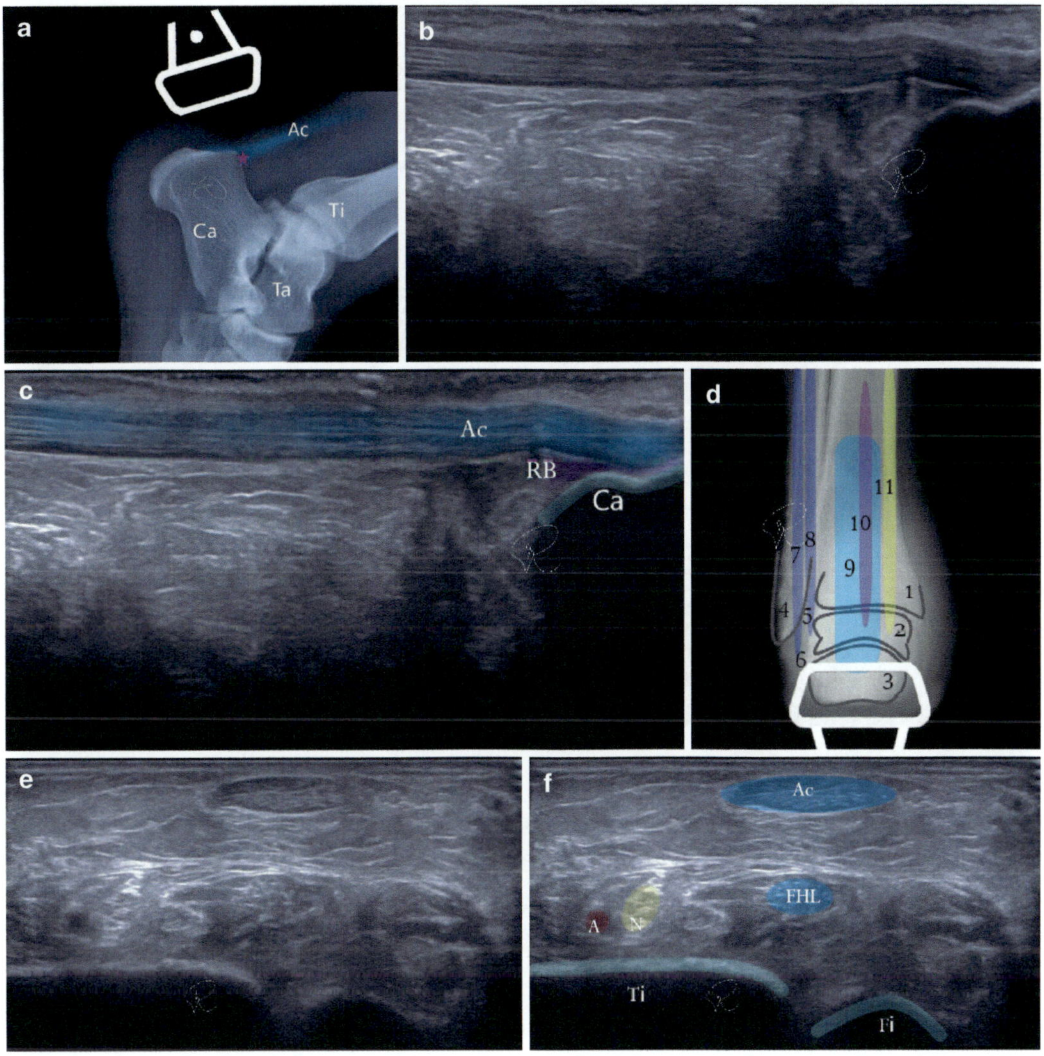

Fig. 7.13 Posterior ankle scanning. The image comprises six panels that illustrate the posterior ankle anatomy through various imaging techniques, including ultrasound, X-ray, and anatomical diagrams. Panel (**a**) presents a lateral X-ray of the ankle, emphasizing key anatomical landmarks with labels: Ac (Achilles tendon), Ca (Calcaneus), Ti (Tibia), and Ta (Talus). It also illustrates the patient's positioning and demonstrates the long-axis probe placement for ultrasound examination of the posterior ankle. Panel (**b**) features an unmarked ultrasound image of the posterior ankle in a long-axis view, serving as a reference for comparison. Panel (**c**) displays the same ultrasound image from panel (**b**), now annotated with labels to identify important structures: Ac (Achilles tendon), RB (retrocalcaneal bursa), and Ca (Calcaneus). This panel emphasizes the relationship between the Achilles tendon and its adjacent bursa, which minimizes friction at the tendon's insertion. Panel (**d**) provides a detailed anatomical illustration of the posterior ankle viewed from an anteroposterior position, with numbered sections indicating significant structures. These include the (1) Tibia, (2) Talus, (3) Calcaneus, (4) Fibula, (5) Ankle joint, (6) Subtalar joint, (7) Peroneus brevis, (8) Peroneus longus, (9) Achilles tendon, (10) Flexor hallucis longus, (11) Tibial nerve. This diagram provides an overview of key musculoskeletal and neurovascular structures relevant to the posterior ankle region, accompanied by a probe image that demonstrates the probe's position in the short-axis view. Panel (**e**) presents an unlabeled ultrasound image of the posterior ankle in a short-axis view at the level of the distal tibiofibular joint. Panel (**f**) shows the same ultrasound image as in panel (**e**), now labeled to indicate key anatomical features: Ac (Achilles tendon), Ti (Tibia), A (Tibial artery), N (Tibial nerve), FHL (Flexor Hallucis Longus), and Fi (Fibula). (© Reza Roghani 2024. All Rights Reserved)

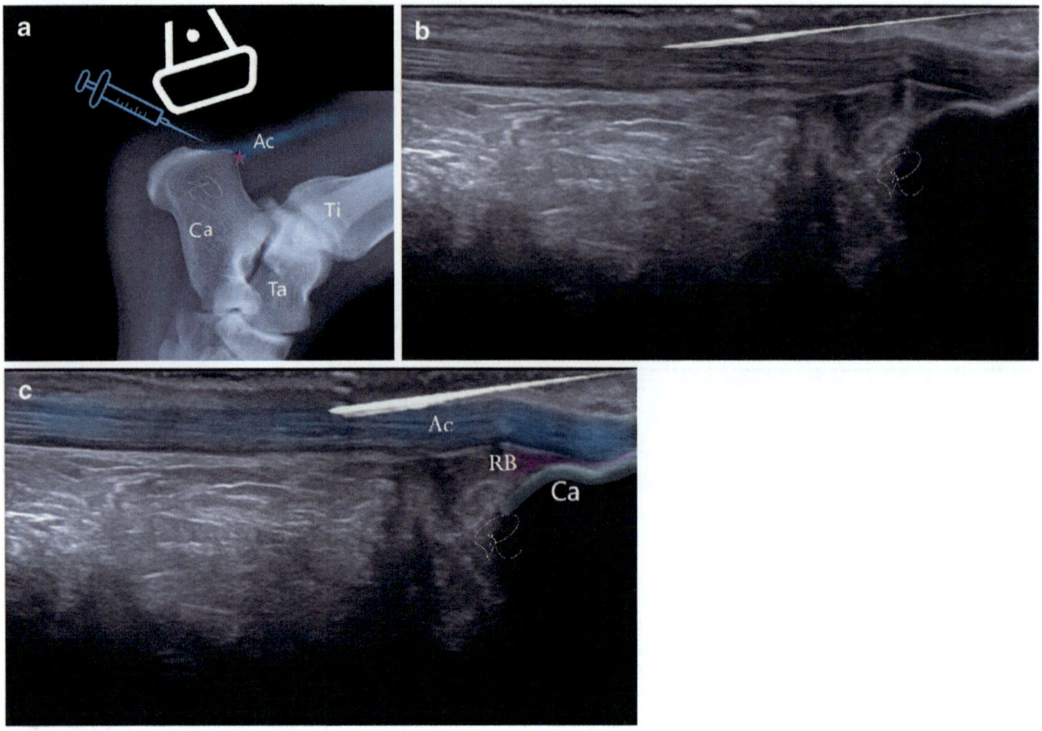

Fig. 7.14 Achilles tendon injection. The image is divided into three panels that depict the process of an Achilles tendon sheath injection. Panel (**a**) presents a lateral X-ray of the ankle, highlighting essential anatomical landmarks with the following labels: Ac (Achilles tendon), Ca (Calcaneus), Ti (Tibia), and Ta (Talus). It also illustrates the probe position and the in-plane needle approach, demonstrating the appropriate patient positioning for an ultrasound-guided posterior ankle evaluation. Panel (**b**) features an ultrasound image in a long-axis view, showcasing the Achilles tendon along with its surrounding structures. The needle is shown advancing towards the tendon sheath. Panel (**c**) offers the same ultrasound image as in panel (**b**) but with added annotations to identify key structures: Ac (Achilles tendon), RB (retrocalcaneal bursa), and Ca (Calcaneus).

redirect the needle to prevent an intratendinous injection, which may elevate the risk of an Achilles tendon rupture. Continuous ultrasound guidance facilitates real-time adjustments, ensuring the needle stays within the peritendinous space and avoids direct contact with the tendon fibers. If resistance continues, it is advisable to withdraw the needle slightly and reposition it before proceeding with the injection. Adhering to proper technique and maintaining careful monitoring enhance safety and efficacy while minimizing the likelihood of complications.

7.5.3.2 Retrocalcaneal Bursitis (Video 7.15)

Retrocalcaneal bursitis is characterized by inflammation and fluid accumulation in the retrocalcaneal bursa, a cushion between the Achilles tendon and the calcaneal bone. Administering an injection in this area can alleviate the patient's discomfort [14].

We recommend using a short-axis view and inserting the needle from a lateral and in-plane aiming for the bursa, as depicted in Fig. 7.15.

7.5.3.3 Subtalar Joint (Video 7.16)

The subtalar joint, also known as the talocalcaneal joint, is a vital structure in foot biomechanics, situated between the talus and calcaneus. It plays a key role in inversion, eversion, and shock absorption during gait. This joint features three articulating facets: the anterior facet, which connects the talus to the anterior facet of the calcaneus; the middle facet, located medially to

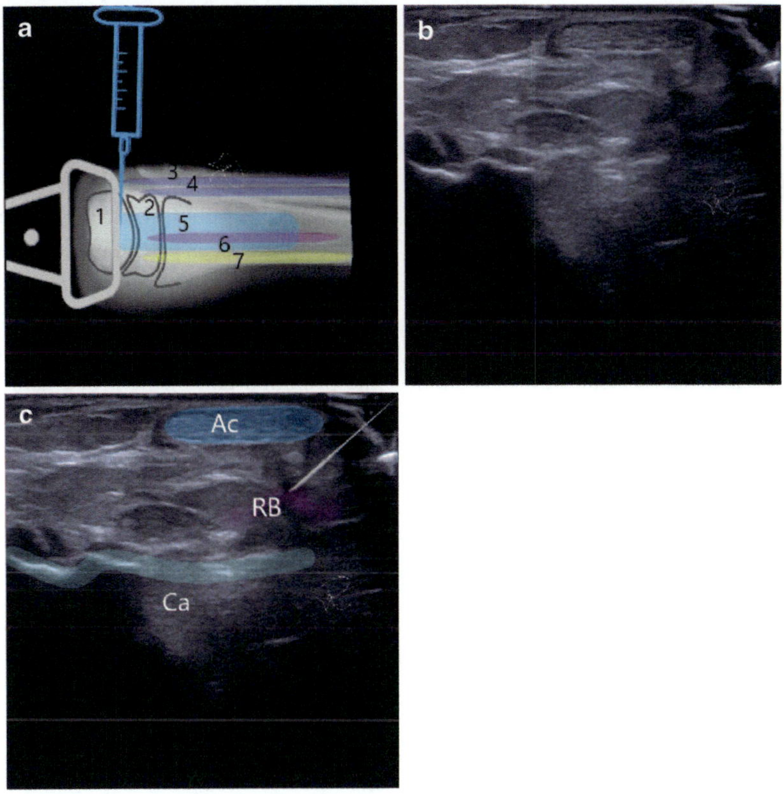

Fig. 7.15 Retrocalcaneal bursa injection. The image features three panels that illustrate an ultrasound-guided retrocalcaneal bursa injection. Panel (**a**) provides a diagram of the ankle in a posterior-anterior view, with anatomical structures clearly labeled: (1) Calcaneus, (2) Talus, (3) Fibula, (4) Peroneus brevis and Peroneus longus, (5) Achilles tendon, (6) Flexor hallucis longus, and (7) Tibial nerve. This diagram provides a contextual overview of the posterior ankle anatomy relevant to the procedure, including probe positioning, needle insertion, and an in-plane approach. Panel (**b**) presents an ultrasound image of the posterior ankle in a short-axis view, displaying the retrocalcaneal bursa and its surrounding structures. Panel (**c**) showcases the same ultrasound image as in panel (**b**) but includes colored overlays to highlight key anatomical structures: Ac (Achilles tendon, blue), RB (retrocalcaneal bursa, purple), and Ca (calcaneus, green). Additionally, the trajectory of the needle toward the bursa is emphasized, promoting accurate delivery of the injectate while minimizing the risk of intratendinous injection. (© Reza Roghani 2024. All Rights Reserved)

provide additional stability; and the posterior facet, the largest and primary articulation between the two bones. These facets are separated by the tarsal sinus and tarsal canal, which contain important ligamentous and vascular structures. Several ligaments stabilize the subtalar joint, including the interosseous talocalcaneal ligament, which serves as the main stabilizer within the sinus tarsi, along with the cervical ligament, which restricts excessive inversion. Additionally, the lateral and medial talocalcaneal ligaments reinforce the joint capsule. The subtalar joint is influenced by extrinsic foot muscles that govern movement and stability; the tibialis posterior and tibialis anterior are responsible for inversion, while the peroneus longus and peroneus brevis facilitate eversion. The flexor hallucis longus also runs near the joint, contributing dynamic support. The neurovascular structures associated with the subtalar joint include the posterior tibial artery and fibular artery, which supply blood to the area, and the medial and lateral plantar nerves, which provide sensory innervation. Clinically, the subtalar joint is frequently affected by conditions such as osteoarthritis, rheumatoid arthritis, post-traumatic arthritis, and instability. Ultrasound-guided injections targeting the subtalar joint can reduce inflammation, enhance mobility, and alleviate pain [15].

Patient position: The patient should be positioned prone on a table, allowing the foot to hang off the edge. A small cushion or towel can be placed under the shin for added comfort and stability.

Probe position: The examiner should carefully place the ultrasound probe on the back of the heel, aligned longitudinally with the Achilles tendon, to scan the posterior ankle in the long axis. This orientation provides a clear view of the tendon fibers, retrocalcaneal bursa, and their relationship to the calcaneus (Fig. 7.16a).

Scanning: In the long-axis (longitudinal) view, the Achilles tendon is a robust fibrillar structure extending from the calcaneal bone to the musculotendinous junction. To visualize the subtalar joint, move the probe laterally until the Achilles tendon is no longer visible. At this stage, three hyperechoic bone cortices become apparent deeper: the calcaneus, talus, and tibia, arranged from bottom to top. The subtalar joint is identified as the space between the calcaneus and talus. For injection, the needle should be inserted from the proximal end of the probe using an in-plane technique, carefully advancing it toward the joint under continuous ultrasound guidance to ensure

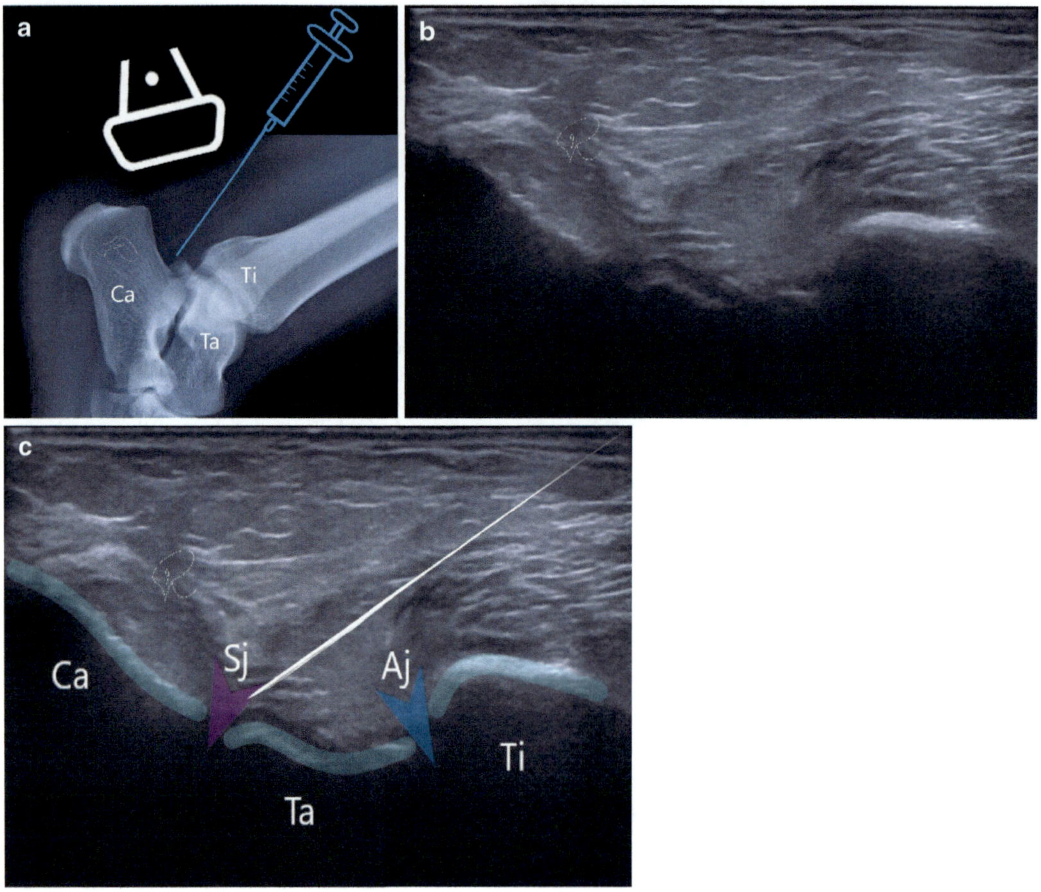

Fig. 7.16 Subtalar joint posterior approach. The image is composed of three panels that illustrate the subtalar joint injection via a posterior approach. Panel (**a**) features a lateral X-ray of the ankle, highlighting key anatomical landmarks with labeled structures: Ac (Achilles tendon), Ca (Calcaneus), Ti (Tibia), and Ta (Talus). This panel also indicates the correct patient positioning for an ultrasound-guided posterior ankle evaluation, the probe's position, and the in-plane needle approach. Panel (**b**) offers an ultrasound image of the ankle and subtalar joint, clearly visualizing the targeted area. Panel (**c**) presents the same ultrasound image as in panel (**b**) and includes labeled structures such as the calcaneus (Ca), talus (Ta), tibia (Ti), subtalar joint (Sj), and ankle joint (Aj), as well as the needle trajectory directed toward the subtalar joint. (© Reza Roghani 2024. All Rights Reserved)

precise placement while avoiding surrounding neurovascular structures (Fig. 7.16b, c).

7.6 Foot

7.6.1 Anatomy

The human foot is an intricate anatomical structure that plays a vital role in supporting the body's weight, maintaining balance, and facilitating mobility. The plantar surface is characterized by multiple layers of soft tissues, including the plantar fascia, intrinsic foot muscles, tendons, ligaments, and neurovascular elements. The plantar fascia, a robust fibrous band, originates from the medial tubercle of the plantar surface of the calcaneus and extends distally, dividing into five slips that insert into the bases of the proximal phalanges. This structure is crucial for upholding the foot's longitudinal arch and mitigating mechanical stress during physical activities such as walking and running. The metatarsophalangeal (MTP) joints, where the metatarsal heads meet the proximal phalanges, operate as hinge joints, permitting flexion, extension, and limited lateral movement. The stability of these joints during gait is enhanced by the joint capsules, which are supported by plantar plates, collateral ligaments, and the deep transverse metatarsal ligament. Sensory innervation to the toes is provided by the interdigital nerves, branches of both the medial and lateral plantar nerves, which traverse the spaces between the metatarsals. These nerves accompany interdigital arteries and veins before branching into proper digital nerves. Notably, compression or entrapment of the interdigital nerves, particularly between the third and fourth metatarsal heads, can result in Morton's neuroma, a prevalent cause of forefoot pain. Advancements in cross-sectional imaging, such as ultrasound, have enabled detailed visualization of the foot's anatomy. In the longitudinal plane, the plantar fascia is seen as a hyperechoic band extending from the calcaneus, where its thickness can be evaluated to identify conditions like plantar fasciitis. The transverse view represents the metatarsal heads as hyperechoic bony structures, with the plantar plates, flexor tendons, and interdigital nerves located superficially. Furthermore, dynamic assessments via ultrasound can assist in diagnosing conditions like MTP joint synovitis, capsular inflammation, or nerve entrapment [16].

7.6.2 Scan

7.6.2.1 Plantar Fascia Scan and Injection (Videos 7.17 and 7.18)

Patient position: The patient is prone on the examination table, with the foot relaxed and held in a neutral position (Fig 7.17a).

Probe position: The ultrasound probe is positioned longitudinally over the plantar aspect of the calcaneus, toward the metatarsal heads.

Scanning: The plantar fascia is a thick fibrous band that extends from the heel bone beneath the fat pad toward the toes (Fig. 7.17b, c). When the probe is rotated at the tendon insertion 90 degrees and sliding distally to detach it from the bone, the entire width of the plantar fascia can be seen in the short axis. This location allows for an in-plane injection from the medial side (Fig. 7.18). The needle tip should be carefully positioned below the plantar facia in its sheet.

7.6.2.2 Metatarsophalangeal (MTP) Joints Injection (Video 7.19)

Patient position: The patient lies supine on the bed with the knee bent 90° and the plantar surface of the foot on the table.

Probe position: Metatarsal bones are the longest and most superficial bones in the foot. Place the probe's long axis over the bone and slide it toward the MTP joint, as shown in Fig. 7.19a.

Scanning: The metatarsal and phalanx bone cortex are hyperechoic structures deep in the image. The interruption between them represents the MTP joints (Fig. 7.19b, c). To inject these joints, it is recommended to position the ultrasound probe on the dorsal aspect of the MTP joint in a longitudinal orientation and then slide it medially to avoid the extensor tendons, insert the needle from either sides of the probe, and approach the joint in-plane.

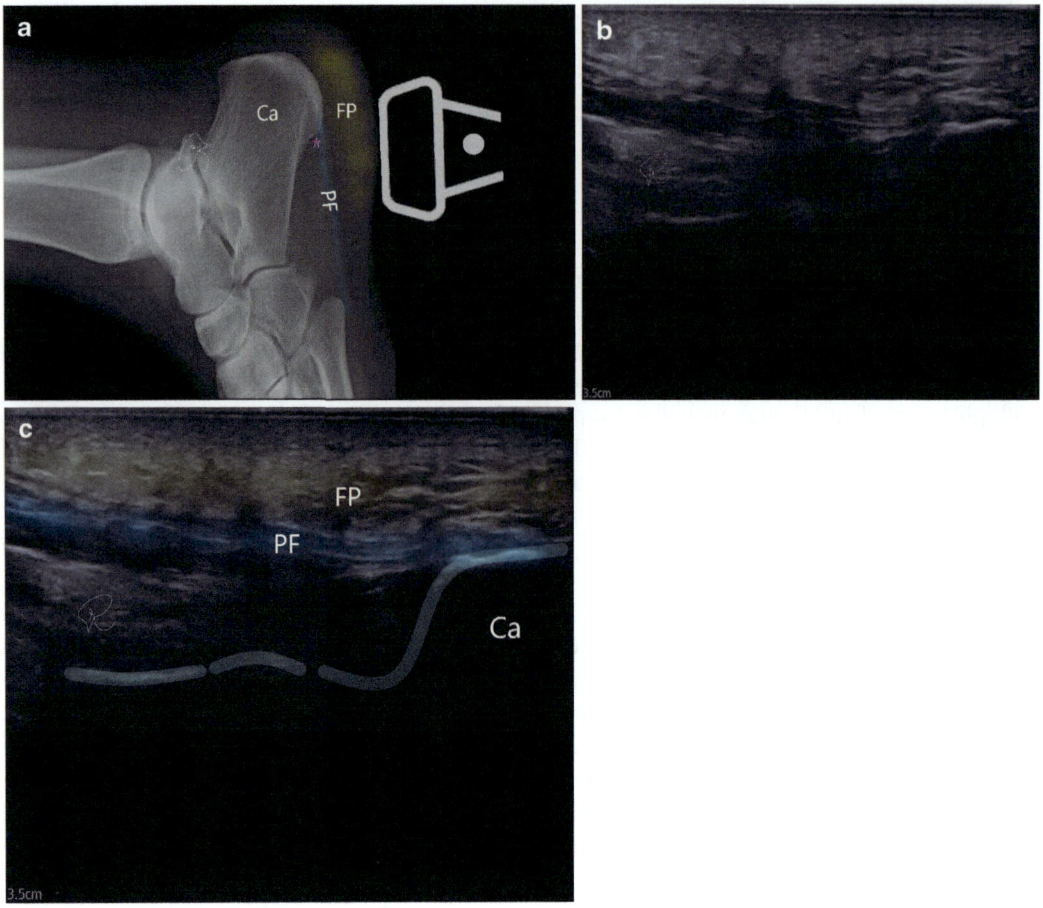

Fig. 7.17 Plantar facia ultrasound scan. The image consists of three panels illustrating the anatomy and ultrasound evaluation of the plantar fascia. Panel (**a**) presents a lateral X-ray of the foot, highlighting key anatomical structures, including the calcaneus (Ca), plantar fascia (PF), and fat pad (FP). It also depicts the probe position in the long axis and marks the target area for injection with a purple asterisk. Panel (**b**) displays an ultrasound image capturing the plantar fascia in its longitudinal view. Panel (**c**) presents the same ultrasound image as panel (**b**) but with labeled structures: the calcaneus (Ca), the plantar fascia (PF) highlighted in blue, and the fat pad (FP) in yellow, providing an apparent anatomical reference for assessment and intervention.

7.6.2.3 The Interdigital Nerve (Video 7.20)

The interdigital nerves are situated deep within the subcutaneous tissues between the metatarsal heads. Morton neuroma is characterized by the compressive neuropathy of these interdigital nerves in the forefoot, which is caused by constant irritation and compression [17].

Patient position: The patient lies prone on the bed with the ankle in maximum plantar flexion.

Examiner and probe placement: The examiner sits at the foot of the bed and places the ultrasound probe transversely on the plantar surface of the foot, specifically on the metatarsal heads (Fig. 7.20a).

Scanning: When conducting the ultrasound examination, the nerve will appear as a honeycomb adjacent to the pulsatile arteries between the metatarsal heads, deep to the plantar fat pad (Fig. 7.20b, c). The interdigital nerve block can be performed in-plane from the plantar surface, as illustrated in Fig. 7.20.

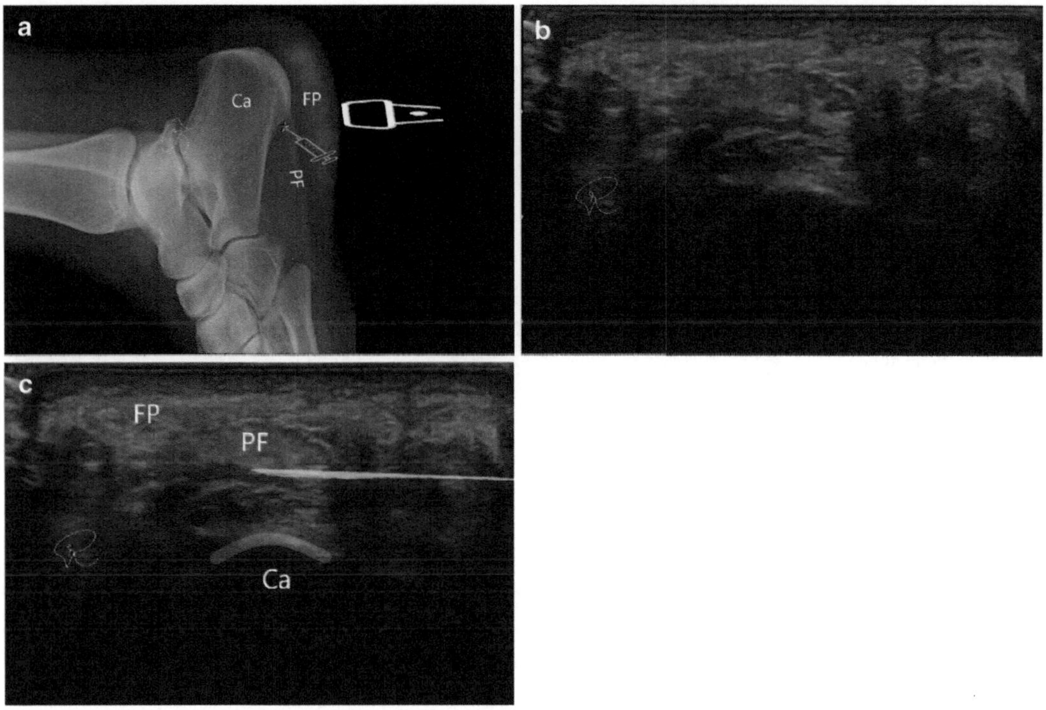

Fig. 7.18 Plantar facia injection. The image is composed of three panels that illustrate the anatomy and ultrasound evaluation of the plantar fascia, as well as an in-plane medial-side approach for injection into its sheath. Panel (**a**) features a lateral X-ray of the foot, highlighting key anatomical structures such as the calcaneus (Ca), plantar fascia (PF), and fat pad (FP). It illustrates the probe position in the short axis and designates the target injection area with a purple asterisk, accompanied by a syringe and the needle, indicating the in-plane injection approach. Panel (**b**) presents an ultrasound image that captures the plantar fascia in a short-axis view. Finally, panel (**c**) displays the same ultrasound image as in panel (**b**), but with the anatomical structures labeled: the calcaneus (Ca), the plantar fascia (PF) marked in blue, and the fat pad (FP) in yellow, along with the trajectory of the needle approaching the plantar fascia sheath, providing a clear anatomical reference for assessment and intervention. (© Reza Roghani 2024. All Rights Reserved)

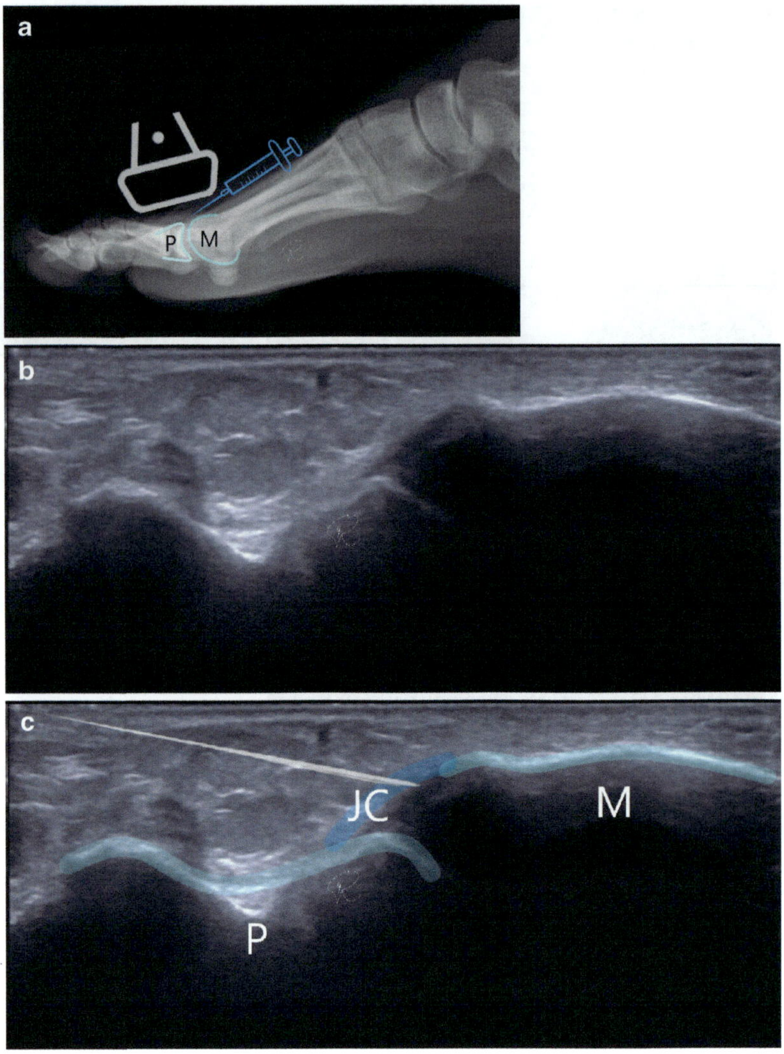

Fig. 7.19 MTP joint injection. The image consists of three panels illustrating the X-ray, ultrasound, and ultrasound-guided injection of the metatarsophalangeal (MTP) joint. Panel (**a**) presents a lateral X-ray view of the foot, with annotations indicating the proximal phalanx (P) and the metatarsal head (M). It also depicts the probe position and the in-plane approach for MTP joint injection. Panel (**b**) displays an ultrasound image of the MTP joint. Panel (**c**) presents the same ultrasound image as panel (**b**) but with labeled structures, including the proximal phalanx (P), metatarsal head (M), joint capsule (JC), and needle trajectory toward the MTP joint. (© Reza Roghani 2024. All Rights Reserved)

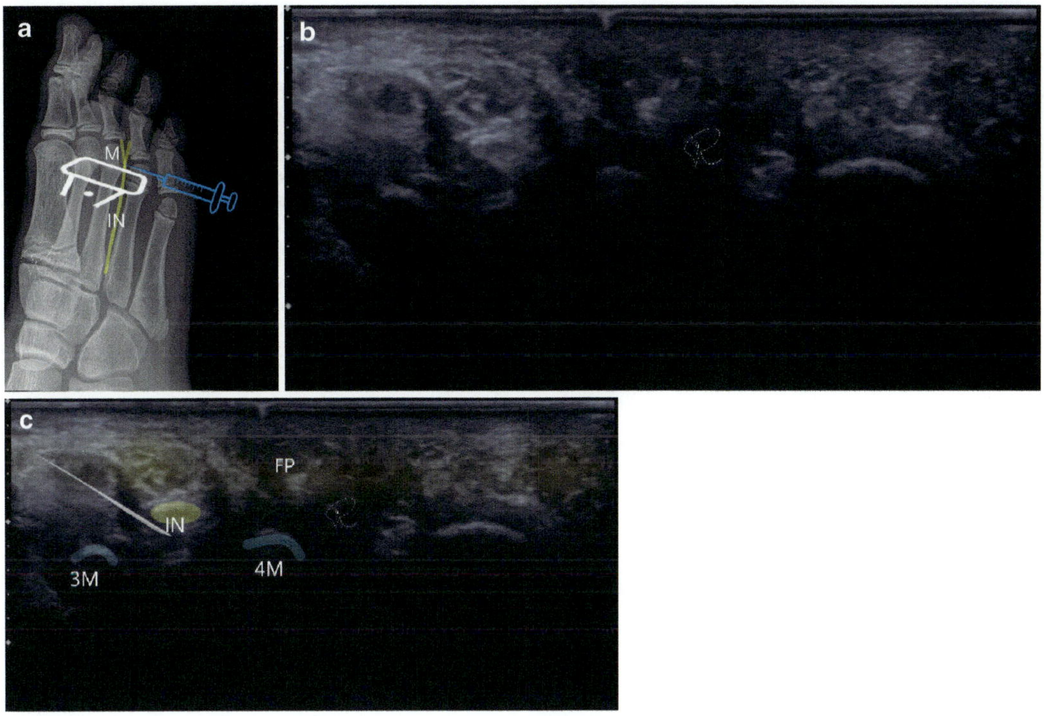

Fig. 7.20 Interdigital nerve scan and injection. The image features three panels illustrating the X-ray, ultrasound, and interdigital nerve block procedure. Panel (**a**) displays an X-ray of the foot, with a probe and syringe indicating the probe's position and the in-plane injection approach for the interdigital nerve block, label M for the metatarsal head, and a yellow line with an IN label for interdigital nerve. Panel (**b**) provides an ultrasound image of the interdigital nerves, clearly visualizing the relevant structures involved in the procedure. Panel (**c**) presents the same ultrasound image as panel (**b**) but with annotations highlighting specific areas: "3M" and "4M" for the third and fourth metatarsal heads, "IN" for the interdigital nerve, and "FP" for the fat pad, thereby delivering a detailed anatomical reference for the nerve block intervention. (© Reza Roghani 2024. All Rights Reserved)

References

1. Anatomy Atlases: Atlas of human anatomy in cross section: section 7. Lower Limb. https://www.anatomyatlases.org/HumanAnatomy/7Section/30.shtml. Accessed 21 Jul 2024.
2. Brockett CL, Chapman GJ. Biomechanics of the ankle. Orthop Trauma. 2016;30(3):232–8. https://doi.org/10.1016/j.mporth.2016.04.015.
3. Furr-Stimming E, Chiou-Tan F, Harrell JS, Zhang H, Taber KH. Procedure-oriented sectional anatomy of the ankle. J Comput Assist Tomogr. 2014;38(6):992–5. https://doi.org/10.1097/RCT.0000000000000126.
4. Kelley LL, Petersen C. Sectional anatomy for imaging professionals. 4th ed. Mosby; 2018.
5. Dreyer MA, Gibboney MD. Anterior tarsal tunnel syndrome. In: StatPearls. StatPearls Publishing; 2024. http://www.ncbi.nlm.nih.gov/books/NBK538488/.
6. Adukia V, Mangwani J, Issac R, Hussain S, Parker L. Current concepts in the management of ankle arthritis. J Clin Orthop Trauma. 2020;11(3):388–98. https://doi.org/10.1016/j.jcot.2020.03.020.
7. Obionu K, Palm H, Astrup Y, Lange NB, Krogsgaard MR. A clinical guide to the medial ligaments of the ankle: anatomy, function, diagnosis of injuries and treatment of instability—a narrative review. Foot Ankle Surg. 2024;30(2):85–91. https://doi.org/10.1016/j.fas.2023.10.010.
8. Omodani T, Takahashi K. Ultrasound findings of the deltoid ligament in patients with acute ankle sprains: a retrospective review. J Orthop Sci. 2023;28(4):843–8. https://doi.org/10.1016/j.jos.2022.05.010.
9. Rodríguez-Merchán EC, Moracia-Ochagavía I. Tarsal tunnel syndrome: current rationale, indications and results. EFORT Open Rev. 2021;6(12):1140–7. https://doi.org/10.1302/2058-5241.6.210031.
10. Ahmed A, Mishra P, Patra B, Ravi PK. Lateral ankle ligaments: an insight into their functional anatomy, variations, and surgical importance. Cureus. 2024;16(2):e53826. https://doi.org/10.7759/cureus.53826.

11. Arshad Z, Bhatia M. Current concepts in sinus tarsi syndrome: a scoping review. Foot Ankle Surg. 2021;27(6):615–21. https://doi.org/10.1016/j.fas.2020.08.013.
12. Giannini S, Buda R, Mosca M, Parma A, Di Caprio F. Posterior ankle impingement. Foot Ankle Int. 2013;34(3):459–65. https://doi.org/10.1177/1071100713477609.
13. Medina Pabón MA, Naqvi U. Achilles tendinopathy. In: StatPearls. StatPearls Publishing; 2024. http://www.ncbi.nlm.nih.gov/books/NBK538149/.
14. Pekala PA, Henry BM, Pekala JR, Piska K, Tomaszewski KA. The Achilles tendon and the retrocalcaneal bursa. Bone Joint Res. 2017;6(7):446–51. https://doi.org/10.1302/2046-3758.67.BJR-2016-0340.R1.
15. Bartonícek J, Rammelt S, Nanka O. Anatomy of the subtalar joint. Foot Ankle Clin. 2018;23(3):315–40. https://doi.org/10.1016/j.fcl.2018.04.001.
16. Ficke J, Byerly DW. Anatomy, bony pelvis and lower limb: foot. In: StatPearls. StatPearls Publishing; 2024. http://www.ncbi.nlm.nih.gov/books/NBK546698/.
17. Munir U, Tafti D, Morgan S. Morton neuroma. In: StatPearls. StatPearls Publishing; 2024. http://www.ncbi.nlm.nih.gov/books/NBK470249/.

Lumbar Spine and Trunk 8

Reza Salman Roghani, John Melendez-Benabe, Jose Juan Diaz, Nicole Schneider, Somayeh Younesian, Padideh Baran, Amirhossein Foroughianyazdi, and Seungwoo Chai

8.1 Introduction

8.1.1 Ultrasound Protocol

Lumbar Spine

- Sagittal (Long Axis)
  - Midline: Spinous process
  - Para Central: Lamina
  - Centrolateral: Facet joint
  - Far Lateral: Transverse process
- Transverse (Short Axis)
  - Lamina View: Intervertebral foramen and nerve root access
  - Interlaminar View: Facet joint, medial branch, and interlaminar access

Sacral Spine

- Sagittal (Long Axis): Caudal epidural access
- Transverse (Short Axis): Caudal epidural access

Trunk

- Thoracic Para Sagittal (Long Axis): Intercostal nerve access
- Trans Abdominal Transverse (Short Axis): (TAP block)
  - Anterior axillary line
  - Mid axillary line
  - Posterior axillary line

Supplementary Information The online version contains supplementary material available at https://doi.org/10.1007/978-3-031-81037-4_8.

R. S. Roghani (✉)
Department of Physical Medicine and Rehabilitation, Larkin Community Hospital, Nova Southeastern University, Miami, FL, USA

J. Melendez-Benabe
Pain Medicine Division, Department of Physical Medicine and Rehabilitation, West Palm Beach VA Healthcare System, US Department of Veterans Affairs, West Palm Beach, FL, USA
e-mail: John.Melendez-Benabe@va.gov

J. J. Diaz
Department of Physical Medicine and Rehabilitation, Larkin Community Hospital, Nova Southeastern University, Miami, FL, USA

Integrative Spine and Sports, Fort Lauderdale, FL, USA

N. Schneider
Dr. Kiran C. Patel College of Osteopathic Medicine, Nova Southeastern University, Fort Lauderdale, FL, USA

S. Younesian
Department of Physical Medicine and Rehabilitation, Broward Health North Hospital, Pompano Beach, FL, USA

P. Baran
Imaging Department, University of Miami, Miami, FL, USA
e-mail: Pxb646@miami.edu

A. Foroughianyazdi
Department of Science, Toronto Metropolitan University, Toronto, ON, Canada

S. Chai
Surgery Department, Robert Packer Hospital, Guthrie Clinic, Sayre, PA, USA

R. S. Roghani, J. J. Diaz (eds.), *Video Atlas of Neuromusculoskeletal Ultrasound*,
https://doi.org/10.1007/978-3-031-81037-4_8

8.2 Sagittal (Long-Axis)

8.2.1 Midline: Spinous Process View

8.2.1.1 Anatomy

The midsagittal anatomy of the lumbar spine offers a comprehensive view of the central structures of the lower back, which is vital for grasping spinal biomechanics, pathology, and interventional procedures. The vertebral bodies are the primary weight-bearing elements, stacked upon one another and separated by intervertebral discs that function as shock absorbers. The spinous processes extend posteriorly from each vertebra as attachment sites for muscles and ligaments. The laminae comprise the posterior portion of the vertebral arch, safeguarding the spinal canal. The interlaminar space, the gap between adjacent laminae, provides access to the epidural space during procedures such as lumbar epidural steroid injections. Within the spinal canal resides the dural sac, encasing either the spinal cord (above the L1-L2 level) or the cauda equina (below L1-L2), alongside cerebrospinal fluid (CSF). The posterior longitudinal ligament (PLL) runs along the back of the vertebral bodies, enhancing spinal stability and restricting excessive flexion. In contrast, the anterior longitudinal ligament (ALL) covers the front of the vertebral bodies, preventing hyperextension. The supraspinous and interspinous ligaments connect the spinous processes, further contributing to posterior spinal stability. Although the facet joints are not directly visible, they are located laterally in a midsagittal view, forming the articulations between the superior and inferior articular processes. The paraspinal muscles, including the erector spinae and multifidus, extend alongside the spine, providing both movement and stabilization (Fig. 8.1) [1]. However, structures anterior to bony elements can be obscured during ultrasound scans, making them difficult to visualize clearly [2].

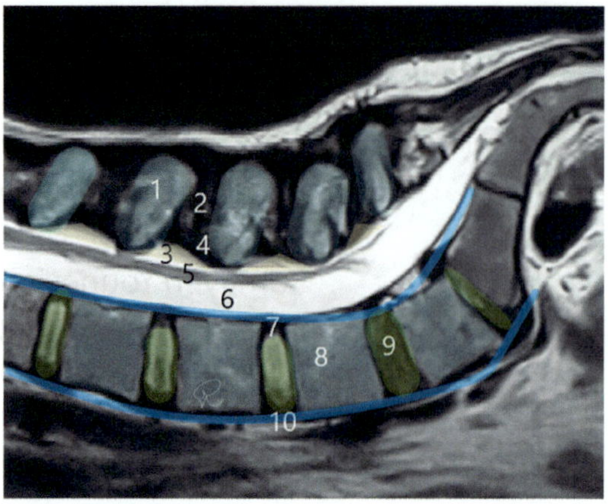

Fig. 8.1 Midsagittal spine cross-section anatomy. This illustration provides a comprehensive overview of a well-labeled mid-sagittal MRI scan of the lumbar spine, focusing on key anatomical structures important for medical analysis. The image utilizes distinct coloring to differentiate various elements: bones are represented in light blue, intervertebral discs in green, and ligaments in blue. This detailed illustration enhances our understanding of spinal anatomy, which is essential for thorough medical evaluation. 1. The spinous process (1) is the bony projection extending posteriorly from each vertebra as an attachment point for muscles and ligaments. 2. The interspinous ligament (2) connects adjacent spinous processes and plays a vital role in maintaining spinal stability. 3. The epidural space (3) is a fat-filled region situated between the dura mater and the vertebral canal. It accommodates nerve roots and blood vessels and is frequently accessed for epidural injections. 4. The ligamentum flavum (4) is a robust elastic ligament that connects the laminae of neighboring vertebrae, facilitating spinal flexibility and supporting posture. 5. The cauda equina (5) comprises a bundle of nerve roots extending from the conus medullaris, responsible for the sensory and motor innervation of the lower limbs and pelvic organs. 6. Cerebrospinal fluid (CSF) (6) encases and buffers the cauda equina within the dural sac, offering protection and metabolic support. 7. The posterior longitudinal ligament (7) is situated along the posterior aspect of the vertebral bodies within the spinal canal, reinforcing disc integrity and restraining excessive flexion. 8. The vertebral body (8) constitutes the large, cylindrical, weight-bearing portion of the vertebra, providing essential structural support. 9. The intervertebral disc (9) is a cushioning structure between the vertebrae, composed of the annulus fibrosus and nucleus pulposus. It allows for flexibility and shock absorption. 10. The anterior longitudinal ligament (10) is a substantial ligament that runs along the anterior aspect of the vertebral bodies, preventing excessive hyperextension of the spine

8.2.1.2 Scan and Injection

Patient Position: The patient should be lying prone on the bed. Placing a pillow under the belly will help separate the spinous processes and improve visualization of the lumbar spine structures.

Probe Position: First, locate and palpate the spinous process in the lumbosacral area, then position the probe along its long axis (Fig. 8.2a).

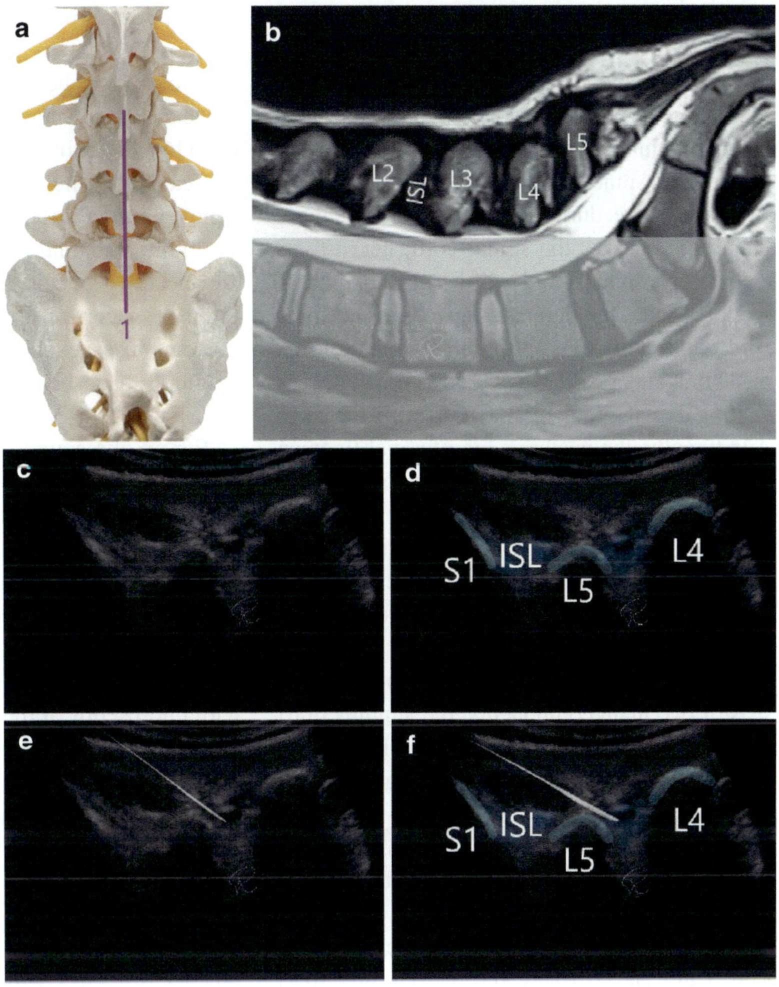

Fig. 8.2 Midsagittal lumbar spine scan: The image comprises six panels illustrating anatomical and imaging perspectives of the mid-sagittal lumbar spine. Panel (**a**) features a posterior view of the lumbar vertebrae, with a red line denoting the midline. Panel (**b**) presents a mid-sagittal MRI scan of the lumbar spine, clearly labeling vertebrae L2 to L5 and interspinous ligament (ISL). Panels (**c**) and (**e**) offer ultrasound images of the lumbar region without annotations. In contrast, Panels (**d**) and (**f**) display corresponding labeled ultrasound images that identify vertebrae L4, L5, and S1, as well as the interspinous ligament (ISL). Panels (**e**) and (**f**) also show the needle trajectory for an interlaminar ligament injection

Scanning: During this scan, you will observe several convex hyperechoic structures, which correspond to the cortices of the spinous process. The most distal structure corresponds to the S1 spinous process, which exhibits an upsloping curvature. Moving proximally, you will encounter structures corresponding to L5 and L4. Between each pair of spinous processes lies the interspinous ligament (Fig. 8.2c, d). Inflammation of this ligament is known as Baastrup's disease [3], which can be effectively managed with steroid injections. To administer the injection, the needle should be inserted from the distal end and advanced in-plane toward the ligament (Fig. 8.2e, f).

8.2.2 Para Central: Lamina View

8.2.2.1 Anatomy

A parasagittal cross-sectional view of the spine at the level of the lamina provides a detailed anatomical perspective, shedding light on the relationship between crucial structures that contribute to spinal stability and function. This slice through the vertebrae reveals several key components. The laminae, which form the posterior part of the vertebral arch, extend from the pedicles and connect to the spinous processes. This bony structure protects the spinal cord within the vertebral canal. In the parasagittal view, the lamina is seen as part of the roof of the spinal canal and is essential for attaining ligaments and muscles. The ligamentum flavum, a strong and elastic ligament anterior to the laminae, connects the adjacent laminas. It runs along the posterior aspect of the spinal canal, helping maintain spinal stability while contributing to the spine's flexibility. Another critical structure is the dural sac, the protective membrane that encases the spinal cord, nerve roots, and cerebrospinal fluid (CSF). In this cross-sectional view, the dural sac envelopes the spinal cord and nerve roots, providing protection and metabolic support. It plays a crucial role in preventing damage to the delicate neural structures. Additionally, the posterior longitudinal ligament runs along the posterior surface of the vertebral bodies and is positioned in front of the spinal cord. Its primary function is to reinforce the intervertebral discs and prevent excessive spine flexion, thus contributing to the overall stability of the vertebral column. The intervertebral disc, situated between adjacent vertebral bodies, consists of two main components: the annulus fibrosus, the outer fibrous layer, and the nucleus pulposus, the inner gel-like core (Fig. 8.3b) [4]. All structures located anterior to the lamina are often obscured during ultrasound scans, making visualization challenging. This limitation typically results from the orientation and positioning of the spine, which can conceal deeper structures from view. Nevertheless, the interlaminar space is a valuable assessment area, mainly when the spine is semi-flexed. This posture enhances the interlaminar space, facilitating a clearer view of deeper structures. Utilizing this space allows for visualizing critical components such as the ligamentum flavum, the dural sac, the posterior aspects of the vertebral bodies, and the intervertebral discs. The capacity to visualize these structures, especially the e, epidural space, is especially beneficial for guiding interventions like epidural steroid injections, nerve blocks, and minimally invasive spinal procedures.

8.2.2.2 Scan and Injection

Patient Position: Lying down on the bed in the prone position. Placing a pillow under the belly will help separate the spinous processes and improve visualization of the lumbar spine structures.

Probe Position: First, locate and palpate the spinous process in the lumbosacral area, then position the probe along its long axis gradually move the probe laterally until the spinous process is no longer visible (Fig. 8.3a).

Scanning: The oblique, relatively flat hyperechoic lamina structures will come into view. From the proximal perspective, you can visualize the L4, L5, and S1 laminas and the interlaminar space that separates them. Additionally, you can observe the ligamentum flavum and the epidural space beneath the laminas (Fig. 8.3c, d) [5].

For an ultrasound-guided injection, insert the needle from the distal end of the probe and smoothly advance it in-plane toward the upper lamina's edge. Proceed to walk the needle off the bone distally until it penetrates the ligamentum flavum (Fig. 8.3e, f). Use a glass syringe to monitor pressure loss at this point. The authors strongly recommend employing a double guide with fluoroscopy at this stage.

8.2.3 Centrolateral: Facet Joint View

8.2.3.1 Anatomy

A parasagittal spine cross-section at the facet joint level offers a comprehensive view of several significant structures within the lumbar or cervical spine. This specific imaging plane slices through the spine slightly off-center, allowing visualization of both bony and soft tissue structures about the facet joint. In this cross-sectional perspective, various key anatomical features can be identified. The inferior articular process is observed as a downward projection from the above vertebra, forming the facet joint's upper component. This process articulates with the superior articular process of the vertebra below. At the core of these structures lies the facet joint, positioned between the inferior and superior articular processes. This synovial joint facilitates controlled motion between adjacent vertebrae, enabling flexion, extension, and rotation. Surrounding this joint is the joint capsule, which contributes to its stability. Additionally, the bony region known as the pars interarticularis can be seen between the superior

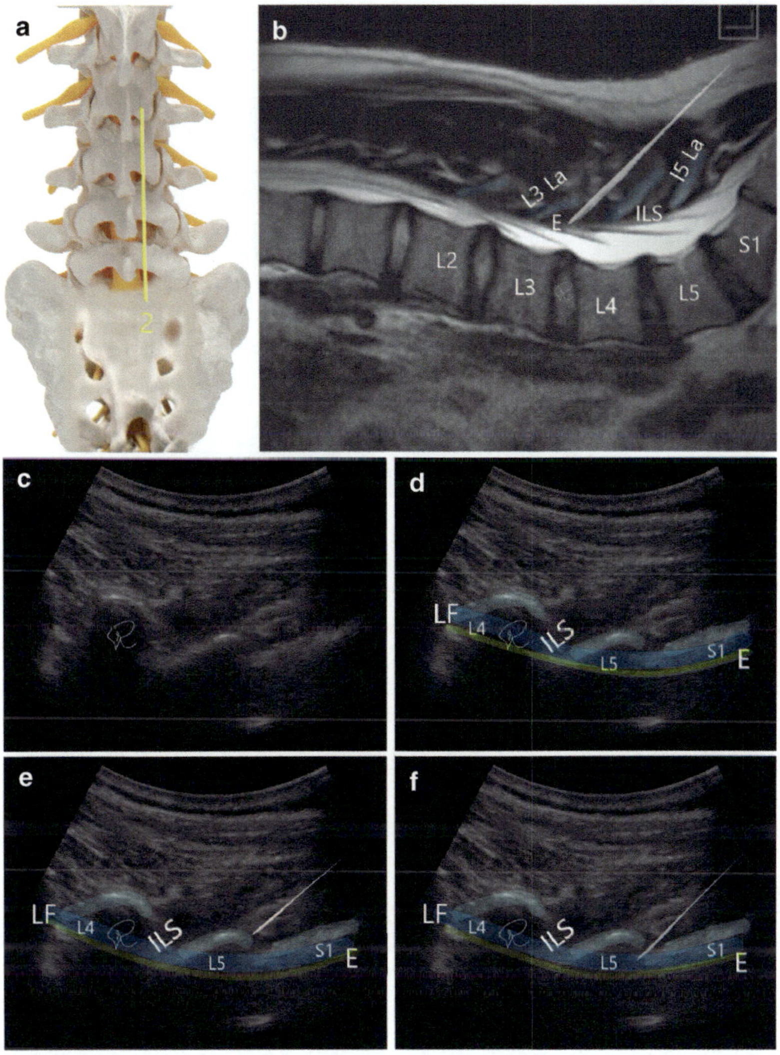

Fig. 8.3 Lumbar spine parasagittal scan; interlaminar view. The image comprises six panels illustrating lumbar spine anatomy and ultrasound imaging. Panel (**a**) depicts a diagram of the lumbar spine, labeling the vertebrae from L1 to S1, with a yellow line indicating the long-axis probe placement. Panel (**b**) presents a sagittal MRI scan highlighting the lumbar vertebrae from L2 to S1 and the lamina, interlaminar space, and epidural space, with a line showing the path to the epidural space. Panel (**c**) displays ultrasound images of the lamina and interlaminar space. Panel (**d**) shows the same image as in (**c**) but with annotations: the lumbar vertebrae (L1 to L5), sacrum (S1), and epidural space (E) are marked with a yellow line, while the interlaminar space (ILS) and ligamentum flavum (LF), highlighted with a thick blue line. Panel (**e**) provides the same image as (**d**), with the needle trajectory touching the inferior pole of the lamina. Finally, Panel (**f**) demonstrates the redirection of the needle tip to the ligamentum flavum

and inferior articular processes; it holds significant importance for spinal stability and is often a common site of injury, particularly in cases of spondylolysis. In this anatomical view, the following structures are also notable: pedicles, vertebral bodies, intervertebral discs, the posterior longitudinal ligament, the dural sac and its contents, and the anterior longitudinal ligament (Fig. 8.4b) [6]. However, all structures anterior to the inferior articular process and pars interarticularis are obscured during ultrasound scans, making them difficult to visualize.

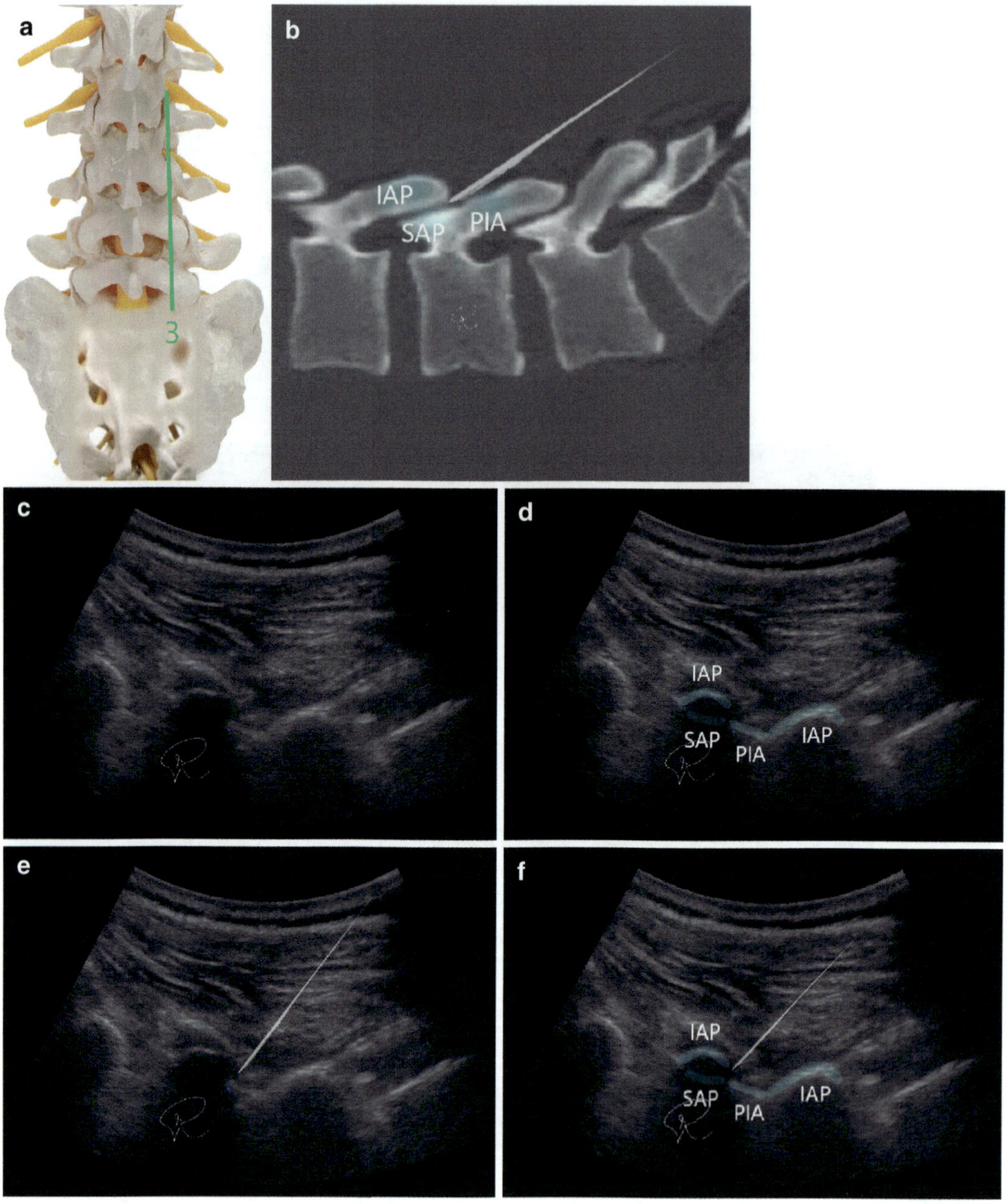

Fig. 8.4 Lumbar spine parasagittal scan; facet joint view. The image is composed of six panels that depict spinal anatomy and long-axis ultrasound imaging at the level of the facet joints. Panel (**a**) features a labeled diagram of the lumbar spine, with a green line indicating the probe's position over the facet joints in a long-axis view. Panel (**b**) showcases a CT scan of the lumbar spine, with labels identifying the Inferior Articular Process (IAP), Superior Articular Process (SAP), and Pars Interarticularis (PIA). Panels (**c**) through (**f**) display ultrasound images of the lumbar region. Panel (**c**) presents an unlabeled ultrasound image of the lumbar spine on the long axis over the facet joints, while Panels (**d**) and (**f**) incorporate labels for the Inferior Articular Process (IAP), Superior Articular Process (SAP), and Pars Interarticularis (PIA). Panels (**e**) and (**f**) contain the same images as Panels (**c**) and (**d**) but additionally illustrate the needle trajectory as it enters the facet joint

8.2.3.2 Scan and Injection

Patient Position: Lying down on the bed in the prone position. Placing a pillow under the belly will help separate the spinous processes and improve visualization of the lumbar spine structures.

Probe Position: Begin by identifying and palpating the spinous process in the lumbosacral region. Once located, position the ultrasound probe along the long axis of the spinous processes for optimal visualization. Then, slide the probe laterally to observe the flat, hyperechoic structures corresponding to the laminae. Continue moving the probe laterally to reveal the multiple humps, which lie more superficially than the laminae but are not as superficial as the spinous processes (Fig. 8.4a).

Scanning: These humps represent the inferior articular processes (IAPs). Typically, the superior articular processes (SAPs) are not visible via ultrasound as they are situated beneath the IAPs. The pars interarticularis is located between two consecutive IAPs (Fig. 8.4c, d) [7, 8]. For facet joint injection in this view, the needle should be inserted from the distal end to approach the lower pole of the IAP and SAP junction in-plane (Fig. 8.4e, f).

8.2.4 Far Lateral: Transverse Process View

8.2.4.1 Anatomy

This axial plane offers a cross-sectional view of the spine at the level of the transverse process, providing a detailed examination of several key anatomical structures. The transverse process extends laterally from each vertebra and is prominently visible, serving as an essential bony landmark for identifying adjacent muscles and structures. Superficial to the transverse process, the erector spinae muscle can be observed; this muscle runs along the spine and is vital for maintaining posture and facilitating spinal movement. Moreover, the psoas muscle is visible deep in the transverse process on either side of the vertebral column. The psoas muscle plays a crucial role in hip flexion and is often considered in the context of spinal and hip pathology. Additionally, the lumbar plexus, situated within the psoas muscle, can be visualized in this plane. This network of nerves is essential for innervating the lower limbs as well as parts of the pelvis and abdomen (Fig. 8.5b) [9].

8.2.4.2 Scan

Patient Position: Lying down on the bed in the prone position. Placing a pillow under the belly will help separate the spinous processes and improve visualization of the lumbar spine structures.

Probe Position: Commence by identifying and palpating the spinous processes within the lumbosacral region. Once palpation confirms their location, orient the ultrasound probe along the long axis of the spinous processes to optimize visualization of these structures near the skin surface. As you sweep the probe laterally, you will visualize the flat, hyperechoic laminae. Continuing laterally, multiple superficial elevations will become apparent, representing the facet joints situated above the laminae yet below the spinous processes level. Further lateral movement reveals another set of distinct, deeper prominences: transverse processes. These structures lie deeper than the facet joints and are vital anatomical landmarks for lumbar plexus evaluations and interventions.

Scanning: Start by identifying S1, the most distal vertebra with its characteristic upsloping contour. Then, move proximally to locate L5 and, subsequently, the L4 transverse process, following the natural alignment of the lumbar spine. The erector spinae muscles are positioned posterior to the transverse processes, forming a key landmark for spinal imaging. The psoas muscle is anterior to the transverse processes, which appears as a hypoechoic structure with internal striations (Fig. 8.5c, d) [10, 11].

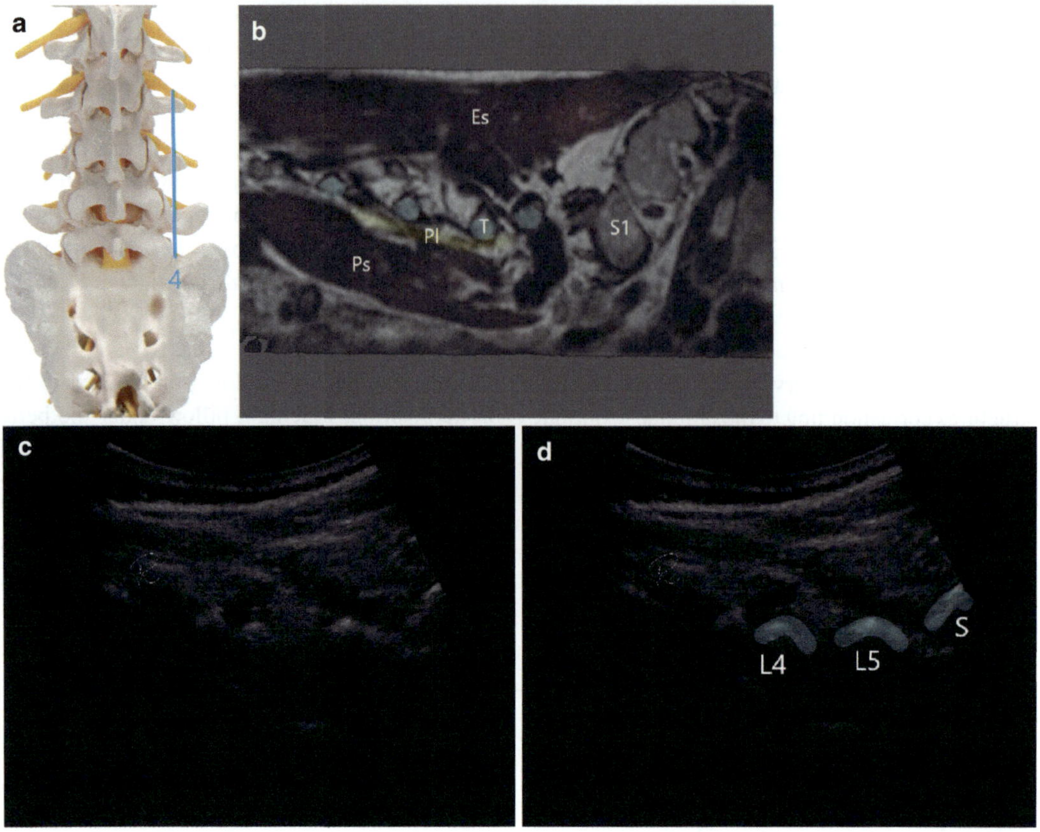

Fig. 8.5 Lumbar spine parasagittal scan; transverse process view. The image consists of four panels illustrating anatomical and ultrasound images of the lumbar spine at the level of the transverse processes in an axial view. Panel (**a**) presents an anatomical model of the lumbar spine, with a blue line indicating the probe position for ultrasound imaging. Panel (**b**) displays a sagittal MRI scan, highlighting key structures, including the erector spinae (Es), psoas muscle (Ps), lumbar plexus (Pl), and sacrum (S1). Panel (**c**) shows an ultrasound image of the lumbar region at the level of the transverse process in a long-axis view without labels. Panel (**d**) is the same ultrasound image as panel (**c**) but annotated with labels identifying the L4 and L5 transverse processes and the sacrum (S)

8.3 Transverse (Short-Axis)

8.3.1 Lamina View

8.3.1.1 Anatomy

The lumbar spine's anatomy at the lamina's level is critical for understanding spine procedures. A cross-sectional perspective reveals several key anatomical elements, including bony landmarks, neural structures, muscles, and connective tissues. The lamina, a flattened segment of the vertebral arch, connects the spinous process to the pedicles, effectively enclosing the vertebral foramen. The spinous process, projecting posteriorly, acts as an attachment site for various ligaments and muscles, while the laterally projecting transverse processes provide additional points for muscle attachment. The facet joints, or zygapophyseal joints, facilitate controlled movement between adjacent vertebrae's superior and inferior articular processes. Neural structures in this region vary depending on the spinal level. Above L1-L2, the spinal cord occupies the vertebral canal, transitioning into the cauda equina below this level—a collection of lumbar and sacral nerve roots. The dura mater encases these neural elements, providing a protective outer layer, while the epidural space around the dura contains adipose tissue and the internal vertebral venous plexus. Muscle groups are vital in providing stability and facilitating movement in the lumbar region. The erector spinae muscles, which include the longissimus, iliocostalis, and spinalis, run bilaterally along the spine, contributing to posture and mobility. The multifidus, a significant stabilizing muscle, is integral to maintaining lumbar stability, while the quadratus lumborum aids in lateral flexion and overall stabilization. In addition to these, muscular structures, ligaments, and soft tissues contribute to the robustness of the lumbar spine. The ligamentum flavum, an elastic connective tissue, links adjacent laminae and is essential for spinal stability, aiding in recovery post-flexion. The interspinous ligament connects adjacent spinous processes to restrict excessive flexion, while the supraspinous ligament extends along the upper tips of the spinous processes, adding further support (Fig. 8.6b) [1, 4]. However, all structures anterior to the lamina are obscured during ultrasound scans, making them difficult to visualize.

8.3.1.2 Scan and Injection

Patient Position: Lying down on the bed in the prone position. Placing a pillow under the belly will help separate the spinous processes and improve visualization of the lumbar spine structures.

Probe position: Begin by locating and palpating the spinous process in the lumbosacral region to establish a reference point. Position the ultrasound probe along the long axis of the spinous process to visualize the alignment of the surrounding spinous processes, which will help identify the desired level. Once the target spinous process is pinpointed, center it on the screen for optimal imaging. Next, rotate the probe 90° to shift from longitudinal to transverse, enabling a cross-sectional assessment of the spinous process and adjacent structures (Fig. 8.6a).

Scanning: When scanning in this view, the image will prominently display a hyperechoic structure that represents the spinous process of the upper vertebral level. Additionally, distinct hyperechoic structures corresponding to the laminae and the pars interarticularis will be visible on each side. Above the lamina and pars interarticularis surrounding the spine, the erector spinae muscles are clearly identifiable, acting as a crucial posterior support structure. More deeply situated and laterally in the image, two further hyperechoic structures can be recognized as part of the posterior body cortex of the vertebra. The intervertebral foramen, located between the pars interarticularis and the vertebral body, allows visualization of the nerve root complex adjacent to the vertebral body (Fig. 8.6c, d) [5, 11]. To effectively block the nerve root, it is recommended to approach it in-plane from the lateral side using a spinal needle. Direct ultrasound guidance allows the practitioner to monitor the needle's path as it approaches the target nerve root closely. Initially, the needle should touch the lamina-pars complex before being maneuvered away from the bone and towards the foramen (Fig. 8.6e, f). At this stage, it is highly recommended to use nerve stimulation or fluoroscopy to confirm the accurate placement of the needle and enhance procedural safety. Nerve stimulation involves delivering low-intensity electrical impulses through the needle to trigger a motor response, which helps to verify the needle's proximity to the nerve root. This method ensures that the needle is sufficiently close to the nerve for effective delivery of anesthetic or corticosteroid while reducing the risk of direct nerve injury. Fluoroscopy provides continuous X-ray imaging, allowing precise needle guidance and nerve root epidural enhancement using contrast materials.

8.3.2 Interlaminar View

8.3.2.1 Anatomy

In this cross-sectional view of the lumbar spine at the facet joint level, the inferior and superior articular processes come together to form the facet joint, a synovial joint encapsulated within a joint capsule. This structure allows for controlled movement while providing stability to the spine. Anteriorly, the vertebral body is the primary weight-bearing component and houses the intervertebral disc, a cushion to absorb mechanical stress. The pedicle functions as a supportive

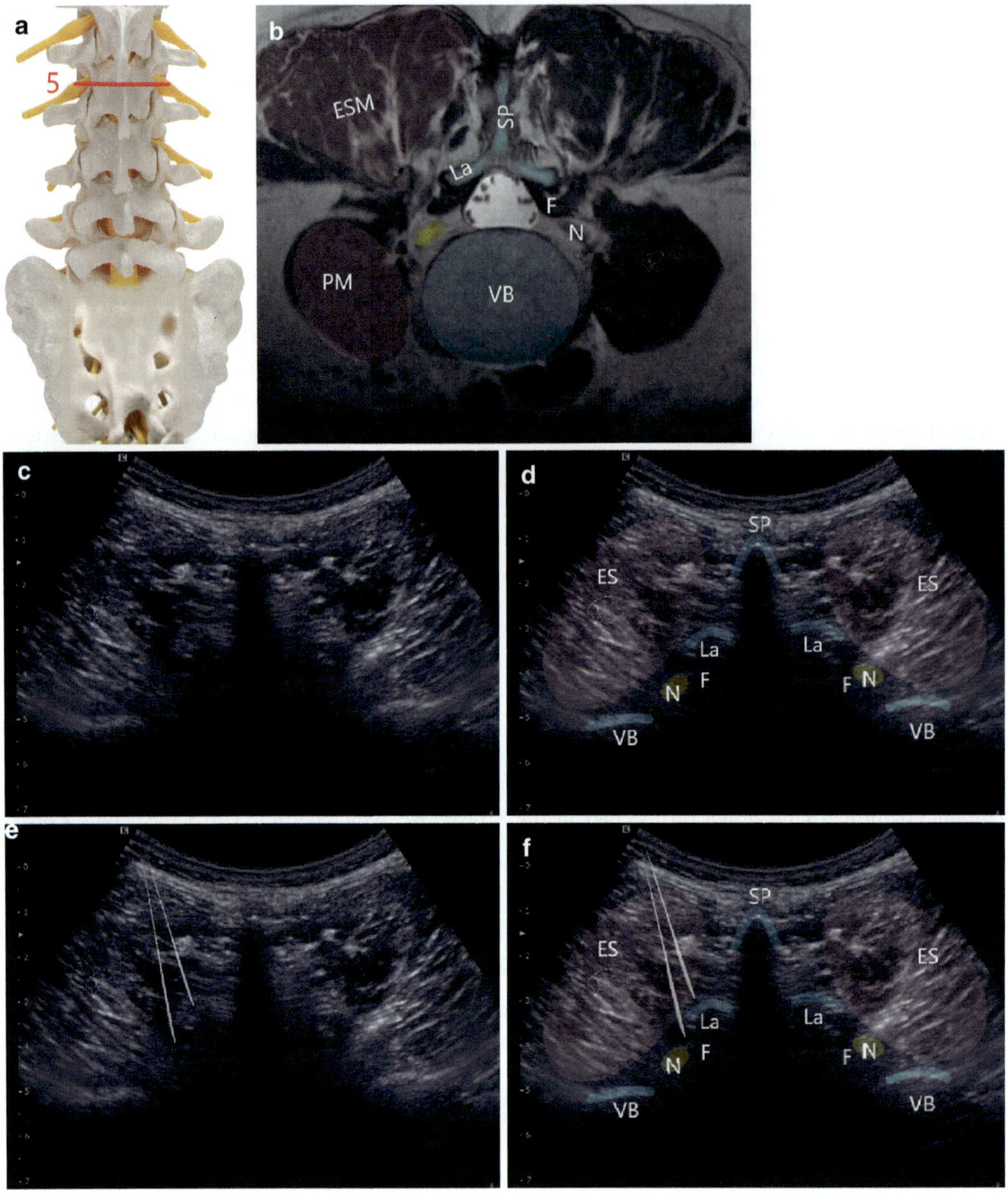

Fig. 8.6 Lumbar spine transverse scan; Lamina and nerve root view. The image set consists of six panels depicting anatomical and ultrasound views of the lumbar spine and surrounding muscles. Panel (**a**) presents a diagram of the lumbar spine, marked with a red line that indicates the vertebra in the axial plane at the lamina level, serving as a reference for proper short-axis probe positioning. Panel (**b**) features a cross-sectional MRI that highlights essential muscles and nerves, labeled as the erector spinae muscle (ESM), multifidus (M), foramen (F), nerve root (N), and vertebral body (VB), providing a detailed visualization of deep lumbar structures. Panels (**c**) and (**e**) show short-axis ultrasound images at the lamina level without annotations, which serve as comparative views for interpretation. Panels (**d**) and (**f**) display corresponding ultrasound images with labeled structures, including the spinous process (SP), erector spinae (ES), vertebral body (VB), foramen (F), and nerve root (N), illustrating the relative positioning of these muscles and nerves. Additionally, panels (**e**) and (**f**) highlight the trajectory of the needle, demonstrating its approach to the lamina before navigating into the foramen. This comprehensive imaging set effectively illustrates the correlation between MRI and ultrasound modalities in identifying lumbar anatomy, enhancing clinical assessments and procedural accuracy

bridge between the vertebral body and the posterior elements, contributing to the structural integrity of the neural arch. Extending laterally, the transverse process is an attachment site for various muscles and ligaments, including the erector spinae muscles, which are vital for spinal extension and stabilization. Anterior to the transverse process lies the psoas muscle, located near the lumbar plexus, playing an essential role in hip flexion and core stability. Several ligamentous structures further reinforce the spine. The ligamentum flavum connects adjacent laminae, providing elasticity and assisting in maintaining spinal alignment. The posterior longitudinal ligament runs along the back of the vertebral bodies, limiting excessive flexion, while the anterior longitudinal ligament offers support against hyperextension. The dural sac, which encases the spinal cord and nerve roots, is also visible in this view, surrounded by cerebrospinal fluid. This anatomical perspective is particularly valuable for guiding interventional procedures such as facet joint injections, medial branch blocks, and radiofrequency ablation. It ensures precise needle placement and minimizes the risk of complications (Fig. 8.7b) [6, 9]. However, all structures anterior to the articular process are obscured during ultrasound scans, making them difficult to visualize.

8.3.2.2 Scan and Injection

Patient Position: position the patient prone on the table with a pillow under their belly.

Probe position: Start by identifying and palpating the spinous process in the lumbosacral region to establish a precise reference point. Position the ultrasound probe along the long axis of the spinous process to confirm the alignment of adjacent spinous processes, facilitating accurate level identification. Once the target spinous process is located, ensure it is centered on the display for optimal imaging. Subsequently, rotate the probe 90° to transition from a longitudinal to a transverse view, allowing for a detailed cross-sectional evaluation of the spinous process and its surrounding anatomical structures. Sweep the probe distally until the shadow of the spinous process becomes undetectable (Fig. 8.7a).

Scanning: In this ultrasound image, two hyperechoic curved structures are identified as the inferior articular processes (IAP) of the superior vertebrae. These structures appear as bright, well-defined lines. Between them is a hypoechoic gap at the midline, which corresponds to the interlaminar space—an important area for accessing the epidural space and conducting various spinal procedures. Adjacent to the IAPs is another hyperechoic structure known as the superior articular process (SAP), which is also bright. A small hypoechoic interruption located between the IAP and SAP indicates the presence of the facet joint, a critical structure when assessing lumbar spine mobility or performing interventions such as facet joint injections. Additionally, there is a transverse process extending laterally and sloping upwards next to the SAP. The angle formed between the transverse process and the SAP is significant as it defines the pathway for the medial branch of the dorsal rami, which is essential for innervating the facet joints. Between the two IAPs on either side, the ligamentum flavum is visible as a thin hyperechoic line that connects adjacent vertebrae, playing a crucial role in maintaining spinal stability and elasticity. Deep to the ligamentum flavum, the epidural space can be observed, which is vital for performing epidural steroid injections intended to alleviate nerve root compression. In the deeper regions of the image, the hyperechoic line of the posterior wall of the vertebral body is visible, providing structural support and serving as a reference point for identifying the anterior elements of the spinal canal. Above the facet joints, the multifidus muscles can be seen as relatively hypoechoic compared to surrounding structures (Fig. 8.7c, d) [11].

Interlaminar epidural injection: Performing an interlaminar epidural block requires precise needle placement. Begin by inserting the needle from the lateral side, directing it toward the medial border of the contralateral inferior articular process (IAP). Navigating carefully around and off the bony structure of IAP is essential to reach the ligamentum flavum. Access to the epidural space can be achieved once the needle tip is positioned near or within this ligament

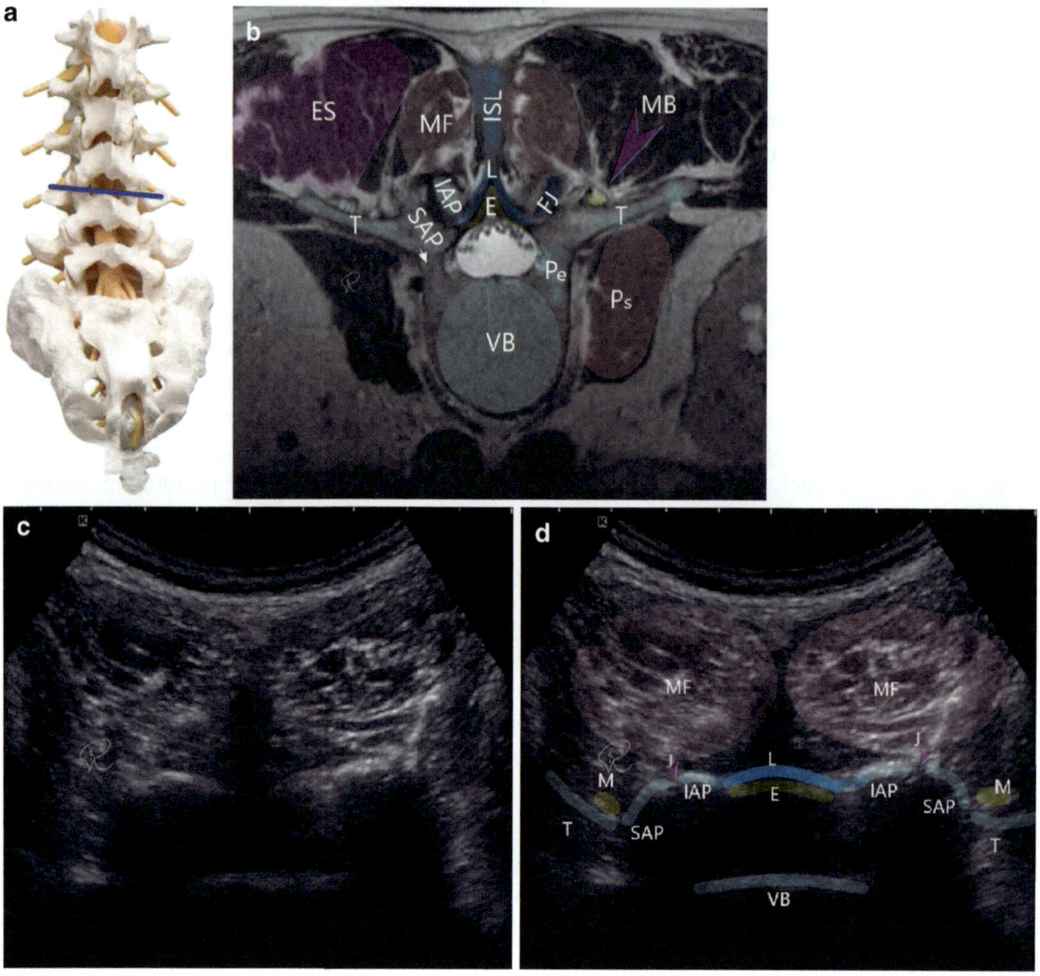

Fig. 8.7 Lumbar spine transverse scan; facet joint and transverse process view. The image is split into two distinct sections, displaying twelve panels that provide detailed anatomical and ultrasound views of the lumbar spine in cross-section at the facet joint level, along with three significant procedures. **Part A:** Panel (**a**) showcases a model of the lumbar spine, where a transverse blue line indicates the short-axis ultrasound probe's position at the facet joint's level. Panel (**b**) presents a cross-sectional axial MRI scan featuring color-coded highlights and labeled anatomical structures. The anatomical components highlighted include the vertebral body (VB), psoas muscle (Ps), pedicle (Pe), transverse process (T), superior articular process (SAP), inferior articular process (IAP), facet joint (FJ/J), epidural space (E), ligamentum flavum (L), interspinous ligament (ISL), multifidus muscle (MF), erector spinae (ES), and the medial branch (MB/M), which is denoted by a violet arrowhead. Panels (**c**) and (**d**) present the lumbar spine ultrasound images in a short-axis view at the facet joint level. In panel (**d**), the anatomical structures identified in panel (**b**) are similarly annotated, with the medial branch labeled simply as "M." Panels (**e**) and (**f**) expand upon the preceding images by incorporating a needle trajectory directed towards the facet joint. **Part B:** The second section of the image consists of six ultrasound scans labeled from (**g**) to (**l**), reflecting the same views as those in panels (**c**) and (**d**) while maintaining consistent color highlights and anatomical annotations. These images depict various procedural needle trajectories. Panels (**g**) and (**h**) illustrate the technique for interlaminar epidural injection, detailing the precise needle approach necessary for accessing the epidural space. Panels (**i**) and (**j**) represent the needle trajectory for the medial branch block, emphasizing the path targeted at the medial branch of the dorsal ramus to alleviate facet joint pain. Lastly, panels (**k**) and (**l**) amalgamate the three procedural approaches—interlaminar epidural injection, medial branch block, and facet joint injection—into a single comprehensive image, showcasing different needle orientations

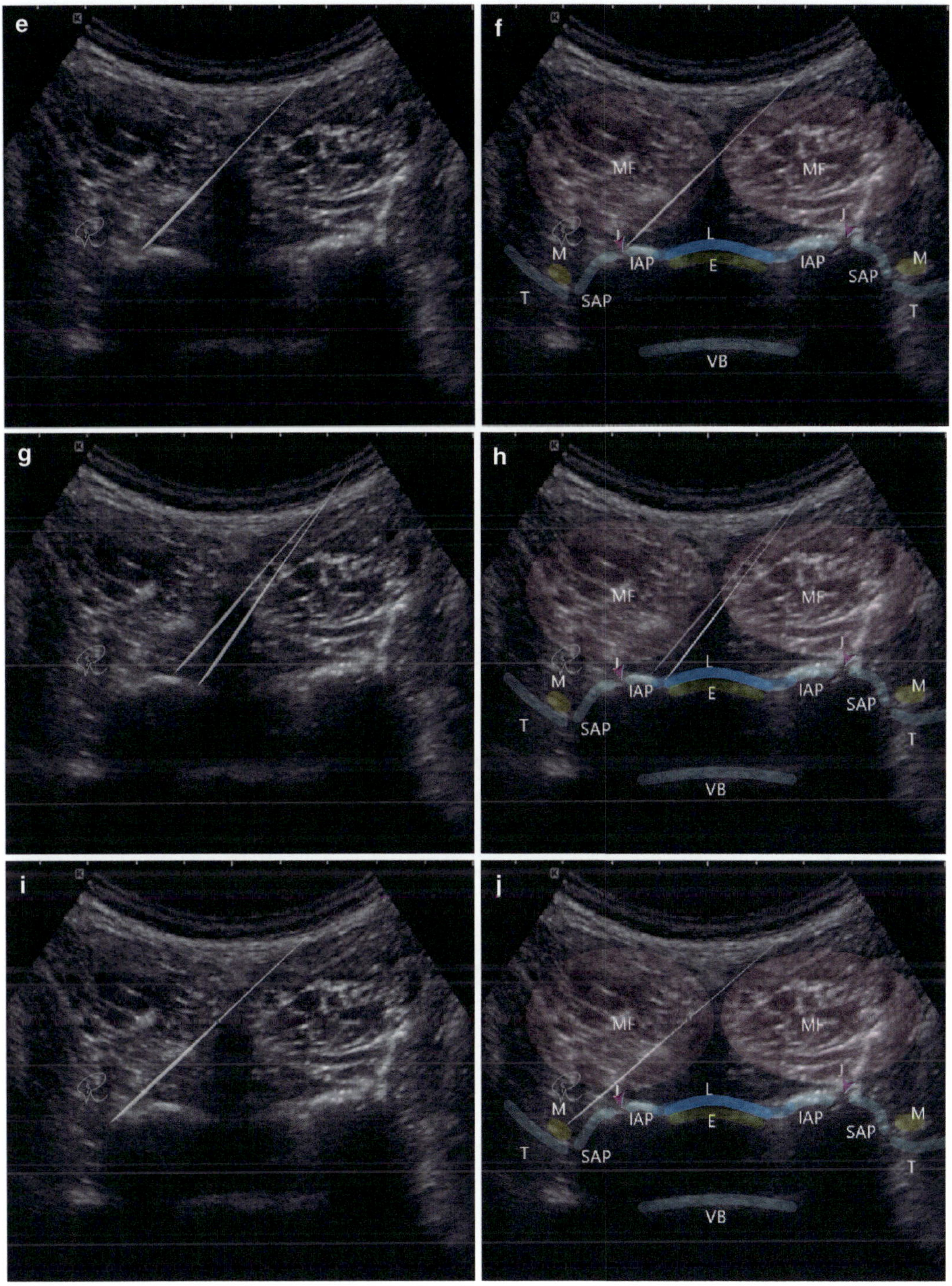

Fig. 8.7 (continued)

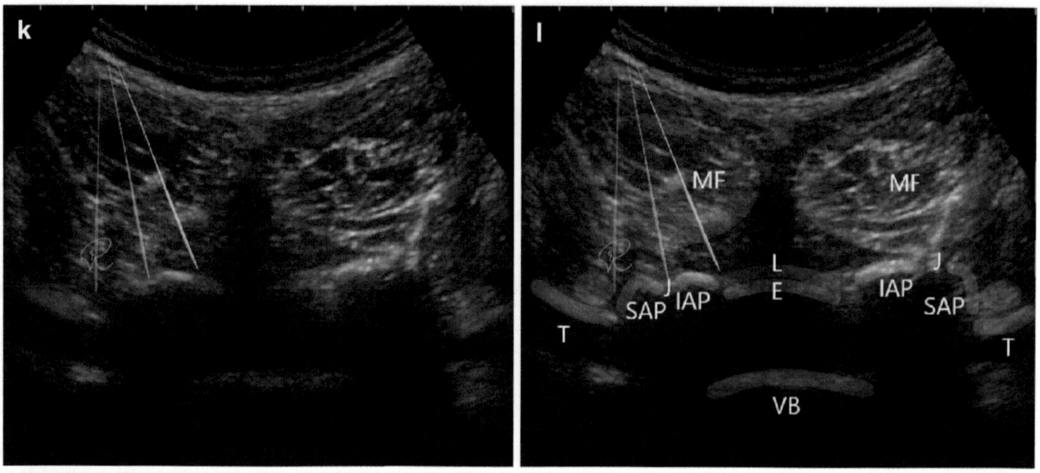

Fig. 8.7 (continued)

(Fig. 8.7e, f). To enhance accuracy and ensure safe needle placement, it is strongly recommended that a glass syringe be used to confirm the correct needle position before proceeding with the injection. Additionally, employing a double guide technique—The use of fluoroscopy during this procedure —can further increase precision.

Facet joint injection: To perform a facet joint injection, insert the needle from the lateral side, ensuring the approach remains in-plane with the ultrasound probe. The needle should be directed toward the contralateral facet joint, concentrating on the specific area of the joint to ensure optimal delivery of the injectate. This technique effectively delivers therapeutic relief to the facet joint and its surrounding structures (Fig. 8.7g, h).

Medial Branch Block: This view is well-suited for performing a medial branch block. To start, insert the needle from the lateral side, approaching the junction of the transverse process and the superior articular process (SAP) on the contralateral side using an in-plane technique. Gently guide the needle towards the medial branch, which usually lies at the junction of the superior articular process (SAP) and the transverse process. Using an in-plane approach provides clear visualization of the needle's path, ensuring precise placement in the targeted area for effective administration of the block.This technique can significantly relieve pain associated with facet joint dysfunction by directly targeting the medial branch nerves (Fig. 8.7i, j).

8.3.3 Sacral Spine Hiatus View

8.3.3.1 Anatomy

The sacral hiatus is located at the base of the sacrum, along the midline. It serves as an access point for caudal epidural injections. This hiatus is formed due to the incomplete fusion of the posterior elements of the sacral vertebrae, resulting in a gap at the distal end of the sacrum. Bordered by the sacral cornua—bony projections extending from the sacrum—on either side, the sacral hiatus leads into the sacral canal, which houses the cauda equina, a collection of spinal nerves at the lower end of the spinal cord. The sacrococcygeal ligament covers the hiatus, and its dimensions and shape may vary among individuals. The most common technique for caudal epidural injection is an inplane ultrasound-guided procedure, in which a needle is inserted just above the coccyx. The needle penetrates the sacrococcygeal ligament to reach the epidural space (Fig. 8.8b) [12].

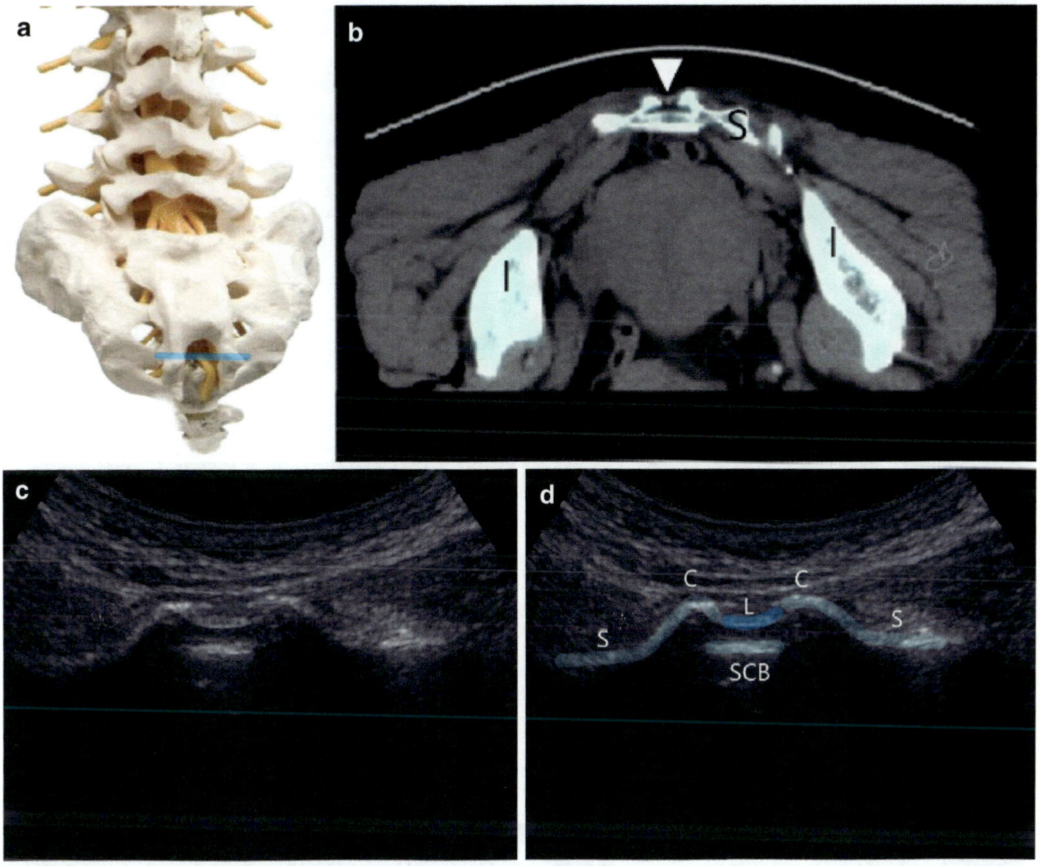

Fig. 8.8 Sacral hiatus scan and caudal epidural injection. This figure comprises two distinct parts, divided into ten panels that comprehensively demonstrate the anatomy and ultrasound imaging of the sacral hiatus. **Part A** encompasses four panels, all presenting the short-axis view of the sacral hiatus. In Panel (**a**), a lumbar spine model is depicted, with a transverse blue line delineating the precise location of the short-axis ultrasound probe over the sacral hiatus. Panel (**b**) provides a cross-sectional CT scan that details various anatomical structures, featuring labels such as I for the iliac bone, S for the sacrum, and an arrowhead indicating the sacral hiatus's location. Panels (**c**) and (**d**) present ultrasound images of the sacral hiatus in a short-axis orientation. Particularly in Panel (**d**), various layers and structures are identified with annotations, including S for the sacrum, C for cornua, SCL (L) for the sacrococcygeal ligament, SCB for the sacral canal base, and SCR for the sacral canal roof. **Part B** contains six panels from e to j that portray long-axis views and supplementary details of the sacral hiatus. In Panel (**e**), a lumbar spine model is again represented, this time with a sagittal blue line that indicates the positioning of the ultrasound probe in reference to the sacral hiatus. Panel (**f**) showcases a midsagittal CT scan, annotated to highlight important anatomical components such as the sacrum (S) and sacrococcygeal ligament (SCL (L)). Panels (**g**) and (**h**) present long-axis midsagittal ultrasound scans of the sacral hiatus, with Panel (h) highlighting and labeling structures such as SCL (L), SCB, and SCR, which clarify the relationship between these anatomical elements. Notably, Panel (**i**) resembles Panel (**f**) but includes the addition of a needle connected to a syringe placed within the sacral hiatus, demonstrating the needle's positioning for procedures within this anatomical region. Finally, Panel (**j**) mirrors Panel (**h**) but illustrates the needle trajectory directed towards the caudal epidural space, offering a clear view of how the needle is maneuvered to reach the epidural space for injections or other medical interventions

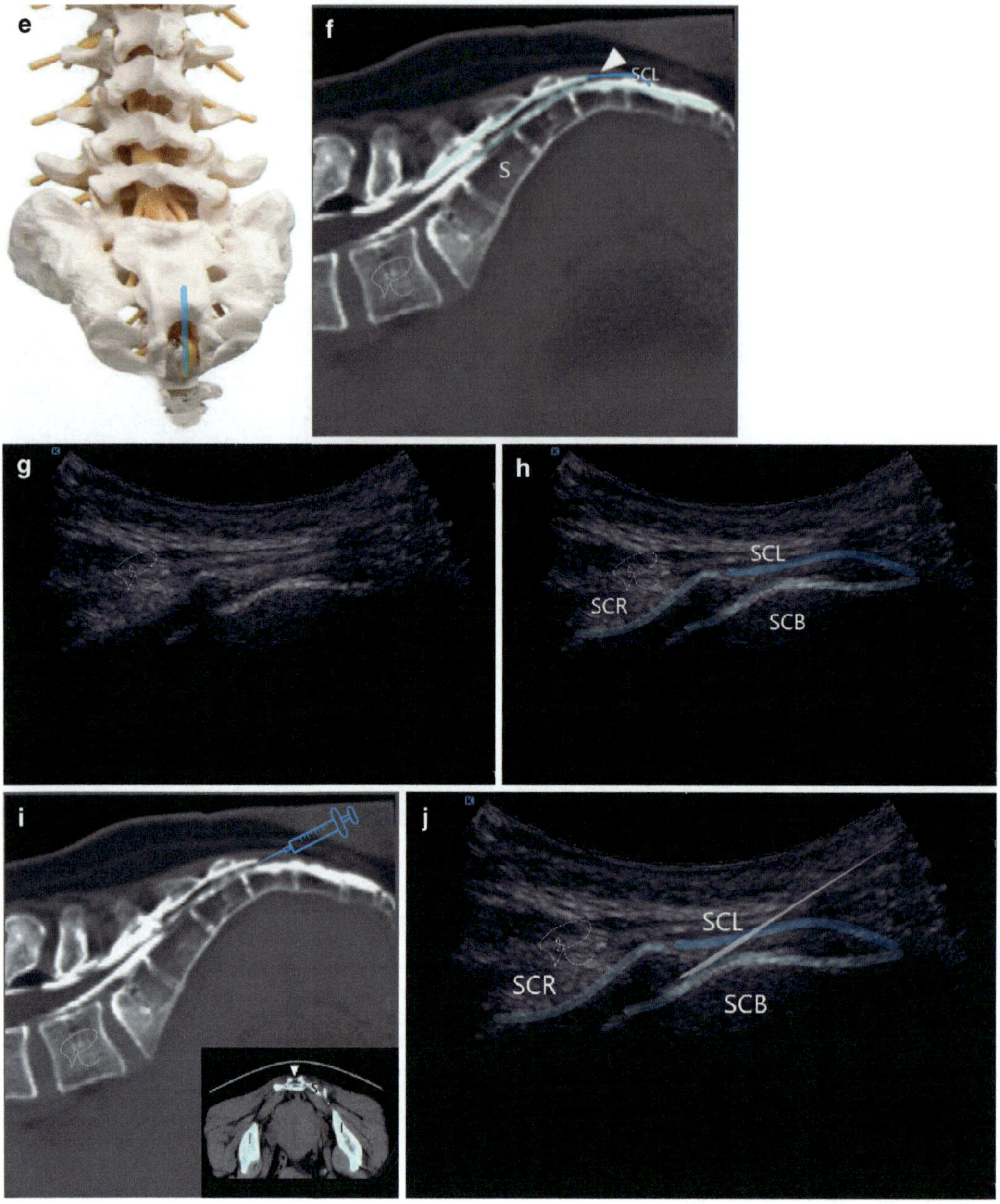

Fig. 8.8 (continued)

8.3.3.2 Scan and Injection

Patient Position: Position the patient in a prone position with a pillow under the pelvis area on the examination table.

Probe position: Position the probe transversely over the sacrum and begin sliding it downward. As the probe moves caudally, two hyperechoic convex structures will appear on the image, separated by a distinct hypoechoic area representing the sacral hiatus. This landmark is crucial for locating the sacral cornua and is an entry point for caudal epidural injections. Adjusting the probe tilt and image depth will enhance the clarity of these anatomical features, facilitating accurate needle placement and increasing the likelihood of procedural success (Fig. 8.8a).

Scanning: The observed humps correspond to the sacral cornua, which are important landmarks for identifying the sacral hiatus. In the ultrasound image, the sacral cornua will be seen on either side of the sacral hiatus, while the sacral bone appears as a continuous hyperechoic structure. Further into the image, a bright hyperechoic line indicates the floor of the sacral canal, marking its anterior boundary.The sacrococcygeal ligament is positioned between the cornua and manifests as a thin, hyperechoic band (Fig. 8.8c, d) [13]. To better define the caudal foramen, rotate the probe 90° to capture a long axis view (Fig. 8.8e, f). In this orientation, the deep hyperechoic line corresponds to the anterior wall of the sacral canal base, while the superficial hyperechoic line reflects the posterior wall of the sacral canal roof. The sacrococcygeal ligament is visible between these two structures, forming the dorsal boundary of the sacral hiatus (Fig. 8.8g, h). For a caudal epidural injection, it is recommended to insert the needle from the distal end of the sacral hiatus and advance it in-plane using ultrasound guidance. The needle should pass through the sacrococcygeal ligament before reaching the base of the sacral canal. Color Doppler imaging will help visualize the spread of the injectate, ensuring that it is not inadvertently injected into vascular structures or bone marrow, particularly in elderly individuals (Fig. 8.8i, j).

8.3.4 Thoracic Para Sagittal (Long-Axis): Intercostal Nerve Access

8.3.4.1 Anatomy

This cross-sectional view offers a comprehensive visualization of the anatomical layers of the thoracic wall, including the ribs, intercostal muscles, intercostal nerves, vasculature, pleura, and lungs, arranged from the outermost to the innermost structures. The intercostal nerve, which originates from the ventral rami of the thoracic nerve root, emerges from the neuroforamen and perforates the posterior intercostal membrane approximately 3 cm laterally. It subsequently enters the subcostal groove of the corresponding rib, where it continues along with the neurovascular bundle. Within the neurovascular bundle, the intercostal nerve is inferior to the intercostal vein and artery, adhering to the typical "VAN" arrangement (vein superiorly, artery in the middle, and nerve inferiorly). The ribs create acoustic shadows in ultrasound imaging, facilitating the identification of the intercostal space and the localization of neurovascular structures. Deep into the neurovascular bundle, the pleura presents as a hyperechoic linear structure, delineating the boundary between the thoracic wall and the lung parenchyma. The lung can be observed as an area exhibiting characteristic artifact patterns, such as A-lines or lung sliding, which vary with respiration (Fig. 8.9b) [12].

8.3.4.2 Scan and Injection

Patient position: Position the patient in a prone position to ensure optimal access to the targeted anatomical structures. This positioning provides a clear ultrasound window for visualizing the intercostal space, neurovascular bundle, and surrounding musculature.

Probe position: To visualize the intercostal short axis, position the probe parallel and approximately 2 inches lateral to the midsagittal line of the spine. This orientation provides a cross-sectional view of the intercostal structures, including the ribs, intercostal muscles, neurovascular bundles, and pleura. Adjust the angle of the probe as necessary to enhance image quality and

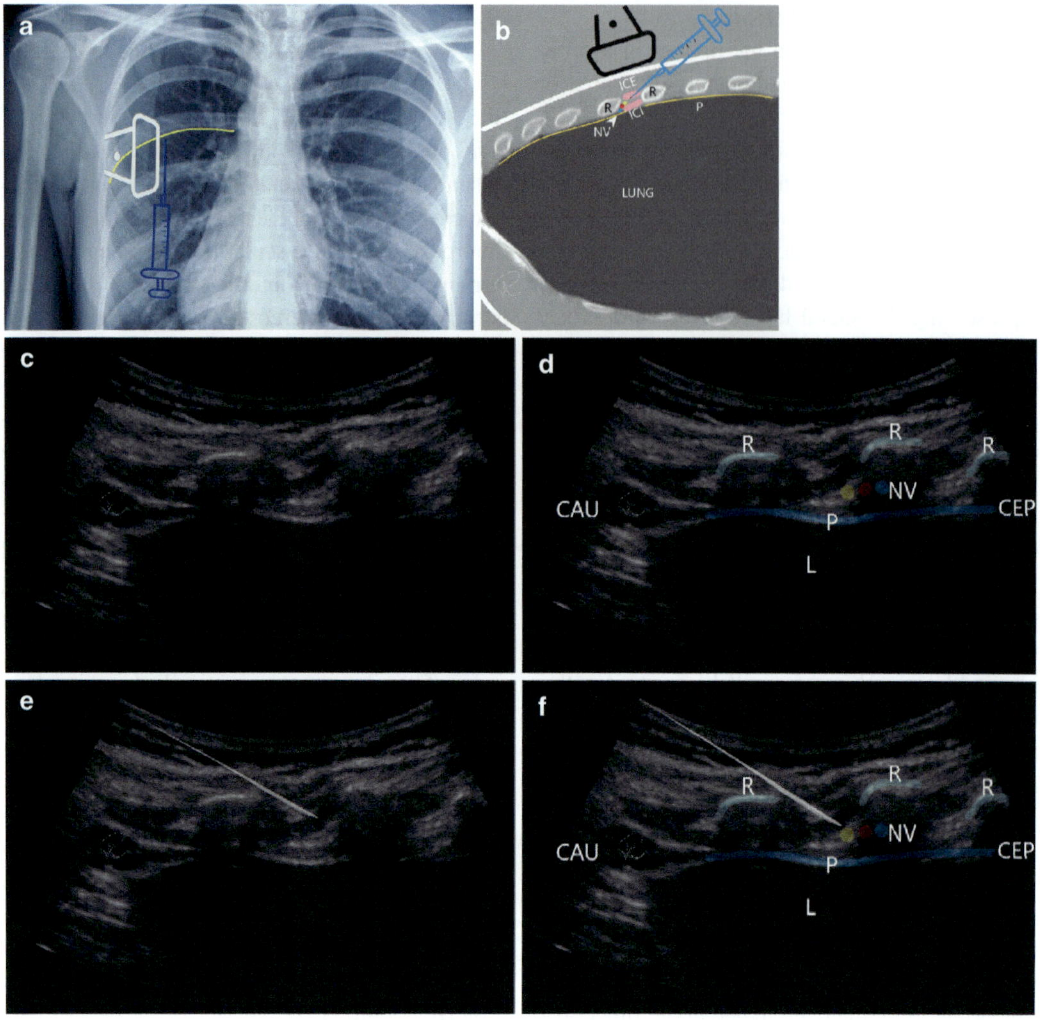

Fig. 8.9 Intercostal scan and nerve block. This composite image set presents a multi-modal approach to visualizing an intercostal nerve and block. Panel (**a**) features a chest X-ray with a highlighted yellow line, indicating an intercostal nerve, a probe for the probe position in a short-axis view of the nerve, and a syringe demonstrating the nerve block in plane procedure. Panel (**b**) offers a cross-sectional anatomical diagram of the chest, with key structures labeled, including the ICE intercostal external muscle, ICI intercostal internal muscle, P pleura, NV neurovascular bundle, R rib, and an illustration of a syringe demonstrating the procedural technique. Panels (**c**) through (**f**) provide ultrasound imaging perspectives of the intercostal space and nerve. Panel (**c**) shows an unlabeled ultrasound image. Panel (**d**) includes annotations identifying crucial landmarks, such as the P for pleura, R for rib, CAU for caudal, CEP for cephalad, and NV for the neurovascular bundle, which is marked with colored small circles: red for artery, blue for vein, and yellow for nerve. Panels (**e**) and (**f**) depict the same images as panels (**c**) and (**d**), but with the added needle trajectory indicating the target for the nerve block

optimize the identification of key anatomical landmarks (Fig. 8.9a).

Scanning: The rib cortices appear as a series of bright, curved lines with posterior acoustic shadowing, which indicates their dense bony structure. Beneath and between the ribs, a distinct bright line delineates the pleura, which can be seen moving with each breath, confirming lung movement. The intercostal neurovascular bundle is located just below the lower border of each rib within the subcostal groove. In this bundle, the vein is positioned most cephalad (toward the head), the artery is located centrally, and the intercostal nerve is the most caudal (toward the feet) structure (Fig. 8.9c, d) [14]. To perform an intercostal nerve block, position the needle in-plane from a caudal approach and carefully advance it toward the nerve while avoiding blood vessels. Accurate needle placement and real-time ultrasound guidance are crucial to ensure effective delivery of anesthetic while minimizing the risk of puncturing blood vessels or injuring the pleura (Fig. 8.9e, f).

8.3.5 Trans Abdominal Plane (Short Axis) (TAP Block)

8.3.5.1 Anatomy

A cross-sectional view of the transversus abdominis plane (TAP) block illustrates the abdominal wall's anatomical layers and their relationships to the neurovascular structures. From the superficial to the deep layers, the primary components include the skin and subcutaneous tissue, followed by three muscle layers: the external oblique (EO), internal oblique (IO), and transversus abdominis (TA). The fascial plane between the transversus abdominis and internal oblique contains the thoracolumbar nerves, making it the optimal site for local anesthetic deposition, TAP block. In terms of muscular anatomy from medial to lateral, the rectus abdominis (RA) is positioned near the midline, transitioning laterally to the oblique muscles (EO, IO, and TA) and further outward to the quadratus lumborum (QL), which forms the posterior abdominal wall. Ultrasound imaging renders these structures distinct hypoechoic muscle layers, separated by hyperechoic fascial planes. The neurovascular structures within the plane are visualized as small hypoechoic or anechoic formations, depending on the visibility of the nerves and vessels (Fig. 8.10b) [15].

8.3.5.2 Scan and Injection

(Fig. 8.10a).

Scanning: The abdominal muscles are visualized in a long-axis orientation during the scanning process. In the midaxillary view, the external oblique (EO) is the most superficial layer, followed by the internal oblique (IO), and the deepest layer is the transversus abdominis (TA). Beneath the transversus abdominis lies the pleura (Fig. 8.10c, d) [16]. At the anterior axillary line level, the rectus abdominis is positioned medially to the oblique muscles. In the posterior axillary line level scan, the latissimus dorsi (LD) and serratus anterior (SA) muscles are observed to be superficial to the oblique muscles. The quadratus lumborum (QL) muscle is posterior to the oblique muscles, while the psoas (Ps) muscle is located deep to the oblique muscles, attached to the anterior surface of the transverse process. The TAP block can be performed at various anatomical levels to achieve differing degrees of analgesia. The subcostal TAP block is administered between the xiphoid process and the anterosuperior iliac spine, following the anterior axillary line. The objective is to inject local anesthetic between the transversus abdominis muscle and the posterior rectus sheath, targeting the T6 to T9 dermatomes and blocking the anterior cutaneous nerves. However, it is important to note that this technique does not provide coverage for the skin lateral to the anterior axillary line (Fig. 8.10e, f). For a more caudal approach, the TAP block can be performed midway between the subcostal region and the iliac crest along the medial axillary line. The needle is inserted laterally and advanced in-plane between the transversus abdominis and internal oblique muscles. This approach offers sensory blockade of the T10 to T12 dermatomes, effectively blocking anterior and lateral cutaneous nerves (Fig. 8.10g, h). In the case of the posterior TAP block, the focus shifts to the anterolateral aspect of the quadratus lumborum (QL) muscle. The probe is initially positioned along the midaxillary line and then moved posteriorly to visualize the transversus abdominis and quadratus lumborum junction, typically at the posterior axillary line. The needle is inserted posteriorly, employing an in-plane technique to approach the junction. This method efficiently covers the T9 to T12 dermatomes and provides anterior and lateral cutaneous nerve blockade (Fig. 8.10i, j).

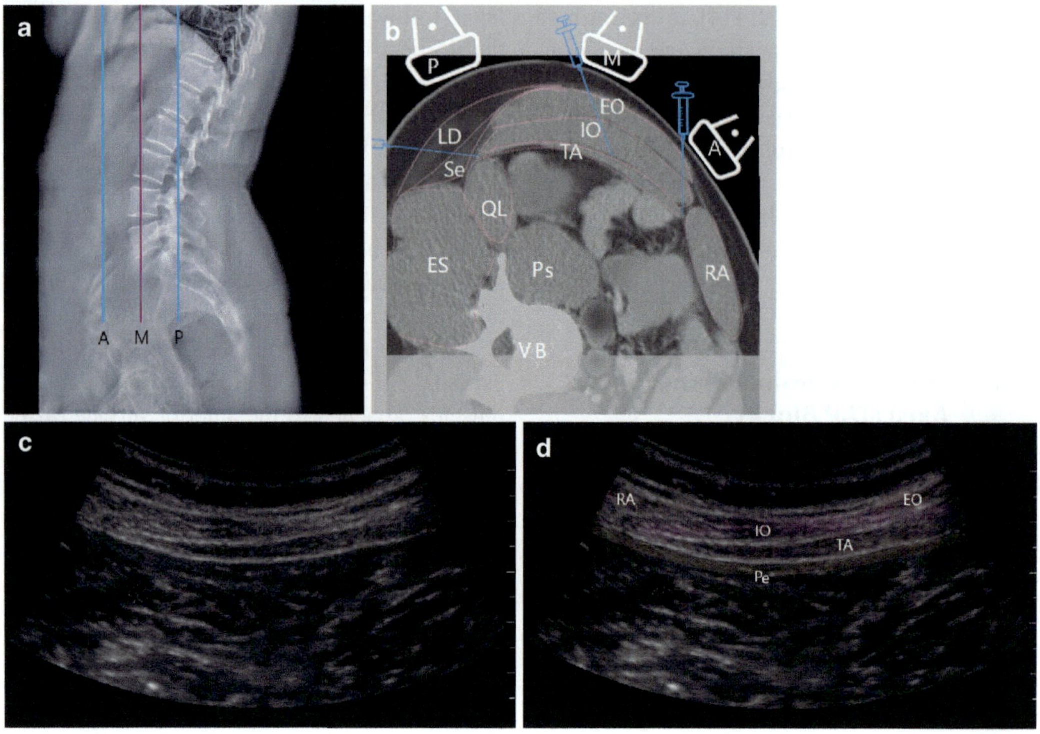

Fig. 8.10 Trans abdominal plane block. The image provides a clear and organized depiction of the transversus abdominis plane (TAP) block, consisting of two distinct parts and ten panels. **Part A** consists of four panels focusing on transabdominal anatomy and corresponding ultrasound imaging. Panel (**a**) features a lateral X-ray view of the abdomen, delineated by three colored lines—A (anterior axillary line), M (mid-axillary line), and P (posterior axillary line)—which serve as key anatomical reference points. Panel (**b**) offers a modified cross-sectional MRI scan of the abdomen, annotated with essential anatomical structures, including the transversus abdominis (TA), internal oblique (IO), external oblique (EO), rectus abdominis (RA), psoas muscle (Ps), quadratus lumborum (QL), erector spinae (ES), vertebral body (V), latissimus dorsi (LD), and serratus muscle (Se). Notably, this MRI image also indicates three distinct probe positions (A, M, P) corresponding to anterior, mi, and posterior axillary lines scanning locations, along with syringe and needle placements that illustrate the in-plane approach. Panels (**c**) and (**d**) exhibit ultrasound scans of the transabdominal plane; panel (**c**) presents an unannotated grayscale ultrasound image captured at the level of the mid-axillary line, while panel (**d**) features the same ultrasound image with labeled structures such as TA, IO, EO, RA, and pleura (Pe), enhanced through color overlays for improved clarity. **Part B** consists of six panels demonstrating the TAP block performed at various levels along the anterior-to-posterior mid-axillary line. Panels (**e**) and (**f**) are modified versions of panels (**c**) and (**d**), specifically highlighting the needle trajectory for the TAP block performed at the anterior axillary line. The subsequent panels (**g**) and (**h**) are the ultrasound scans showcasing the TAP block at the mid-axillary line, with panel (**h**) highlighting the three muscle layers, EO, IO, and TA. Panel (**i**) displays an unlabeled grayscale ultrasound image representing the posterior axillary line level, with a visible needle trajectory for the TAP block. Finally, panel (**j**) is an annotated version of panel (**i**), which identifies multiple anatomical structures, including TA, IO, EO, QL, transverse process (TP), LD, serratus muscle (Se), lumbar plexus (LP), and psoas muscle (Ps), utilizing color overlays to distinguish these features. This detailed collection of images is an essential reference for practitioners performing TAP blocks. It links anatomical landmarks with ultrasound imaging techniques, improving needle placement accuracy and the effectiveness of anesthetic delivery

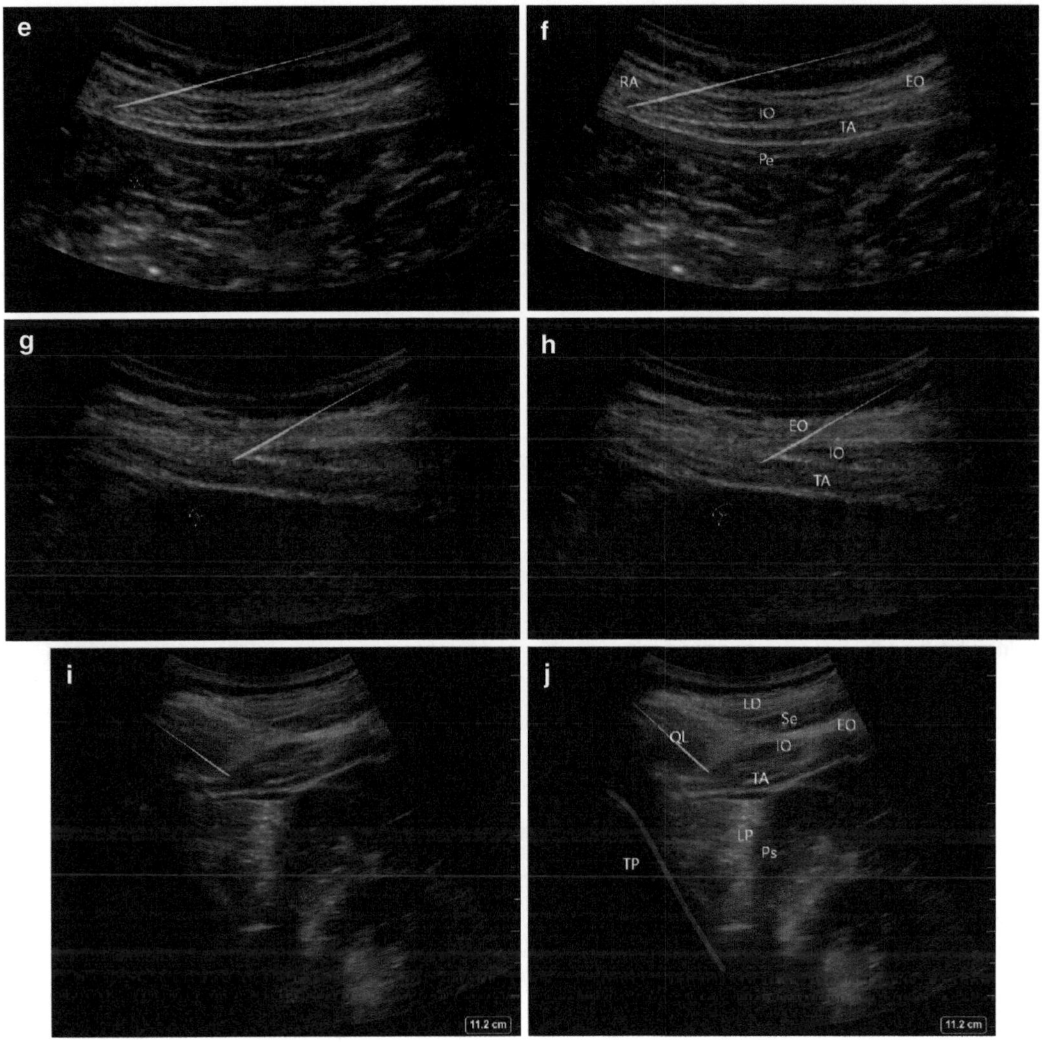

Fig. 8.10 (continued)

References

1. Winegar BA, Kay MD, Taljanovic M. Magnetic resonance imaging of the spine. Pol J Radiol. 2020;85:e550–74. https://doi.org/10.5114/pjr.2020.99887.
2. Grogan SP, Mount CA. Ultrasound physics and instrumentation. In: StatPearls. StatPearls Publishing; 2024. http://www.ncbi.nlm.nih.gov/books/NBK570593/.
3. Philipp LR, Baum GR, Grossberg JA, Ahmad FU. Baastrup's disease: an often-missed etiology for back pain. Cureus. 2016;8(1):e465. https://doi.org/10.7759/cureus.465.
4. Sollmann N, Fields AJ, O'Neill C, Nardo L, Majumdar S, Chin CT, Tosun D, Han M, Vu AT, Ozhinsky E, Shah LM, Harris RE, Lobo R, Anderst W, Herzog R, Psioda MA, Standaert CJ, Price RT, Lotz JC, et al. Magnetic resonance imaging of the lumbar spine: recommendations for acquisition and image evaluation from the BACPAC Spine Imaging Working Group. Pain Med. 2022;24(Suppl 1):S81–94. https://doi.org/10.1093/pm/pnac130.
5. Chin KJ, Karmakar MK, Peng P. Ultrasonography of the adult thoracic and lumbar spine for central neuraxial blockade. Anesthesiology. 2011;114(6):1459–85. https://doi.org/10.1097/ALN.0b013e318210f9f8.
6. Almeer G, Azzopardi C, Kho J, Gupta H, James SL, Botchu R. Anatomy and pathology of facet joint. J Orthop. 2020;22:109–17. https://doi.org/10.1016/j.jor.2020.03.058.
7. Shi W, Tian D, Liu D, Yin J, Huang Y. The comparison of measurement between ultrasound and computed tomography for abnormal degenerative facet joints. Medicine. 2017;96(31):e7680. https://doi.org/10.1097/MD.0000000000007680.
8. Wong MJ, Rajarathinam M. Ultrasound-guided axial facet joint interventions for chronic spinal pain: a narrative review. Can J Pain. 2023;7(2):2193617. https://doi.org/10.1080/24740527.2023.2193617.
9. Singh O, Al Khalili Y. Anatomy, back, lumbar plexus. In: StatPearls. StatPearls Publishing; 2024. http://www.ncbi.nlm.nih.gov/books/NBK545137/.
10. Santhosh SA, Bhoi D, Thangavel K, Soni L. Ultrasound-assisted transverse process line as a guide for performing lumbar neuraxial block. Saudi J Anaesth. 2023;17(1):133–5. https://doi.org/10.4103/sja.sja_462_22.
11. Yoo S, Kim Y, Park S-K, Ji S-H, Kim J-T. Ultrasonography for lumbar neuraxial block. Anesth Pain Med. 2020;15(4):397–408. https://doi.org/10.17085/apm.20065.
12. Sattar MH, Guthrie ST. Anatomy, back, sacral vertebrae. In: StatPearls. StatPearls Publishing; 2024. http://www.ncbi.nlm.nih.gov/books/NBK551653/.
13. Opfermann P, Kraft F, Obradovic M, Zadrazil M, Schmid W, Marhofer P. Ultrasound-guided caudal blockade and sedation for pediatric surgery: a retrospective cohort study. Anaesthesia. 2022;77(7):785–94. https://doi.org/10.1111/anae.15738.
14. Lopez-Rincon RM, Hendrix JM, Kumar V. Ultrasound-guided intercostal nerve block. In: StatPearls. StatPearls Publishing; 2024. http://www.ncbi.nlm.nih.gov/books/NBK555900/.
15. Flynn W, Vickerton P. Anatomy, abdomen and pelvis: abdominal wall. In: StatPearls. StatPearls Publishing; 2024. http://www.ncbi.nlm.nih.gov/books/NBK551649/.
16. Mavarez AC, Hendrix JM, Ahmed AA. Transabdominal plane block. In: StatPearls. StatPearls Publishing; 2024. http://www.ncbi.nlm.nih.gov/books/NBK560527/.

Index

R. S. Roghani, J. J. Diaz (eds.), *Video Atlas of Neuromusculoskeletal Ultrasound*,
https://doi.org/10.1007/978-3-031-81037-4

GPSR Compliance

The European Union's (EU) General Product Safety Regulation (GPSR) is a set of rules that requires consumer products to be safe and our obligations to ensure this.

If you have any concerns about our products, you can contact us on ProductSafety@springernature.com

In case Publisher is established outside the EU, the EU authorized representative is:

Springer Nature Customer Service Center GmbH
Europaplatz 3
69115 Heidelberg, Germany

Batch number: 10732809

Printed by Printforce, the Netherlands